HEALTH AND HEALTH CARE CONCERNS AMONG WOMEN AND RACIAL AND ETHNIC MINORITIES

RESEARCH IN THE SOCIOLOGY OF HEALTH CARE

Series Editor: Jennie Jacobs Kronenfeld

Recent Volumes:

Volume 23: Health Care Services, Racial and Ethnic Minorities and Underserved Populations, 2005

Volume 24: Access, Quality and Satisfaction with Care: Concerns of Patients, Providers and Insurers, 2007

Volume 25: Inequalities and Disparities in Health Care and Health: Concerns of Patients, Providers and Insurers, 2007

Volume 26: Care for Major Health Problems and Population Health Concerns: Impacts on Patients, Providers, and Policy, 2008

Volume 27: Social Sources of Disparities in Health and Health Care and Linkages to Policy, Population Concerns and Providers of Care, 2009

Volume 28: The Impact of Demographics on Health and Healthcare: Race, Ethnicity, and Other Social Factors, 2010

Volume 29: Access to Care and Factors that Impact Access, Patients as Partners in Care and Changing Roles of Health Providers, 2011

Volume 30: Issues in Health and Health Care Related to Race/Ethnicity, Immigration, SES and Gender, 2012

Volume 31: Social Determinants, Health Disparities and Linkages to Health and Health Care, 2013

Volume 32: Technology, Communication, Disparities and Government Options in Health and Health Care Services, 2014

Volume 33: Education, Social Factors, and Health Beliefs in Health and Health Care Services, 2015

Volume 34: Special Social Groups, Social Factors and Disparities in Health and Health Care, 2016

RESEARCH IN THE SOCIOLOGY OF HEALTH CARE
VOLUME 35

HEALTH AND HEALTH CARE CONCERNS AMONG WOMEN AND RACIAL AND ETHNIC MINORITIES

EDITED BY

JENNIE JACOBS KRONENFELD

Sociology Program, Sanford School of Social and Family Dynamics, Arizona State University, USA

emerald PUBLISHING

United Kingdom – North America – Japan
India – Malaysia – China

Emerald Publishing Limited
Howard House, Wagon Lane, Bingley BD16 1WA, UK

First edition 2017

British Library Cataloguing in Publication Data
A catalogue record for this book is available from the British Library

ISBN: 978-1-78743-150-8 (Print)
ISBN: 978-1-78743-149-2 (Online)
ISBN: 978-1-78743-178-2 (Epub)

ISSN: 0275-4959 (Series)

Printed and bound by CPI Group (UK) Ltd, Croydon, CR0 4YY

CONTENTS

PART III
HEALTH CARE PRACTITIONERS AND HEALTH AND HEALTH CARE

PART IV
RACIAL AND ETHNIC MINORITIES AND HEALTH AND HEALTH CARE

LIST OF CONTRIBUTORS

Kathryn Freeman Anderson	Department of Sociology, University of Houston, Houston, TX, USA
Denise L. Anthony	Department of Sociology, Dartmouth College, Hanover, NH, USA
Mikaila Mariel Lemonik Arthur	Department of Sociology, Rhode Island College, Providence, RI, USA
Shawn Bauldry	Department of Sociology, Purdue University, West Lafayette, IN, USA
Allison Pope Burger	Southern New Jersey Perinatal Cooperative, Pennsauken, NJ, USA
Tracey Chantler	London School of Hygiene & Tropical Medicine (LSHTM), London, UK
Claudia Chaufan	School of Health Policy and Management, York University, Toronto, Canada
William C. Cockerham	Department of Sociology, University of Alabama at Birmingham, Birmingham, AL, USA
Lisa A. Cubbins	Department of Sociology, University of Washington, Seattle, WA, USA
Patricia Drentea	Department of Sociology, University of Alabama at Birmingham, Birmingham, AL, USA
Alicia Fernandez	School of Medicine, University of California, San Francisco, CA, USA
Michael Seth Friedson	Department of Sociology, University of Wisconsin-Whitewater, Whitewater, WI, USA

Rob Haile	Oxford County Public Health and Emergency Services, Woodstock, Canada
Bryant W. Hamby	Department of Sociology, University of Alabama at Birmingham, Birmingham, AL, USA
Megan M. Henley	Social and Behavioral Sciences, Colorado Mesa University, Grand Junction, CO, USA
Mi-Kyung "Miki" Hong	Institute for Health & Aging, University of California San Francisco, San Francisco, CA, USA
Jacob Chao-Lun Huang	School of Humanities, Religion, and Social Sciences, Fresno Pacific University, Fresno, CA, USA
Katrina Kimport	ANSIRH, University of California San Francisco, San Francisco, CA, USA
Jennie Jacobs Kronenfeld	Sociology Program, Sanford School of Social and Family Dynamics, Arizona State University, AZ, USA
Nancy S. Landale	Department of Sociology and Demography, Pennsylvania State University, University Park, PA, USA
Heidi Larson	London School of Hygiene & Tropical Medicine (LSHTM), London, UK
Shelley Lees	London School of Hygiene & Tropical Medicine (LSHTM), London, UK
Lilian Magalhães	Department of Occupational Therapy, Federal University of Sao Carlos, Sao Paulo, Brazil
Karthikeyan Meganathan	Department of Family and Community Medicine, University of Cincinnati, Cincinnati, OH, USA
Miriam Naiman-Sessions	Department of Sociology, Carroll College, Helena, MT, USA

Aggie J. Noah	School of Social Transformation, Arizona State University, Tempe, AZ, USA
Pauline Paterson	London School of Hygiene & Tropical Medicine (LSHTM), London, UK
Louise Marie Roth	School of Sociology, University of Arizona, Tucson, AZ, USA
Brenly Rowland	ANSIRH, University of California San Francisco, San Francisco, CA, USA
Debbie Laliberte Rudman	School of Occupational Therapy, University of Western Ontario, London, Canada
Magdalena Szaflarski	Department of Sociology, University of Alabama at Birmingham, Birmingham, AL, USA
Emily Walton	Department of Sociology, Dartmouth College, Hanover NH, USA
Nicole Maki Weller	Department of Sociology, Indiana University Kokomo, Kokomo, IN, USA
Rose Jane Wilson	London School of Hygiene & Tropical Medicine (LSHTM), London, UK

ABOUT THE AUTHORS

Kathryn Freeman Anderson is Assistant Professor in the Department of Sociology at the University of Houston. She received her Ph.D. in Sociology from the University of Arizona. Her research lies at the intersection of the sociology of health and illness, urban sociology, race/ethnicity, and organizations. Her work is generally focused on understanding the social sources of health disparities in the United States. In particular, she examines the role of race/ethnicity and urban neighborhood dynamics to analyze how these factors may affect individual health. Her work on racial inequality, neighborhoods, and health is published in *Social Problems*, *Population Review*, and *Race and Social Problems*.

Denise Anthony is Vice Provost for Academic Initiatives and Professor of Sociology at Dartmouth College. She is also a faculty affiliate at The Dartmouth Institute for Health Policy and Clinical Practice. Anthony's research explores issues of cooperation, trust, and privacy in a variety of settings, from health care delivery to micro-credit borrowing groups to online groups such as Wikipedia and Prosper.com. Her current work examines the use of information technology in health care, including effects on quality, on the organization of health care, as well as the implications for the privacy and security of protected health information. Her multi-disciplinary research has been funded by grants from the National Science Foundation and others, and published in sociology as well as in health policy and computer science journals, including among others the *American Sociological Review*, *Social Science and Medicine*, *Journal of the American Medical Association*, *Health Affairs*, and *IEEE Pervasive Computing*.

Shawn Bauldry is Assistant Professor of Sociology at Purdue University. His research interests include health disparities, particularly related to the education-health gradient, and multigenerational processes shaping health. In addition, he works on the development of structural equation models.

Allison Pope Burger is Evaluation Specialist at the Southern New Jersey Perinatal Cooperative, a state-licensed nonprofit. Allison collaborates with Program Coordinators to implement survey research and write reports for partners and funders. Highlights of her research include making data-driven recommendations for the Salem Health and Wellness Foundation's adoption of teen pregnancy and STI prevention programs in Salem County, New Jersey. Her report served as a national model. She has also conducted several rounds of client satisfaction surveys and focus group research for Camden Healthy Start, a program aimed at reducing infant mortality in one of America's most impoverished cities. She holds a Master's Degree in Sociology from Rutgers University, where her studies focused on Environmental Sociology and Public Health.

Tracey Chantler has been involved in research relating to vaccines and immunization for 15 years. She also has significant experience of coordinating community health and immunization programs in Haiti, which included supervising and training health workers in vaccination. Dr. Chantler's research in this field spans pediatric clinical vaccine trials, organizational, qualitative, and mixed methods research in the United Kingdom related to the delivery of vaccine programs, vaccine trial participation, public engagement, acceptance of new vaccines, as well as longer term ethnographic fieldwork related to community engagement, vaccine trials, and ethics in western Kenya. In post-doctoral work, Dr. Chantler studied the role and value of reciprocal monitoring in clinical trials, and has been part of a multi-disciplinary research team developing a mobile health self-monitoring system for patients with heart failure. As part of this research, Dr. Chantler conducted home visits, to observe how patients were integrating use of this system into their daily lives, and do talk to them about their experiences of adopting technology for self-monitoring.

Claudia Chaufan is Associate Professor of Health Policy and Global Health at York University, Toronto. Her interdisciplinary background spans medicine, sociology/critical political economy, and philosophy. She practiced medicine in her native Argentina and later shifted to a career in academic sociology. Her research and intellectual interests include the political economy of health/global health, comparative health policy, the medicalization of social problems, the sociology of genomics, the health and social effects of neocolonialism and capitalist globalization, power/discourse, and the scholarship of teaching and learning. She has published in *Social Science & Medicine*, *Critical Public Health*, and the *International Journal of Health Services*, among other academic outlets; is editorial board member and ad hoc reviewer of several peer-reviewed journals; and is a long-time member/activist/supporter of US Physicians for a National Health Program.

William C. Cockerham, Ph.D., is Distinguished Professor and Chair of the Department of Sociology at the University of Alabama at Birmingham. His most recent books are *Sociology of Mental Disorder*, 10th edition (Routledge, 2017) and *Medical Sociology*, 14th edition (Routledge, 2017); he is also Associate Editor-in-Chief of the seven-volume *International Encyclopedia of Public Health*, 2nd edition (Academic Press, 2017) and co-editor of a special issue of the *American Journal of Preventive Medicine* (January, 2017).

Lisa A. Cubbins, Ph.D., is Sociologist and an independent consultant. Previously, she was a senior research scientist at Battelle Health and Analytics. She has also held faculty positions at the University of Washington and the

University of Cincinnati. She specializes in social stratification, immigrant health, and risky behaviors and HIV. She has led and collaborated on NIH- and other federally-funded studies of social issues in health.

Patricia Drentea, Ph.D., is Associate Professor in the Department of Sociology at the University of Alabama at Birmingham. She studies how ascribed statuses, such as gender and race, determine physical and mental health both directly and indirectly through employment and family status, economic inequality, and differential life chances. Her work is published recently in journals such as *Society and Mental Health, Aging and Mental Health,* and *The Gerontologist*. She is working on the book on *Families and Aging* with Rowman and Littlefield.

Alicia Fernandez, MD, is Professor of Medicine, University of California, San Francisco. Her research is on health care disparities in chronic disease with a strong focus on Latinos and diabetes. Dr. Fernandez' efforts were supported in part by NIH K24DK102057.

Michael Friedson is Assistant Professor in the Department of Sociology, Criminology & Anthropology at the University of Wisconsin-Whitewater. His research interests include the relationship between crime, policing, and poverty, as well as the effects of poverty on childhood health. He has published research articles in academic journals such as *The Annals of the American Academy of Political and Social Science* and *Child Abuse & Neglect: The International Journal*.

Rob Haile, M.Sc., is a Public Health Planner for Oxford County Public Health & Emergency Services in Woodstock, Ontario. He conducts planning and evaluation for the County's health promotion and health protection programs, and performs ongoing research on various local topics of interest to assess community wants, needs, and assets. Rob applies a critical lens in his research to examine how social, cultural, and environmental contexts impact certain marginalized communities.

Bryant W. Hamby, M.A., is Doctoral Candidate in Sociology at the University of Alabama at Birmingham. His research focuses on the social determinants of health, with recent publications in *Communist and Post-Communist Studies* and the *American Journal of Preventive Medicine*.

Megan M. Henley is an Assistant Professor of Sociology at Colorado Mesa University. Her primary research interests are gender, knowledge, family, and reproduction. Her research focuses on doulas (labor support people) and how they legitimate their role within the medical and non-medical birth realms. Her current research looks at mothers who hire doulas and how they learn about the benefits of doula support. Dr. Henley collaborated on the development of the Maternity Support Survey, a cross-national survey of doulas, childbirth educators, and labor and delivery nurses in the United States and Canada. She specifically created questions having to do with doulas and their sources of knowledge. She has used the survey data both in her own research and in collaborative papers with other members of the Maternity Support Research Team.

Mi-Kyung "Miki" Hong is health Services Researcher with formal training in epidemiology and health management and policy. She is a tobacco control scholar and has published journal articles that relay the conflicts of interest between academic scientists and the tobacco industry. Miki is interested in medical effectiveness research as it relates to policy and lawmaking. She has served as a task force member with the California Health Benefits Review Program, a body that responds to requests from the California State legislature to provide independent analysis of the medical, financial and public health impacts of proposed health insurance benefit mandates and repeals in California state. Miki received her BA from Columbia University and an MPH and an executive MHSA from the University of Michigan.

Jacob Chao-Lun Huang (Ph.D. in Sociology, University of North Texas) is Assistant Professor of Sociology at Fresno Pacific University. His research focuses on how health behaviors impact health outcomes for elderly Asian Americans in the United States. He is currently conducting a research that explores perceptions of health services and immigration experiences for Hmong elderly. In addition, he has a great passion for employing sociological insights into community services. His publications include "Using Data in Service of Community Transformation" (adopted in *Out of Nazareth: Christ-Centered Civic Transformation in Unlikely Places*, pp. 244–282, Skyforest, CA: Urban Loft Publishers, 2017) and "NGOs in Asia: A Case Study of the Mennonite Social Welfare Foundation in Taiwan" (adopted in *Nongovernmental Organization Case Studies in Leadership*, Dubuque, IO: Kendall Hunt Publishing Company, forthcoming).

Katrina Kimport is Assistant Professor in the Department of Obstetrics, Gynecology & Reproductive Science and research Sociologist in the Advancing New Standards in Reproductive Health (ANSIRH) program at the University of California, San Francisco. Her research focuses on the (re)production of inequality, with a particular emphasis on gendered and sexuality-based inequality. Dr. Kimport's work has been published in the *Journal of Health and Social Behavior*, *Gender & Society*, and *Journal of Sex Research*. She is the author of *Queering Marriage: Challenging Family Formation in the United States* (2014, Rutgers University Press) and, with Jennifer Earl, PhD, of *Digitally Enabled Social Change: Activism in the Internet Age* (2011, MIT Press).

Nancy S. Landale, Ph.D., is a Liberal Arts Research Professor of Sociology and Demography at Pennsylvania State University. Professor Landale's research focuses on family patterns and health outcomes of racial and ethnic minorities in the United States. She is currently investigating the health and development of Mexican children of immigrants, with an emphasis on links between immigration and assimilation processes, family contexts and multiple dimensions of health. Professor Landale has also written extensively about the roles of migration and assimilation in the family patterns and infant health outcomes of Puerto Ricans; early family formation patterns; and the financial and non-financial contributions of fathers. Professor Landale teaches in the areas of social demography and the family.

Heidi Larson, MA, PhD, is Anthropologist and Director of The Vaccine Confidence Project (VCP); Associate Professor, Department of Infectious Disease Epidemiology, LSHTM; Associate Clinical Professor, Department of Global Health, University of Washington; and Chatham House Centre on Global Health Security Fellow. Dr. Larson previously headed Global Immunisation Communication at UNICEF, chaired GAVI's Advocacy Task Force, and served on the WHO SAGE Working Group on vaccine hesitancy. The VCP is a WHO Centre of Excellence on addressing Vaccine Hesitancy. Dr. Larson's research focuses on the analysis of social and political factors that can affect uptake of health interventions and influence policies. Her particular interest is on risk and rumor management from clinical trials to delivery – and building public trust. She served on the FDA Medical Countermeasure (MCM) Emergency Communication Expert Working Group, and is Principle Investigator of the EU-funded (EBODAC) project on the deployment, acceptance and compliance of an Ebola vaccine trial in Sierra Leone.

Shelley Lees, Ph.D., is Associate Professor in Anthropology of Gender, Violence and HIV. The main focus of Dr. Shelley Lees' research is exploring gender, violence, and HIV. Through anthropological research conducted with participants in HIV and GBV trials in Tanzania, which aim to empower women, Dr. Lees is exploring what impact such trials have on Tanzanian women's power. With 20 years of working and living in Tanzania, she is developing an in-depth understanding of changes in Tanzanian women's power, and how this is impacted on by scientific endeavors, such as the trials, as well as social and economic development. Further to this, Dr. Lees is interested in understanding women's power in relation to concepts of uncertainty and hope. She is also exploring the role on anthropology in clinical and community-based trials, especially to reveal broader ethical considerations of trials. For this purpose, Dr. Lees is leading anthropological research into an Ebola Virus Disease trial in Sierra Leone.

Mikaila Mariel Lemonik Arthur is Associate Professor and Chair of Sociology at Rhode Island College, where she teaches courses primarily in research methods and the sociology of law. Her research focuses on organizational issues in higher education and on social science pedagogy.

Lilian Magalhães is Adjunct Professor at Federal University of São Carlos, Brazil. Dr. Magalhães also holds an Emeritus Professor status at Western University in London, Ontario, Canada. Her research interests focus on emancipatory practices, community engagement, and visual methodologies. Dr. Magalhães has secured national and international funding to support projects in investigating the living and working conditions of undocumented immigrant workers. Dr. Magalhães has been applying innovative visual methods such as photovoice and body mapping to her projects, which afford interesting venues to convey participants' narratives.

Karthikeyan Meganathan is Data Analyst at the University of Cincinnati. He is involved in the design, data management, and statistical analysis of diverse groups of clinical, population-based, and healthcare-related projects conducted by investigators from University of Cincinnati, Cincinnati Children's Hospital, and Cincinnati Veterans Affairs. His experience and areas of interest also include analyses of data from publicly available national surveys as well as national registries.

Miriam Naiman-Sessions is Adjunct Professor of Sociology at Carroll College. Her primary research interests are gender, health, family, and emotions. Her previous research analyzed the associations between medical interventions and women's emotional experiences during birth. Her most recent research examines the link between hospital characteristics and women's birth outcomes. Dr. Naiman-Sessions collaborated on the development of the Maternity Support Survey, a cross-national survey of doulas, childbirth educators, and labor and delivery nurses in the United States and Canada. She has used the survey data in collaborative papers with other members of the Maternity Support Research Team.

Aggie J. Noah, Ph.D., is Assistant Professor in Asian Pacific American Studies & Justice and Social Inquiry in School of Social Transformation at the Arizona State University. Her research and teaching interests are in understanding the influence of social contexts, often operationalized as neighborhoods and activity spaces, on immigrants' well-being using the demographic perspective. Specifically, she investigates how the complex interplay of social inequalities at the individual, family, and contextual levels influences immigrants. Her recent work has been published in *Demography*, *Demographic Research*, *Journal of Marriage and Family*, and *Journal of Family Theory and Research*.

Pauline Paterson, Research Fellow, BSc, MSc, Ph.D., MBA, is Co-Director of The Vaccine Confidence Project team with Dr Heidi Larson. She has been researching issues of public confidence in immunizations since 2010. Specific research activities include qualitative analysis of parental reasons for not vaccinating their child with influenza vaccine in England, analysis of concerns surrounding HPV vaccine in India and Japan, and a systematic review on public trust in vaccination. Dr. Paterson is a member of the National Institute for Health Research (NIHR), Health Protection Research Unit (HPRU) in immunization in partnership with Public Health England. She has also researched HIV risk perception in sub-Saharan Africa, and feasibility and acceptability of PrEP in Kenya, and carried out a systematic review on conceptualizations of uncertainty and risk, and implications for uptake and use of biomedical HIV prevention technologies in sub-Saharan Africa. Dr. Paterson has a Ph.D. in Epidemiology, an MBA, and an MSc in Environmental Technology from Imperial College London.

Louise Marie Roth is Associate Professor of Sociology at the University of Arizona. Her primary research interests are gender, family, organizations, and law. Her previous research analyzed gender inequality in pay and performance evaluations in finance, medicine, and among scientists. Her more recent research focuses on the effects of tort laws and reproductive rights laws on reproduction and childbirth. With an inter-university research team, she developed a survey of Maternity Support Workers (doulas, childbirth educators, and labor and delivery nurses) to study their experiences with maternity care in the United States and Canada. In this research, she examined doulas' and nurses' views of each other, the frequency with which doulas and nurses witness ethical violations during childbirth, and maternity support workers' views of reproductive rights across the spectrum from abortion to birth.

Brenly Rowland is Senior Research Analyst at UCSF-ANSIRH, where she supports multiple research projects with study development, project management, and interviewing. Her past experiences include working as a sex educator, volunteering as a counselor at an abortion clinic, and leading workshops on domestic violence prevention and contraceptive options in Nicaragua. Ms. Rowland received her BA in Medical Anthropology from Hampshire College.

Debbie Laliberte Rudman, PhD, OT Reg.(Ont.), is Associate Professor in the School of Occupational Therapy and the Health and Rehabilitation Sciences Graduate Program (Occupational Science field) in the Faculty of Health Sciences at Western University. She applies critically oriented qualitative approaches to examine how everyday occupations (encompassing the range of activities people need and want to do in order to maintain and optimize their lives, families and communities) and identities of individuals and collectives, particularly of groups who experience social and economic marginalization, are situated within sociocultural, political, economic, and historical conditions. Dr. Rudman's work attends to the sociopolitical and discursive shaping of social issues and inequities, such as long-term unemployment and the extension of working lives, and raises awareness of the implications of re-configurations for how social issues come to be addressed and negotiated by individuals and through services.

Magdalena Szaflarski is Assistant Professor in the Department of Sociology at the University of Alabama at Birmingham. Her research interests include immigrant mental health, religion and HIV, and medical cannabis use. She has led a NIH-funded study of religious organizations' responses to HIV and is currently a co-investigator/social scientist on a study of cannabidiol oil in patients with epilepsy, sponsored by the State of Alabama (Carly's Law).

Emily Walton is Assistant Professor at Dartmouth College. As the U.S. population continues to be shaped by immigration in the 21st century, her research aims to add complexity to the way scholars and policymakers understand the meanings of race and place. Her early work investigated co-ethnic neighborhood concentration, focusing on resilience and providing insight into factors that can promote health and well-being in disadvantaged communities. More recently, she has turned her attention toward understanding social interactions in multiethnic communities, asking how individuals with different backgrounds and identities may come together in transformative interaction.

Nicole Maki Weller is Assistant Professor of Sociology at Indiana University Kokomo. Professor Weller's research focuses on reproductive health across the life course ranging from adolescent risky sexual health behaviors to exploring the determinants and outcomes stemming from the infertility experience. Her previous work on the interaction between parity status and health-seeking behaviors for infertility was published in *Population Review* and considered whether parity status would influence health-seeking behaviors for infertility. She has co-authored a manuscript that examined the impact of infertility and utilization of infertility services on self-rated health outcomes for women. This research was published in the *Journal of the Indiana Academy of the Social Sciences*. The project presented in this edited volume was funded in part from a Research Faculty Fellowship and a Research Grant from Indiana University Kokomo. In addition to her research on infertility, Professor Weller has explored the front-end of reproductive health and has explored the relationship between sex education on adolescent sexual behaviors. She has published in the *Journal of Health Behavior* and *Policy Review* on the rates of unprotected sexual debut as a condition of the sex education content received. Her current research project is an examination of sex education content and perceptions of sexual violence. In addition to this research agenda, Professor Weller facilitates the Medical Sociology Concentration for the Department of Sociology at Indiana University Kokomo.

Rose Wilson is currently conducting a Ph.D. on understanding vaccination uptake among pregnant women in Hackney, London, within the Vaccine Confidence Project at the London School of Hygiene & Tropical Medicine (LSHTM). Previous to this, Rose worked as a Research Assistant at the school During this time, she worked on a systematic review commissioned by the World Health Organisation (WHO), on the effectiveness of interventions to address vaccine hesitancy. She also co-authored an article published in *Human Vaccines & Immunotherapeutics* and two technical reports for the Center for Strategic and International Studies (CSIS) on the issue of HPV vaccine acceptance in Japan. The reports offer advice to the Japanese government on how to overcome vaccine hesitancy surrounding the human papillomavirus (HPV) vaccine. Rose holds an MA in Social Anthropology of Development from the London School of Oriental and African Studies (SOAS).

PART I
INTRODUCTION TO VOLUME

HEALTH, HEALTH CARE, AND WOMEN AND RACIAL AND ETHNIC MINORITIES

Jennie Jacobs Kronenfeld

ABSTRACT

This chapter provides both an introduction to the volume and a brief review of literature on women, gender, and health and health-care services as well as racial/ethnic minorities in the same areas.

The chapter argues for the importance of greater examination of women, issues of gender, and racial and ethnic minorities in health and health-care services.

The chapter reviews the issues of women and racial and ethnic minorities and previews this book.

Keywords: Women; gender and health care; ethnic minorities; racial minorities

This chapter provides an introduction to Volume 35 in the *Research in the Sociology of Health Care series, Health and Health Care Concerns Among Women and Racial and Ethnic Minorities*. The beginning of this chapter will

Health and Health Care Concerns among Women and Racial and Ethnic Minorities
Research in the Sociology of Health Care, Volume 35, 3–10

ISSN: 0275-4959/doi:10.1108/S0275-495920170000035001

review some of the more important material about women, gender, and health and health care and racial and ethnic minorities. The second part of this chapter will review the overall contents of the volume and the structure of the volume.

WOMEN, GENDER, AND HEALTH AND HEALTH CARE

Throughout the 20th century and into the new century, an important feature of mortality trends has been that women live longer than men (Rieker, Bird, & Lang, 2010). This was not always true in the more distant past. At one point in time, binary approaches to differences in health between men and women often tried to determine which was the weaker sex or which gender was more advantaged. Part of the complexity is that although women have better mortality experiences, they have higher morbidity rates and in later years of life report a diminished quality of life (National Center for Health Statistics, 2009). Understanding these differences is complex, as there are some variations across countries and other social factors. One of the most important of these is socioeconomic status and another is racial and ethnic differences. Altogether, these also impact differences between men and women both in the United States and in many other countries in the world.

One approach to understanding of differences between men and women in health and health outcomes is the constrained choice model developed by Bird and Rieker (2008) in their book, entitled *Gender and Health*. In this multilevel model, they conclude health is not only an individual responsibility but is also one shared by decision makers at multiple levels. The model argues that individuals make everyday choices that create health outcomes. These choices are made within the context of family, employment settings, and community. There is also a relationship with biological processes, such as stress responses, and all these go together to create health outcomes, both morbidity and mortality.

A different review article has examined gender and health care (Anspach, 2010). This review points out that the health-care system is a deeply gendered institution, and because of that, it often impacts men and women differently. They also note, as have many other authors, that women are more likely to seek medical treatment than men, and because of this, they become the principal consumers of health care. Often the care women receive is somewhat different from what men receive, and documenting these types of differences was an important topic of research as part of the resurgence of the feminist movement in the 1960s and 1970s in the United States, with many researchers pointing out that definitions of health and illness are impacted by social context including in the past differences in providers with nurses generally being women and physicians more often being men. This has changed greatly in the United States in the past 30 years, so that there are now many more women physicians, although nursing is still very heavily a female dominated field.

In addition to differences by gender in providers of care, differences have been noted in communication styles between men and women providers and linked also to the sex of patients. For some health problems, especially cardiovascular problems, women have been treated less aggressively than men (Lutfey & McKinlay, 2009). Some of this stems from an older, now discredited idea that heart disease is more important for men than for women. Other factors are that some procedures have been viewed as more risky for women, women often present with different symptoms and other cultural assumptions about gender and disease (Anspach, 2010). Importantly, in the past few decades, research on gender and health care has been modifying away from an exclusive focus on gender to broadening the approach to include the intersection of gender with race, class, and other forms of inequality. The constrained choice model already discussed is one example of this type of work. The chapters in this volume in many cases help to contribute to these more complex understandings of issues of gender, often linked in with other social factors such as social class and race/ethnicity.

RACE AND ETHNICITY

In the early years of sociology within the United States, there was a major focus both on social class differences, to the extent that data were available and to an early consideration of both racial and ethnic issues within the United States. From a health care and medical sociology perspective, these types of differences in recent years have become redefined as disparities with the growth of federal government efforts in health, and there has been more focus on race/ethnicity. I have already discussed some of this material in greater depth in an earlier volume within this series (Kronenfeld, 2012). If studies focus on race/ethnicity and ignore social class issues, it is too easy to conclude that differences are linked either specifically to race/ethnicity or even to biological differences that may be linked to race and ethnicity (Issacs & Schroeder, 2004).

In a review article, Takeuchi, Walton, and Leung (2010) argue that there is an important role played by segregation as a social process. It contributes to differential exposure to many particular environments and contexts and these different opportunity structures and community structures may influence health by shaping social processes. Similarly, a recent review article about the Hispanic paradox by Dubowitz, Bates, and Acevado-Garcia (2010) points out how the sociopolitical context and patterns of migration contribute to health and to the paradox that Hispanics/Latinas have higher life expectancies than would be expected based on their higher representation among the poor. The more factors researchers consider in trying to understand the complexity between health differences, immigration, race/ethnicity, and socioeconomic status, the more confusing and conflicting results researchers sometimes find.

Perhaps some of the studies in this volume will add to better understanding as well as the growing complexity of this confusing literature along with the literature on sex and gender within health and health care.

REVIEW OF CONTENTS OF THE VOLUME

This volume is divided into four sections. The first section is the introduction to this volume and contains only this chapter. The second section is on women and reproductive related health and health care concerns and includes four chapters related to this topic. In the first chapter, Freidson and coauthors Arthur and Burger examine the relationship of pregnancy intentions to breastfeeding duration. They point out that previous research has found that whether pregnancies are wanted, unwanted, or mistimed influence breastfeeding behavior. Using national survey data from the United States, they find that pregnancy timing matters most for sustaining breastfeeding for durations past 6 months and that differences in rates of breastfeeding discontinuation between mothers with wanted, unwanted, and mistimed pregnancies are most pronounced in the 3–7 months post-partum period. In addition, they find that Medicaid recipients (but not non-recipients) are less likely to exclusively breastfeed for 6 months when their pregnancies are mistimed. In the next chapter in this section, Kimport and Rowland discuss insurance in abortion care and the role of poverty. They point out that, partly due to legal restriction on insurance coverage, most women seeking abortions pay out-of-pocket for care. Because most abortion patients are low income, these costs can constitute a hardship. They interviewed 22 abortion facility administrators, representing 64 clinical sites in 21 states that varied in their legal allowance of public and private insurance coverage for abortion, about their facility's insurance practices and experiences. Accepting private insurance carried risks, including non-payment because costs fell within patients' deductibles. Different facilities used workarounds to protect their facility from non-payment and enable patients to use their private insurance. The third chapter in this section looks at the patient–health-care worker relationship and how it affects patient views toward vaccination during pregnancy. Wilson and her coauthors use the theory of relational autonomy with its emphasis that persons are socially embedded, with decisions being made within social relationships, to explore how the health-care professional–patient relationship can affect pregnant women's decisions to accept pertussis and influenza vaccines. They conducted in-depth interviews with 40 pregnant and recently pregnant women, as well as 10 health-care professional within the National Health Service (NHS) in Great Britain. Their findings indicate that advice from friends and family can greatly influence a pregnant woman's vaccination decisions. If close relationships with patients are formed, health-care professional advice is more likely to be trusted.

With support from health-care professionals, patients feel competent, empowered to make the right decision, and are more likely to vaccinate. The last chapter in this section examines a different reproductive health concern, health-seeking behaviors for infertility. This chapter by Weller also looks at insurance coverage for infertility and examines state-level mandates for this within the United States. The behavioral model of health services utilization is used in this chapter to examine the relationship between state-level mandates that insurance providers cover infertility service on the rates of health seeking behaviors (HSB) for infertility among a nationally representative sample of women. Fifteen US states have such mandates. The rates of health-seeking behaviors for infertility were higher among women residing in states with state-level mandates.

The third section in this volume includes three chapters related to health care practitioners and health and health care. In the first chapter, Naiman-Sessions and her colleagues examine emotional burnout among maternity support workers. They use data from a study of about 800 labor and delivery nurses in the United States and Canada, along with around 1200 doulas in the same locations. Multivariate ordinary least squares (OLS) regression models examine the effects of work–family conflict, overwork, emotional intelligence, witnessing unethical mistreatment of women in labor, and practice characteristics on emotional burnout. Work–family conflict, feelings of overwork, witnessing a higher frequency of unethical mistreatment, and working in a hospital with a larger percentage of cesarean deliveries are associated with higher levels of burnout among master's of social works (MSWs). Higher emotional intelligence is associated with lower levels of burnout, and the availability of hospital wellness programs is associated with less burnout among L&D nurses. In the second chapter, Chaufan, Hong, and Fernandez examine how clinicians make sense of structural barriers to diabetes care among US Latinos with limited English proficiency (LEP). The chapter focuses on how clinicians assisting low-income US Latino patients with diabetes and LEP made sense of language-discordant care in the context of the social determination of health. They interviewed 14 physicians in an urban teaching hospital. Participants believed that language barriers undermine the quality of the clinical encounter and diabetes outcomes, were eager to serve disadvantaged patients, and were well-schooled in the social determination of health and its role in diabetes inequalities. The last chapter in this section by Anderson looks at racial residential segregation and the distribution of auxiliary health-care practitioners across urban space. They point out that recent studies have shown inequities in the distribution of a wide variety of health-related organizations across urban neighborhoods, but relatively little attention has been given to the distribution of health-care facilities in particular. The chapter considers how segregation is related to the distribution of several auxiliary health-care practitioners in a series of spatial regression models of zip codes across the United States using data from the 2010 U.S. Census and County Business Patterns. She finds that both Black and Latino segregation are negatively related to the density of a number of auxiliary health-care practitioners, including mental health providers, dentists, physical/occupational/speech therapists, chiropractors, optometrists, podiatrists, and miscellaneous health-care practitioners. However, this association is reduced (in certain instances to non-significance) with the inclusion of socioeconomic indicators, chiefly the percent of college educated individuals and the unemployment rate of the zip code. This association is reduced for both Black and Latino segregation, with a larger reduction in the size of the effects for Latino segregation.

The last section in this volume has six chapters, all related to racial and ethnic minorities and health and health care. One focuses on Black men, one on Asian Americans, and one on Mexican Americans, while the other chapters look across some racial and/or ethnic differences. The first chapter by Szaflarski and her colleagues examines issues of nativity, race–ethnicity, and dual diagnosis among US adults. This chapter investigates disparities in dual diagnosis (comorbid substance-use and depressive/anxiety disorders) among US adults by nativity and racial–ethnic origin and socioeconomic, cultural, and psychosocial factors that may account for the observed disparities using two waves of the National Epidemiological Survey on Alcohol and Related Conditions. Racial–ethnic categories included African, Asian/Pacific Islander, European, Mexican, Puerto Rican, and other Hispanic/Latino. Substance-use and depressive/anxiety disorders were assessed per diagnostic and statistical manual-VI (DSM-VI). The prevalence of dual diagnosis was low but varied by nativity, with the highest rates among Europeans and Puerto-Ricans born in US states, and the lowest among Mexicans and Asians/Pacific Islanders. The nativity and racial–ethnic effects on likelihood of having dual diagnosis remained significant after all adjustments.

In the second chapter by Haile, Rudman, and Magalhaes, the hypertension experiences of Black men are examined. This chapter explores how Black men make sense of their hypertension and how they negotiate this condition within their everyday lives, illuminating how racism and power dynamics embedded within their environments affect their experiences living with hypertension. Critical race theory tenets were used along with a narrative design to obtain stories of hypertension experiences of a small sample of men in Ontario Canada. Participants' experiences with discrimination, isolation, and migration raise awareness of how power relations embedded within social, political, and historical contexts can affect hypertension experiences. The next chapter by Huang discusses the influence of health-care utilization and social characteristics on health outcomes among elderly Asian Americans. Using the Andersen health behavioral model, the chapter examines if there is a reciprocal relationship between health-care utilization and health outcomes, and how social characteristics play their role in this relationship between US born and foreign born elderly Asian Americans with data from the US National Health Interview Survey (NHIS) 1998–2012. Results show a reciprocal relationship between health outcomes and health-care utilization. Also, predisposing characteristics had a direct effect on health outcomes, and enabling resources had an indirect effect on health outcomes via health-care utilization. In addition, living in the West had both direct and indirect effects on health outcomes.

Noah and Landale examine behavioral functioning among Mexican-origin children, with a focus on parental legal status and neighborhood context. Their chapter investigates the influence of parental legal status and neighborhood characteristics on Mexican-origin children's behavioral functioning using a multilevel approach with data from the Los Angeles Family and Neighborhood Study and 2,000 decennial census. The multilevel results show the importance of considering parental legal status. Mexican children of unauthorized mothers are more likely to exhibit internalizing and externalizing problems than all other groups of Mexican children. Furthermore, neighborhood-concentrated disadvantage is significantly associated with internalizing behavior problems, and neighborhood-concentrated affluence is significantly associated with externalizing behavior problems.

The next chapter in this section by Walton and Anthony contextualizes race and ethnic differences in care-seeking. The chapter deals with past data demonstrating that racial and ethnic minorities utilize less health care than their similarly situated White counterparts in the United States, and the speculation that these actions may stem in part from less desire for care. Using data from a 2005 national survey of community-dwelling Medicare beneficiaries ($N = 2{,}138$), they examine racial and ethnic variation in intentions to seek care, grounding analyses in the behavioral model of health-care utilization. They find that Latino, Black, and Native American older adults express greater preferences for seeking health care compared to Whites. Worrying about one's health, having skepticism toward doctors in general, and living in a small city rather than a metropolitan area, but not health need, socioeconomic status, or health-care system characteristics, explain some of the racial and ethnic variation in care-seeking preferences. They show that even after comprehensively accounting for factors known to influence disparities in utilization, elderly racial and ethnic minorities express greater desire to seek care than Whites.

The last chapter in the volume is by Cockerham and colleagues and examines changing patterns of female smoking by comparing workers and full-time homemakers by class, race, and community type in the United States at two points in time, 1979 and 2014. Results show that smoking is most prevalent among homemakers in small communities. This outcome supports earlier studies citing smoking as a major causal factor for the decline in female life expectancy among less-educated White women in certain low-income and rural counties in the United States. The premise that female smoking is strongly associated with the workplace appears to be no longer true. Similarly, Black women in 1979 had 67% higher odds of smoking, but by 2014 they had 49% lower odds of smoking showing a significant racial reversal in cigarette use. This suggests Black women have been more receptive than White women to smoking avoidance and cessation over time.

REFERENCES

Anspach, R. R. (2010). Gender and health care. In C. E. Bird, P. Conrad, A. M. Fremont, & S. Timmermans (Eds.), *Handbook of medical sociology* (5th ed.). Nashville, TN: Vanderbilt University Press.

Bird, C. E., & Rieker, P. R. (2008). *Gender and health: The effects of constrained choices and social policies*. New York, NY: Cambridge University Press.

Dubowitz, T., Bates, L. M., & Acevado-Garcia, D. (2010). The Latino health paradox: Looking at the intersectionality of sociology and health. In C. E. Bird, P. Conrad, A. M. Fremont, & S. Timmermans (Eds.), *Handbook of medical sociology* (5th ed.). Nashville, TN: Vanderbilt University Press.

Issacs, S. L., & Schroeder, S. A. (2004). Class – The ignored determinant of the nation's health. *New England Journal of Medicine*, *351*(11), 1137–1142.

Kronenfeld, J. J. (2012). Health care system issues and race/ethnicity, immigration, SES and gender as sociological issues linking to health and health care. In J. J. Kronenfeld (Ed.), *Issues in health and health care related to race/ethnicity, immigration, SES and gender. Research in the Sociology of Health Care* (Vol. 30). London, UK: Emerald Press.

Lutfey, K. E., & McKinlay, J. B. (2009). What happens along the diagnostic pathways to CHD treatment? Qualitative results concerning cognitive processes. *Sociology of Health and Illness*, *31*(7), 1077–1092.

National Center for Health Statistics (NCHS). (2009). *Health, United States, 2008, with chartbook*. Hyattsville, MD: NCHS.

Rieker, P. R., Bird, C. E., & Lang, M. E. (2010). Understanding gender and health: Old patterns, new trends and future directions. In C. E. Bird, P. Conrad, A.M. Fremont, & S. Timmermans (Eds.), *Handbook of medical sociology* (5th ed.). Nashville, TN: Vanderbilt University Press.

Takeuchi, D. T., Walton, E., & Leung, M. (2010). Race, social contexts and health: Examining geographic spaces and places. In C. E. Bird, P. Conrad, A. M. Fremont, & S. Timmermans (Eds.), *Handbook of medical sociology* (5th ed.). Nashville, TN: Vanderbilt University Press.

PART II
WOMEN AND REPRODUCTIVE RELATED HEALTH AND HEALTH CARE CONCERNS

THE RELATIONSHIP OF PREGNANCY INTENTIONS TO BREASTFEEDING DURATION: A NEW EVALUATION

Michael Seth Friedson, Mikaila Mariel Lemonik Arthur and Allison Pope Burger

ABSTRACT

Past research suggests that whether pregnancies are wanted, unwanted, or mistimed may influence breastfeeding behavior. The purpose of this chapter is to develop a more precise understanding of this relationship. Specifically, this chapter asks three questions: first, do pregnancy intentions matter most in sustaining breastfeeding for long or for short durations postpartum; second, at what time postpartum are rates of breastfeeding discontinuation most differentiated by pregnancy intentions; and third, how does poverty (measured here by Medicaid receipt) moderate the relationship between pregnancy intentions and breastfeeding duration.

Logistic regression analysis of survey data from a national sample representative of US mothers is used to determine the relationship of pregnancy intentions to whether breastfeeding continues for various durations and through various intervals after birth. Interaction terms between pregnancy intentions and mother's Medicaid status are used to test for relationships specific to poor or nonpoor mothers between pregnancy intentions and breastfeeding duration.

Health and Health Care Concerns among Women and Racial and Ethnic Minorities
Research in the Sociology of Health Care, Volume 35, 13–37

ISSN: 0275-4959/doi:10.1108/S0275-495920170000035002

Results show that pregnancy timing matters most for sustaining breastfeeding for durations past 6 months and that differences in rates of breastfeeding discontinuation between mothers with wanted, unwanted, and mistimed pregnancies are most pronounced in the 3–7 months postpartum period. In addition, findings show that Medicaid recipients (but not nonrecipients) are less likely to exclusively breastfeed for 6 months when their pregnancies are mistimed.

The literature on fundamental causes of health disparities typically suggests that poverty impairs access to resources necessary for effective planning to achieve desirable health outcomes. This study's results, however, show that planning of pregnancies is more critical for poor mothers to sustain exclusive breastfeeding. Further research is needed to explain this relationship. The results also suggest that policy interventions to help mothers with unplanned pregnancies to sustain breastfeeding should target the period from 3 to 7 months postpartum.

These findings can help shape policies for facilitating the continuation of breastfeeding for durations recommended by health authorities and advance our understanding of the effects of poverty on health behaviors.

Keywords: Breastfeeding; health disparities; poverty; planning; health behavior

Successful breastfeeding may be difficult, and requires planning, work, and resources. An expansive body of prior research shows that pregnancy intentions matter for breastfeeding initiation and persistence, and medical experts have established clear recommendations for minimum durations of breastfeeding and of exclusive breastfeeding. Yet the literature has not made clear to what extent pregnancy planning and timing matter for persistence to the recommended duration of breastfeeding or when the differentiation between those who persist and those who do not is most likely to occur. Thus, this chapter seeks to pinpoint whether pregnancy planning matters for sustaining breastfeeding to different durations, and to compare rates of discontinuation of breastfeeding at different points postpartum among women with planned, unwanted, and mistimed pregnancies. Furthermore, prior research has shown that poverty impairs planning across a wide range of behaviors. This chapter thus examines whether a similar pattern can be found for breastfeeding behavior by exploring the interaction between poverty and pregnancy planning in relationship to breastfeeding outcomes. The findings of this research will facilitate the development of policy interventions deployed at the time postpartum that makes the greatest impact on breastfeeding persistence, as well as those that can specifically enhance poor women's ability to sustain breastfeeding. More broadly, this chapter advances our understanding of the circumstances under which people are able to make decisions that they believe – or public health standards suggest – will benefit their own and their children's health.

The prevalence of breastfeeding has increased over the past few decades (Avishai, 2007; Blum, 1999), and the vast majority of children experience at least some breastfeeding. Nationally, as of 2014, 79.2% of children were ever breastfed, with 49.4% still being breastfed at 6 months and 26.7% at 12 months (National Center for Chronic Disease Prevention and Health Promotion, 2014). Exclusive breastfeeding rates are, unsurprisingly, much lower: 40.7% of children were exclusively breastfed at 3 months and 18.8% at 6 months, and 19.4% of breastfed infants receive formula within the first 2 days postpartum (National Center for Chronic Disease Prevention and Health Promotion, 2014). Currently, health experts recommend that mothers breastfeed exclusively for the first 6 months of a child's life and that breastfeeding should continue in conjunction with the introduction of other foods for at least a year, with some recommendations encouraging even longer durations of breastfeeding (American Academy of Pediatrics, n.d.; World Health Organization, 2015).

These recommendations are based on a considerable body of findings on the significant benefits which accrue to breastfed children, including reductions in obesity (Seipel & Shafer, 2013; Stein & Kuhn, 2009) and behavioral problems (Heikkilä, Sacker, Kelly, Renfrew, & Quigley, 2011), improved cognitive performance (Stein & Kuhn, 2009), and reductions in infections and infant deaths (Stein & Kuhn, 2009). Breastfeeding has benefits for mothers as well, including quicker cessation of uterine bleeding, reduced risk of breast and ovarian cancer and osteoporosis, weight loss, and protection against conception (Stein & Kuhn, 2009). However, these findings are not as conclusive as once thought (Colen & Ramey, 2014; Evenhouse & Reilly, 2005; Rippeyoung, 2013; Seipel & Shafer, 2013; Wolf, 2007). For example, a randomized controlled trial of breastfeeding versus formula-feeding in Belarus found no effect of breastfeeding duration or exclusivity on obesity at 6.5 years of age (Kramer et al., 2009).

FACTORS AFFECTING BREASTFEEDING DURATION

A variety of personal, demographic, medical, and social factors act to promote or inhibit breastfeeding. The strongest consensus is around the effects of age, education, and marriage. Older mothers have higher rates of breastfeeding (Kost, Landry, & Darroch, 1998; Lee, Elo, McCollum, & Culhane, 2009; Ruowei, Darling, Maurice, Barker, & Grummer-Strawn, 2005; Taylor & Cabral, 2002; Taylor, Risica, Geller, Kirtania, & Cabral, 2006). More educated mothers are more likely to breastfeed and to sustain breastfeeding (Jacknowitz, 2008; Kost et al., 1998; Ruowei et al., 2005; Taylor & Cabral, 2002; Taylor et al., 2006), as are married mothers (Kost et al., 1998; Peters, Wehkamp, Felderbaum, Krüger, & Linder, 2006; Ruowei et al., 2005; Taylor & Cabral, 2002; Taylor et al., 2006). Living with the child's father also increases breastfeeding, but marriage has a much stronger impact than does cohabitation (Gibson-Davis & Brooks-Gunn, 2007; Jacknowitz, 2008; Lee et al., 2009).

There is substantial evidence about the effects of income, poverty, and employment on breastfeeding. Higher-income individuals are more likely to initiate and sustain breastfeeding (Kost et al., 1998), though this effect diminishes as breastfeeding duration increases (Ruowei et al., 2005). Poverty can matter beyond just the income effect. For example, housing issues can affect breastfeeding: mothers with unstable housing or a lack of privacy at home are less likely to breastfeed and to sustain breastfeeding (Lee et al., 2009; Peters et al., 2006). Working-class mothers have particular issues around privacy for breastfeeding, especially given limited physical space in the typical working-class residence (Blum, 1999). Additionally, the health risks of poverty, including those associated with maternal health, are greater for women than for men due to women's lower wages and lesser control of household resources (Jacobson, 1993; Ruspini, 2001).

Receiving public assistance tends to reduce breastfeeding (Jacknowitz, 2008; Lee et al., 2009), and women receiving support from WIC – the supplemental nutrition program for pregnant women, new mothers, and young children – are less likely to breastfeed. This is not solely an income effect: women who are eligible for but do not receive WIC are more likely to breastfeed (Ruowei et al., 2005). One study indicates that WIC may discourage breastfeeding by providing free formula (Lee et al., 2009), at least prior to recent reforms (Whaiey et al., 2012).

Despite the fact that most mothers initiate breastfeeding after giving birth, far fewer persist in breastfeeding over a longer duration. Indeed, quitting before the first month postpartum has passed is quite typical (Kimbro, 2006). The need to return to working outside the home, especially in the early postpartum period, is associated with lower breastfeeding initiation and persistence (Arora, McJunkin, Wehrer, & Kuhn, 2000; Kost et al., 1998; Cooklin, Rowe, & Fisher, 2012; Gibson-Davis & Brooks-Gunn, 2007; Jacknowitz, 2008; Lucas & McCarter-Spaulding, 2012; Smith et al., 2013), especially among women with administrative or manual jobs (Kimbro, 2006), and women who seek to combine breastfeeding with employment face many obstacles (Avishai, 2007; Johnston & Esposito, 2007). However, if a woman persists in breastfeeding after the return to work, especially beyond the first 2 months of her return, she is more likely to continue for the long term (Kimbro, 2006; Murtagh & Moulton, 2011). Current U.S. law and policy do not provide sufficient protection for breastfeeding among employed mothers (Kogan, Singh, Dee, Belanoff, & Grummer-Strawh, 2008; Mulford, 2012; Murtagh & Moulton, 2011).

For educated, professional women, breastfeeding is a "project," requiring substantial financial investment in breastfeeding equipment and products as well as lactation consultants (Avishai, 2007). Middle- and upper-class women often have the resources to engage in this project, at least where workplace demands do not conflict with it, but poor and working-class women do not have the resources to approach breastfeeding in this fashion. Yet the fact "that white, middle-class women in the United States do not themselves breastfeed much beyond 6 months, when the recommendation is to continue for a year at least, suggests that even resources and will are not enough to comply with medical guidelines" (Hausman, Smith, & Labbok, 2012, p. 6). Furthermore, longer-duration breastfeeding is associated with a substantial drop in employment, working hours, and income for mothers (Rippeyoung & Noonanb, 2012b)

Negative pregnancy outcomes, including low-birth-weight babies and premature births, tend to be associated with lower rates and durations of breastfeeding (Kost et al., 1998; Taylor & Cabral, 2002) – though one study found that prematurity did not reduce breastfeeding initiation but did shorten duration (Heikkilä et al., 2011) – and full-term births are more likely to result in breastfeeding that lasts past the third month (Taylor et al., 2006). Studies have found that second and subsequent children are less likely to be breastfed (Buckles & Kolka, 2014; Kost et al., 1998), but among those with prior pregnancies who do breastfeed, breastfeeding tends to be sustained for a longer period (Lee et al., 2009).

A large volume of literature has considered the role of race and ethnicity in breastfeeding behavior. Typically, such studies find that breastfeeding is highest for Whites (Jacknowitz, 2008; Taylor & Cabral, 2002) or Latinas (Ruowei et al., 2005) and lowest for Blacks (Kost et al., 1998; Ruowei et al., 2005). Some research suggests, however, that racial differences in breastfeeding are spurious (Dodgson, 2012). Research is unclear about the effects of foreign-born status on breastfeeding (Kimbro, 2006; Lee et al., 2009), but a number of studies have found that acculturation makes mothers less likely to breastfeed (Kimbro, 2006; Kimbro, Lynch, & McLanahan, 2008; Kogan et al., 2008).

THE ROLE OF PLANNING

Research has found that poverty reduces individuals' ability to engage in certain kinds of future-oriented planning. In particular, poverty increases the salience of financial concerns and increases individuals' engagement in solving their most salient problems, but also encourages behaviors that entail borrowing against the future to solve present problems (Shah, Mullainathan, & Shafir, 2012). This sense of urgency may particularly imperil poor people's ability to engage in proactive health-related planning (Dumas, Robataille, & Jette, 2014).

Unstable environments, such as those created by poverty, can significantly impact planning, decision-making, and follow-through (Kidd, Palmeri, & Aslin, 2013). This process, called ego depletion, results when the cognitive resources used to make decisions and engage in self-control are overused (Baumeister, Bratslavsky, Muraven, & Tice, 1998). In order for a pregnancy to be planned, not only do women have to have the more general financial, social, and cognitive resources to engage in planning, but they also need to feel that they have control over their contraceptive and sexual behaviors, which many women – especially young, low-income women – do not (Kendalla et al., 2005).

Planning plays an important role in fertility outcomes. Researchers distinguish between pregnancies which occur when intended; those which were mistimed, in other words wanted pregnancies that occurred earlier than would have been desirable; and those that are unwanted or unintended entirely (D'Angelo, Gilbert, Rochat, Santelli, & Herold, 2004). Currently, 31% of American pregnancies are mistimed and 20% are unwanted; 60% of these unplanned pregnancies end in live birth (Guttmacher Institute, 2015). Five percent of women of childbearing age experience a mistimed or unwanted pregnancy annually, as do more than half of women in their lifetimes. The inclusion of the mistimed category in retrospective research is crucial (Besculides & Laraque, 2004), as nearly a third of mothers who say their pregnancy was unintended during gestation will say it was intended subsequent to delivery (Joyce, Kaestner, & Korenman, 2000). Women who do not effectively or consistently use contraceptives are more likely to experience unplanned pregnancies (Dehlendorf, Rodriguez, Levy, Borrero, & Steinauer, 2010), and may consider these pregnancies to be mistimed when reluctant to classify them as unwanted (Kendalla et al., 2005, p. 308).

Overall, mistimed pregnancies result in more negative outcomes (such as premature birth and low birth weight) than do intended pregnancies, and unwanted pregnancies result in more negative outcomes than do those that are mistimed (Kost et al., 1998). Women with unintended pregnancies have less social and paternal support and score lower on measures of self-efficacy (Maxson & Miranda, 2011), which are important factors in promoting the ability to plan. When pregnancies are not planned, women are less likely to express the intention to breastfeed, even before giving birth (Dye, Wojtowycz, Aubry, Quade, & Kilburn, 1997). Mothers with intended pregnancies are considerably more likely to breastfeed and to sustain breastfeeding (D'Angelo et al., 2004; Peters et al., 2006), while those with unintended pregnancies are particularly less likely to breastfeed (D'Angelo et al., 2004; Marsiglio & Mott, 1988), and this relationship is found globally (Hromi-Fiedler & Pérez-Escamilla, 2006; Rudzik, 2012). Among mistimed pregnancies, the more severely the pregnancy is mistimed, the lower the likelihood of breastfeeding (Pulley, Klerman, Tang, & Baker, 2002).

Some analyses have suggested that the relationship between breastfeeding and the wantedness of a pregnancy is spurious – for instance, that older, lower-income, or Black mothers are both more likely to have unwanted pregnancies and less likely to breastfeed (Marsiglio & Mott, 1988). Breastfeeding decisions are typically made early in the childbearing process (Arora et al., 2000), while unwanted pregnancies are typically recognized later in the pregnancy (Kost & Lindberg, 2015). Wantedness has strong effects on birth outcomes, which are then in turn related to breastfeeding and to other health outcomes in later life (Hummer, Hack, & Raley, 2004; Kost & Lindberg, 2015). Furthermore, wantedness is strongly related to relational factors like intimate partner violence and the sustaining of unhealthy relationships that may affect breastfeeding (Donovan, 1995; Mauldon, Foster, & Roberts, 2015; Roberts et al., 2014). A propensity score analysis shows that controlling for propensity to have a severely mistimed or unwanted pregnancy reduces the significance of the relationship between intention and health behaviors/outcomes, but intention still matters (Kost & Lindberg, 2015).

The following analysis seeks to go beyond these existing findings in specifying a more precise relationship between pregnancy intentions, poverty status, and breastfeeding duration. In light of recommendations that breastfeeding be sustained for at least a year after birth, we ask whether pregnancy intentions are associated with maintaining breastfeeding for this longer duration or only for shorter periods. Given the considerable commitment and resources needed to continue breastfeeding for longer periods, it is possible that planning is particularly relevant in regard to breastfeeding over extended durations. We next attempt to specify when, within the first year after birth, pregnancy intentions matter most in differentiating between mothers who continue and cease breastfeeding. Finally, we investigate how poverty shapes the relationship between her pregnancy intentions and breastfeeding behavior. Given past findings indicating that poverty reduces the efficacy of planning, we ask if pregnancy intentions matter less in shaping breastfeeding outcomes for mothers in poverty, and whether poverty status is related to these outcomes independently of its interaction with pregnancy intentions.

DATA AND METHODS

Outcome, Predictor, and Control Variables

Breastfeeding duration, pregnancy intention, and control variables are derived from the 2006–2010 and 2011–2013 cycles of the National Survey of Family Growth (NSFG), administered by the Centers for Disease Control and Prevention (National Center for Health Statistics, 2015). The NSFG sample is designed to be representative of the US household population between the ages of 15 and 44. The present study's cases consist of all live births by women in the NSFG sample for which any breastfeeding was reported and the mother lived with the child for at least 1 year, thus ensuring that the mother was not prevented, by physical separation from the child, from breastfeeding for the maximum duration of 1 year investigated here.

The outcome variables are self-reported metrics of the duration of any and of exclusive breastfeeding. Pregnancies are classified according to whether any breastfeeding was reported for more than 6 weeks, more than 13 weeks (3 months), more than 26 weeks (6 months), and at least 52 weeks (1 year) after birth. Inspection of the data reveals that breastfeeding is most commonly stopped within 6 weeks, at 3 months, at 6 months, and at 52 weeks after birth. The outcome variables thus allow for classification of subjects according to whether they continue breastfeeding past empirically common thresholds for cessation, and whether breastfeeding is sustained for the minimum of 1 year currently recommended by public health organizations and research (American Academy of Pediatrics, n.d.; World Health Organization, 2015). Cases are additionally classified according to whether exclusive breastfeeding is continued for at least 6 months from birth, a commonly recommended period for exclusive breastfeeding (Ahnquist, Wamala, & Lindstrom, 2012; Boyas, 2013).

The main predictor variable is a self-reported metric of pregnancy intentions. Cases are classified according to whether the mother considered the pregnancy to be: (a) unwanted; (b) wanted but occurring too soon; or (c) wanted, combining those specifying that their wanted pregnancies took place at the right time or too late. (These categories are labeled as "unwanted," "too soon," and "timing ok" respectively when discussing results.) This follows existing conventions in the literature on pregnancy intentions (D'Angelo et al., 2004; Maxson & Miranda, 2011).

The regressions control for a range of demographic and health factors that, according to past research, may influence breastfeeding behavior. Subjects are classified by educational attainment, race and ethnicity, and nativity/foreign-born status. Controls are also included for age at conception; whether subjects were experiencing their first pregnancies; whether subjects were married at both conception and birth (stable relationship), married at birth but not conception (new relationship), or unmarried at birth; and whether delivery took place via Cesarean section, at a low birth weight (< 5 pounds 9 ounces), or before reaching full term (< 39 weeks postconception). Regressions also include a predictor indicating the calendar year of the child's birth, to account for time trends in breastfeeding behavior.

Analytic Strategy

The first section of the analysis investigates the relationship between the duration of any breastfeeding and pregnancy intentions. Proportions of the population in each pregnancy intention group that continue breastfeeding for more than 6 weeks, more than 13 weeks, more than 26 weeks, and at least 52 weeks are estimated and compared. This makes it possible to ascertain whether aggregate differences in the duration of breastfeeding by pregnancy intentions apply in the immediate aftermath of birth, over the longer run, or both. The breastfeeding outcomes are then regressed on the pregnancy intention and control variables, to determine if differences in these outcomes by pregnancy intentions are robust to such controls.

The most robust differences by pregnancy intentions in breastfeeding duration emerge over the longer run, in the populations continuing to breastfeed for more than 26 weeks and at least 52 weeks. On the basis of these findings, the analysis seeks to pinpoint the period in the first year after birth when differences between pregnancy intention groups in the discontinuation of breastfeeding are most acute. To make this possible, a series of regressions predicts the likelihood that those who already breastfed through a given interval will continue through the next interval. First, a subsample including all those who breastfed for at least 7 weeks is used to regress whether the breastfeeding duration equaled at least 14 weeks (i.e., more than 3 months) on the predictor and control variables. Second, a subsample including all those who breastfed for at least 14 weeks is used to regress whether the breastfeeding duration equaled at least 27 weeks (i.e., more than 6 months) on the predictor and control variables. Finally, a subsample including all those who breastfed for at least 27 weeks is used to regress whether the breastfeeding duration equaled at least 52 weeks (i.e., 1 year) on these variables. This makes it possible to determine the interval(s) after birth when pregnancy intentions are most influential in determining the likelihood of continuing to breastfeed, thus paralleling mortality analyses that not only determine cumulative deaths over the life course from particular causes, but proportions of survivors to particular ages who succumb by subsequent ages to such causes (Woloshin, Schwartz, & Welch, 2008). It becomes possible thereby to specify when such causes have their greatest impact in producing premature death (or cessation of breastfeeding), and to target interventions aimed at abating their effects at that time.

The second section of the analysis asks whether the relationship between pregnancy intentions and exclusive breastfeeding duration is specific to disadvantaged or nondisadvantaged mothers. A series of four regressions of the exclusive breastfeeding outcome is used for this purpose. First, as a baseline, this outcome is regressed on the pregnancy intention and control variables used in the analysis of any breastfeeding. An indicator of the mother's disadvantage status, consisting of whether Medicaid helped to pay for the child's birth, is next added to the regression as a predictor variable. Data on whether Medicaid helped pay for the birth is only available for births occurring within 5 years from when the mother was interviewed, thus reducing the sample size from 10,725 to 3,909 pregnancies. No other reliable indicator of the mother's disadvantage status at the time of birth is available in the data set. The third regression of exclusive breastfeeding duration calculates coefficients for the pregnancy intention variables separately for Medicaid recipients and nonrecipients.

Finally, an indicator of the mother's employment and maternity leave status at birth is added to these regressions. Maternal employment may interfere with the continuation of exclusive breastfeeding. Controlling for employment/leave status therefore helps to assure that relationships in prior regressions involving Medicaid status are not artifacts of greater unemployment rates among Medicaid recipients. An indicator of employment/leave status is only available in the 2006–2010 NSFG cycle; controlling for it thus further constricts sample size.

The data set contains multiple pregnancies for some surveyed mothers. However, results are similar to those reported below when they are re-estimated with samples that are limited to one pregnancy per mother, thus suggesting that these results are not artifacts of clustering of pregnancies by mother (contact author for details). It should also be noted that Model 2 through Model 4 of exclusive breastfeeding (below) only use data for a single pregnancy of most mothers (due to missing indicators of Medicaid receipt and employment and maternity leave status). Finally, key findings regarding the study's main predictor variable (pregnancy intentions) are supported in preliminary models that add random effects by mother, run with a recently introduced feature of STATA (melogit procedure with survey commands).

FINDINGS

Any Breastfeeding

The estimated proportions of all breastfeeding mothers, classified by pregnancy intentions, who continue to breastfeed for various durations are shown in Fig. 1. Results are given for breastfeeding for at least 7, 14, 27, and 52 weeks after birth. A consistent pattern characterizes the distribution of results by pregnancy intentions for each duration. The highest proportion continues breastfeeding in the "timing ok" group, while the lowest proportion continues in the "too soon" group. The difference between the proportions in the "timing ok" and "too soon" groups is highly significant ($p < 0.01$) for each timespan shown. The difference between the "timing ok" and "unwanted" groups does not reach a baseline level of significance ($p < 0.10$) for breastfeeding to 7 weeks but is highly significant ($p < 0.02$ or stronger) for the other durations.

Results of logistic regressions of these breastfeeding outcomes on pregnancy intentions and a set of controls are provided in Table 1. The outcome variables in these regressions equal zero if a subject has stopped breastfeeding and one if she has continued breastfeeding. Odds ratios greater than one thus indicate that a regressor is associated with an increased likelihood of the continuation

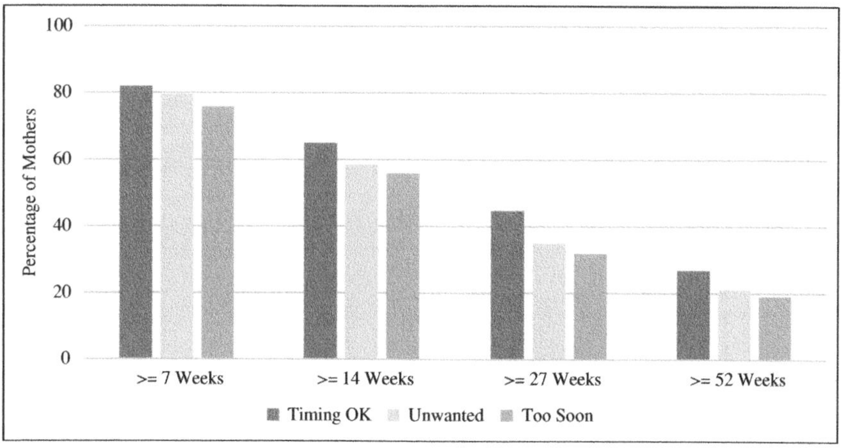

Fig. 1. Estimated Proportions of Mothers Who Continue Any Breastfeeding, by Pregnancy Intentions and Time Elapsed since Birth. *Note*: The percentages in this figure are of mothers who initiated breastfeeding. Breastfeeding durations reported in months by the data source are converted to weeks by multiplying months by 4.333.

of breastfeeding, while those less than one indicate a reduced likelihood of such continuation. In these regressions, becoming pregnant "too soon" remains significant ($p < 0.05$ or stronger) relative to the default category of "timing ok" in predicting a reduced likelihood of the continuation of breastfeeding to 27 or 52 weeks. It no longer, however, reaches a baseline level of significance ($p < 0.10$) in predicting the continuation of breastfeeding to 7 or 14 weeks. Likewise, having an "unwanted" pregnancy only reaches a baseline level of significance ($p < 0.10$) in predicting a reduced likelihood of breastfeeding to 27 weeks.

The results in Fig. 2 provide greater clarity regarding when the cumulative disparities in Fig. 1 are generated. While Fig. 1 shows the percentages of all breastfeeding mothers who continue to breastfeed for specific durations, Fig. 2 shows the percentages – among those breastfeeding for a specific duration – who continue breastfeeding for a greater length of time. For example, the bars in Fig. 2 labeled "7–14 weeks" show the percentages, among those breastfeeding for 7 weeks, who continue to breastfeed for 14 weeks.

The greatest differences by pregnancy intentions in the survival of breastfeeding are visible in the interval from 14 weeks to 27 weeks after birth. Among correctly timed pregnancies, nearly 69% of those who breastfeed to 14 weeks continue for 27 weeks, versus about 57% among pregnancies occurring too soon. In contrast, the percentages in each pregnancy intention category are practically identical of those breastfeeding for at least 27 weeks who continue until

Table 1. Logistic Regressions of the Continuation of Any Breastfeeding.

Cells Show Odds Ratio (Std. Error)	Duration of Breastfeeding (from Birth)			
	>= 7 Weeks	>= 14 Weeks	>= 27 Weeks	>= 52 Weeks
Timing				
Too soon	0.972 (0.102)	0.905 (0.088)	0.760 (0.061)***	0.831 (0.073)**
Unwanted	1.070 (0.127)	0.919 (0.082)	0.806 (0.092)*	0.850 (0.115)
Timing OK (default)	–	–	–	–
Ed. Attainment at Birth				
No high school diploma	0.869 (0.122)	0.884 (0.089)	0.971 (0.092)	1.015 (0.118)
Age 18 or under	1.121 (0.171)	1.341 (0.192)**	1.253 (0.179)	1.326 (0.235)
HS diploma (default)	–	–	–	–
Race/Ethnicity				
Non-Latina Black	1.249 (0.172)	1.174 (0.137)	1.064 (0.152)	0.965 (0.166)
Non-Latina other	1.132 (0.319)	1.099 (0.189)	1.015 (0.148)	1.075 (0.216)
Latina	1.352 (0.200)**	1.132 (0.165)	0.965 (0.130)	1.059 (0.152)
Non-Latina White (default)	–	–	–	–
Mother Born Outside US				
Yes	1.747 (0.252)***	1.508 (0.205)***	1.660 (0.201)***	1.759 (0.231)***
No (default)	–	–	–	–
First Pregnancy				
Yes	0.873 (0.072)	0.996 (0.069)	0.965 (0.070)	1.020 (0.083)
No (default)	–	–	–	–
Marital Status				
Married at conception & birth	1.529 (0.173)***	1.444 (0.139)***	1.586 (0.159)***	1.335 (0.139)***
Married at birth Only	0.958 (0.139)	0.921 (0.137)	1.002 (0.152)	0.847 (0.173)

Unmarried at birth (default)	–	–	–	–
Birth Method				
Cesarean	0.653 (0.067)***	0.660 (0.057)***	0.647 (0.062)***	0.639 (0.066)***
Vaginal (default)	–	–	–	–
Full Term				
Yes	1.153 (0.111)	1.153 (0.104)	1.254 (0.108)**	1.422 (0.142)***
No (default)	–	–	–	–
Low Birth Weight				
Yes	1.110 (0.166)	1.024 (0.121)	0.979 (0.129)	0.871 (0.135)
No (default)	–	–	–	–
Mother's Age at Conception	1.052 (0.012)***	1.056 (0.010)***	1.041 (0.010)***	1.051 (0.011)***
Year of Child's Birth	0.990 (0.010)	0.984 (0.007)**	1.003 (0.008)	1.014 (0.008)*
F-value	9.05***	7.94***	14.21***	15.50***
N	10742	10742	10742	10742

Note: The educational attainment variable distinguishes between subjects over age 18 who received a high school diploma before or during the month of the child's birth, those over age 18 who had not received a high school diploma, and those ages eighteen and under. Breastfeeding durations reported in months by the data source are converted to weeks by multiplying months by 4.333.

$^{*}p < 0.10$, $^{**}p < 0.05$, $^{***}p < 0.01$.

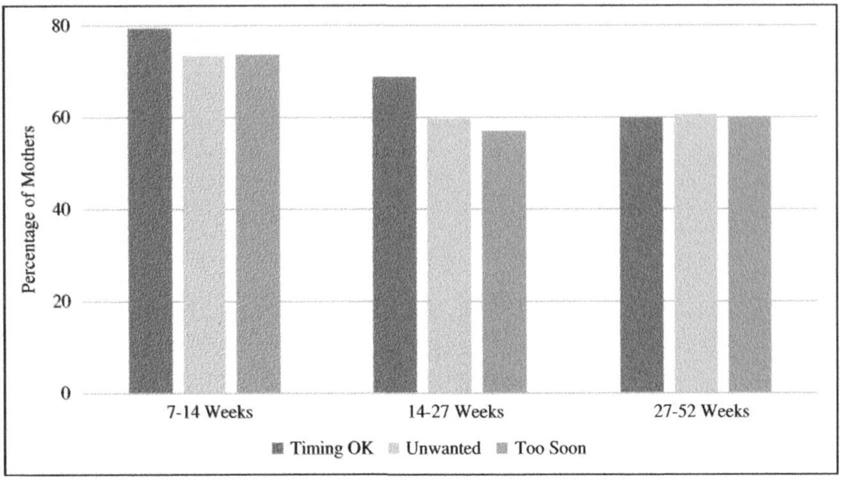

Fig. 2. Survival of Breastfeeding through Intervals after Birth, by Pregnancy Intentions. *Note*: The figure shows the percentages, among mothers breastfeeding at the start of each period, who were continuing to breastfeed at its end. Breastfeeding durations reported in months by the data source are converted to weeks by multiplying months by 4.333.

52 weeks. The disparities between the "timing ok" and other pregnancy intention categories are highly significant ($p < 0.02$ or stronger) for the 7 to 14 and 14 to 27 week intervals, but do not reach a baseline significance level ($p < 0.10$) for the 27 to 52 week interval.

The regressions in Table 2 add a set of controls to pregnancy intentions in predicting the survival of breastfeeding through the intervals shown in Fig. 2. With these controls, becoming pregnant "too soon" remains highly significant ($p < 0.01$) relative to the default category of "timing ok" in predicting a reduced probability of the survival of breastfeeding through the 14 to 27 week interval. Likewise, having an "unwanted" pregnancy achieves a baseline significance level ($p < 0.10$) in predicting such a reduced probability in this interval. For the other intervals, however, the pregnancy intention categories lack significance in predicting survival of breastfeeding. In the interval from 27 to 52 weeks, the odds ratios for "too soon" and "unwanted" approximate one, again confirming the lack of differentiation in the survival of breastfeeding between the pregnancy intention categories during this interval. These findings show that the disparities by pregnancy intentions in the survival of breastfeeding to 52 weeks displayed in Fig. 1 and Table 1 are primarily the products of differences in breastfeeding continuation that appear in the first 7 months.

Table 2. Logistic Regressions of the Survival of Breastfeeding through Intervals after Birth.

Cells Show Odds Ratio (Std. Error)	Interval (from Birth)		
	7–14 Weeks	14–27 Weeks	27–52 Weeks
Timing			
Too soon	0.896 (0.107)	0.716 (0.078)***	1.052 (0.132)
Unwanted	0.843 (0.096)	0.782 (0.115)*	1.014 (0.181)
Timing OK (default)	–	–	–
Mother's Ed. Attainment at Birth			
No high school diploma	0.917 (0.126)	1.071 (0.121)	1.058 (0.141)
Age 18 or under	1.470 (0.248)**	1.068 (0.206)	1.189 (0.289)
High school diploma (default)	–	–	–
Race/Ethnicity			
Non-Latina Black	1.084 (0.144)	0.924 (0.179)	0.885 (0.158)
Non-Latina other	1.073 (0.202)	0.948 (0.180)	1.155 (0.304)
Latina	0.978 (0.175)	0.822 (0.105)	1.213 (0.194)
Non-Latina White (default)	–	–	–
Mother Born Outside US			
Yes	1.261 (0.203)	1.583 (0.216)***	1.421 (0.217)**
No (default)	–	–	–
First Pregnancy			
Yes	1.121 (0.100)	0.944 (0.097)	1.058 (0.119)
No (default)	–	–	–
Marital Status			
Married at conception & birth	1.286 (0.156)**	1.442 (0.197)***	0.852 (0.113)
Married at birth only	0.914 (0.165)	1.116 (0.235)	0.745 (0.179)
Unmarried at birth (default)	–	–	–
Birth Method			
Cesarean	0.731 (0.078)***	0.765 (0.085)**	0.823 (0.093)*
Vaginal (default)	–	–	–
Full Term			
Yes	1.110 (0.115)	1.253 (0.121)**	1.386 (0.168)***
No (default)	–	–	–
Low Birth Weight			
Yes	0.956 (0.134)	0.953 (0.174)	0.804 (0.152)
No (default)	–	–	–
Mother's Age at Conception	1.048 (0.012)***	1.011 (0.014)	1.036 (0.013)***
Year of Child's Birth	0.982 (0.009)**	1.021 (0.010)**	1.023 (0.010)**
F-value	3.52***	8.00***	3.49***
N	8573	6625	4428

Note: See the note in Table 1 regarding the educational attainment variable. Breastfeeding durations reported in months by the data source are converted to weeks by multiplying months by 4.333.
$^*p < 0.10$, $^{**}p < 0.05$, $^{***}p < 0.01$.

Exclusive Breastfeeding

While the analysis so far has considered the durability of any breastfeeding, results in Table 3 examine the duration of exclusive breastfeeding. This table summarizes four logistic regression models of exclusive breastfeeding until at least 6 months after birth. Model 1 includes the same predictors as in Table 1 and Table 2; Model 2 adds an indicator of whether Medicaid paid for the child's delivery; Model 3 calculates the effects of pregnancy intentions separately for Medicaid recipients and nonrecipients; and Model 4 adds controls for maternity leave status.

Results for Model 1 show that becoming pregnant too soon is highly significant ($p < 0.01$) in predicting a reduced probability of exclusive breastfeeding for 6 months. The "too soon" variable drops out of statistical significance in Model 2, due primarily to inflation of its standard error (via reduced sample size) rather than change in its odds ratio.

Model 3 indicates that getting pregnant too soon reduces the likelihood of exclusive breastfeeding only among Medicaid recipients. In this model, the odds ratio of the "too soon" variable roughly equals one for Medicaid nonrecipients. Thus, there is little difference in the likelihood that nonrecipients who became pregnant too soon versus at the right time will exclusively breastfeed for 6 months. In contrast, among Medicaid recipients, those getting pregnant too soon are estimated have odds which are 56.3% of those getting pregnant at the right time to exclusively breastfeed, and this relationship is highly significant ($p = 0.018$).

In Model 4, the difference for Medicaid recipients between getting pregnant too soon versus at the right time retains a baseline level of significance ($p = 0.079$). Furthermore, postestimation testing reveals that the difference between the odds ratio of "too soon" for Medicaid recipients and the odds ratio of "too soon" for nonrecipients (controlling for Medicaid receipt) is significant at the $p < 0.05$ level in Model 3 and at the $p < 0.10$ level in Model 4. This provides evidence of a relationship specific to Medicaid recipients between getting pregnant too soon and reduced odds of the exclusive breastfeeding outcome.

In all models, having an unwanted pregnancy is estimated to reduce the likelihood of exclusive breastfeeding for 6 months. This relationship achieves statistical significance ($p < 0.01$) among Medicaid nonrecipients after controlling for maternity leave status in Model 4. However, postestimation testing of this model shows that the difference between the odds ratio of "unwanted" for Medicaid recipients and the odds ratio of "unwanted" for nonrecipients (controlling for Medicaid receipt) is not significant ($p = 0.287$). Thus it cannot be concluded that the effect of unwanted pregnancies in reducing the likelihood of the exclusive breastfeeding outcome is specific to nonrecipients rather than applicable to the general population.

Table 3. Logistic Regressions of Exclusive Breastfeeding until 6 Months after Birth.

Cells Show Odds Ratio (Std. Error)	Model 1	Model 2	Model 3	Model 4
Timing				
Too soon	0.766 (0.073)***	0.767 (0.133)		
Unwanted	0.826 (0.101)	0.719 (0.163)		
Timing OK (default)	–	–		
Medicaid x				
Too soon			0.563 (0.135)**	0.616 (0.168)*
Unwanted			0.648 (0.183)	0.660 (0.221)
Timing OK (default)			–	–
No Medicaid x				
Too soon			0.991 (0.199)	1.128 (0.271)
Unwanted			0.759 (0.257)	0.411 (0.136)***
Timing OK (default)			–	–
Mother's Ed. Attainment at Birth				
No high school diploma	0.999 (0.112)	1.188 (0.182)	1.179 (0.180)	0.911 (0.204)
Age 18 or under	1.189 (0.205)	1.925 (0.540)**	2.007 (0.558)**	0.845 (0.351)
High school diploma (default)	–	–	–	–
Race/Ethnicity				
Non-Latina Black	1.565 (0.234)***	1.006 (0.187)	0.993 (0.187)	0.839 (0.209)
Non-Latina other	1.372 (0.240)*	1.619 (0.394)*	1.617 (0.399)*	1.152 (0.402)
Latina	1.507 (0.232)***	1.467 (0.340)	1.439 (0.331)	0.823 (0.248)
Non-Latina White (default)	–	–	–	–
Mother Born Outside US				
Yes	1.171 (0.154)	1.056 (0.207)	1.056 (0.207)	1.143 (0.293)
No (default)	–	–	–	–
First Pregnancy				
Yes	0.984 (0.093)	1.162 (0.184)	1.171 (0.188)	1.277 (0.247)
No (default)	–	–	–	–
Marital Status				
Married at conception & birth	1.107 (0.099)	1.188 (0.187)	1.196 (0.185)	1.258 (0.258)
Married at birth only	0.866 (0.153)	0.535 (0.160)**	0.507 (0.150)**	0.545 (0.223)
Unmarried at birth (default)	–	–	–	–
Birth Method				
Cesarean	0.785 (0.077)**	0.716 (0.114)**	0.713 (0.114)**	0.525 (0.097)***
Vaginal (default)	–	–	–	–

Table 3. (*Continued*)

Cells Show Odds Ratio (Std. Error)	Model 1	Model 2	Model 3	Model 4
Full Term				
Yes	1.054 (0.104)	0.816 (0.122)	0.821 (0.122)	1.070 (0.222)
No (default)	–	–	–	–
Low Birth Weight				
Yes	1.110 (0.190)	0.849 (0.216)	0.849 (0.216)	0.948 (0.348)
No (default)	–	–	–	–
Mother's Age at Conception	1.017 (0.011)	1.037 (0.015)**	1.037 (0.015)**	1.048 (0.022)**
Year of Child's Birth	0.994 (0.008)	0.994 (0.027)	0.994 (0.027)	1.048 (0.050)
Medicaid Paid for Delivery				
Yes		0.995 (0.147)	1.142 (0.205)	1.002 (0.248)
No (default)		–	–	–
Maternity Leave				
Took leave				0.479 (0.085)***
No leave – Not needed				0.424 (0.182)**
No leave – Not offered				0.840 (0.313)
No leave – Other reason				0.635 (0.159)*
Not employed (default)				–
F-value	3.61***	3.35***	3.29***	3.12***
N	10725	3909	3909	2646

Note: See the note in Table 1 regarding the educational attainment variable. Breastfeeding durations reported in weeks by the data source are converted to months by dividing months by 4.333.
$^{*}p < 0.10$, $^{**}p < 0.05$, $^{***}p < 0.01$.

Control Variables

Breastfeeding for each duration in Table 1 becomes more probable if the mother was born outside of the US and if she was married at conception and birth (versus being unmarried). These relationships are consistently highly significant ($p < 0.01$) for all breastfeeding durations in the table and correspond with the findings of prior research. In contrast, marriage occurring during pregnancy is not statistically significance in predicting the probability of breastfeeding for any duration in the table. A Caesarean birth consistently decreases the odds of breastfeeding for each duration ($p < 0.01$), while a full-term pregnancy increases the likelihood of breastfeeding for the two longest durations ($p < 0.05$ or stronger).

Results in Table 2 show that marriage before conception promotes breastfeeding to a year through increasing the likelihood of breastfeeding in the first 7 months after birth. Indeed, while the odds ratio for "married at conception and birth" is greater than one and statistically significant ($p < 0.05$ or stronger) from 7 to 14 weeks and from 14 to 27 weeks after birth, it is less than one and lacks significance in the 27 to 52 week interval. In contrast, mother's birthplace remains significant ($p < 0.05$) in increasing odds of breastfeeding through the 27 to 52 week interval.

The chances of exclusive breastfeeding decrease for Cesarean births ($p < 0.05$), as is the case for any breastfeeding (Table 1). Marriages between conception and birth depress odds of exclusive breastfeeding ($p < 0.05$ in Model 2 and Model 3), suggesting that they may tend to create instability detrimental to maintaining such exclusivity. Most indicators that the mother was employed at birth, regardless of whether she took maternity leave, are statistically significant (versus being unemployed) in reducing the odds of the exclusive breastfeeding outcome (Model 4). Relationships between mother's birthplace and the exclusive breastfeeding outcome lack significance, in contrast to those for any breastfeeding.

CONCLUSION

The prior literature has made it clear that planning has effects on breastfeeding persistence, and the medical field has established clear guidelines for breastfeeding duration, but prior research has not established when in the postpartum period is the most crucial turning point. This chapter establishes that it is in the period from 3 to 7 months postpartum that the most significant differences, by pregnancy intentions, in breastfeeding persistence appear. Future research should thus focus on this 3 to 7 month period in order to determine what kinds of social support mothers are lacking in this period. The beginning of this period is a typical endpoint for maternity leave, suggesting that the return to work remains a key factor in limiting persistence. The models of exclusive breastfeeding suggest there may be a breastfeeding advantage to unemployment. Future studies should thus further examine the effects of workplace policies, such as maternity leave and support for pumping breastmilk.

While effects of planning are concentrated from 14 to 27 weeks postpartum, stable marriages (before conception) consistently promote breastfeeding in the first 27 weeks after birth. Marital status can be a source of social support throughout the breastfeeding experience, and its protective role in the earliest months postpartum can help facilitate sustained breastfeeding. However, breastfeeding can exacerbate the gendered division of labor among couples

(Avishai, 2007; Rippeyoung & Noonanb, 2012a). Future research should apply structural equation modeling to analyze reciprocal relationships between breastfeeding and marriage.

Prior literature has established that planning can be very difficult for those living in poverty, so a special concern in this study was whether poor and nonpoor groups differ in terms of the relationship between planning and exclusive breastfeeding persistence. The findings show that pregnancy timing makes a statistically significant difference only for those living in poverty and that such timing makes a greater difference for poor than nonpoor mothers. In order to achieve desirable breastfeeding outcomes, mothers lacking economic resources may particularly benefit from taking a more deliberate approach to their pregnancies. Furthermore, financial incentives for sustaining exclusive breastfeeding (i.e., the cost savings of breastmilk over formula) may be amplified for poor mothers. Reforms to WIC, implemented in October 2009 (Whaiey et al., 2012), increase incentives for poor mothers to sustain exclusive breastfeeding. Most pregnancies in the sample, however, predate these reforms, and those to which these reforms do apply cannot fully account for the relationship shown here of pregnancy timing to breastfeeding duration among poor mothers (contact authors for details). It is important to note that this relationship is seen when examining exclusive breastfeeding, and that the study did not investigate the interaction of planning and poverty status with regard to any breastfeeding. Exclusive breastfeeding requires more planning and commitment than does any breastfeeding, which likely accentuates the effects of timing on persistence.

This study is limited in its ability to empirically demonstrate what accounts for the relationship of pregnancy intentions to breastfeeding persistence among poor mothers, which is a key subject for future research. However, the existence of this relationship suggests that there are substantial payoffs (in terms of ability to sustain breastfeeding) to family planning among those living in poverty. Additionally, it contributes to the broader literature on socioeconomic disparities in health outcomes. While such research typically suggests that planning will be difficult for poor people because of their diminished access to health resources and limited efficacy within the healthcare system (see Link & Phelan, 1995; Phelan, Link & Tehranifar, 2010), this chapter suggests that the payoffs to such planning may be far greater for people living in poverty. Many other studies of health behaviors focus on areas where access to health resources and knowledge are vital. Breastfeeding, in contrast, is a health behavior where medicalized – as opposed to folk – knowledge is not as central and incentives (e.g., financial savings; perceived benefits to child and maternal health) are especially great. The results here suggest the need for additional research to refine our understanding of the role of planning in health disparities, particularly why and how people make decisions about health behaviors that they think – or that public health standards suggest – might benefit their own and their children's health.

These findings have important policy implications. Policy interventions that facilitate breastfeeding and reduce the impact of workplace demands on postpartum mothers could play an important role in facilitating sustained breastfeeding (Jacknowitz, 2008; Kogan et al., 2008; Lubold & Roth, 2012; Mulford, 2012; Murtagh & Moulton, 2011; Smith et al., 2013). Global evidence suggests that such policies are possible – indeed, breastfeeding is nearly universal in Sweden, which utilizes social benefits such as extended parental leave to facilitate it (Hausman, 2012). The findings also suggest that policy interventions that enhance women's ability to plan and time their pregnancies could facilitate sustained breastfeeding, especially among women living in poverty. However, policymakers need to take care to craft policies that can enhance breastfeeding among disadvantaged mothers without further burdening them. Efforts to increase breastfeeding do have the potential to increase surveillance and medicalization of disadvantaged women (Armstrong, 2000; Avishai, 2007; Bridges, 2012).

REFERENCES

Ahnquist, J., Wamala, S. P., & Lindstrom, M. (2012). Social determinants of health: A question of social or economic capital? Interaction effects of socioeconomic factors on health outcomes. *Social Science & Medicine*, *74*(6), 930–939. doi:10.1016/j.socscimed.2011.11.026.

American Academy of Pediatrics. (n.d.). FAQs. Retrieved from https://www2.aap.org/breastfeeding/faqsBreastfeeding.html

Armstrong, E. (2000). Lessons in control: Prenatal education in the hospital. *Social Problems*, *47*(4), 583–605.

Arora, S., McJunkin, C., Wehrer, J., & Kuhn, P. (2000). Major factors influencing breastfeeding rates: Mother's perception of father's attitude and milk supply. *Pediatrics*, *106*(5), e67–e71. Retrieved from http://pediatrics.aappublications.org/content/106/5/e67.full.pdf

Avishai, O. (2007). Managing the lactating body: The breast-feeding project and privileged motherhood. *Qualitative Sociology*, *30*(1), 135–152.

Baumeister, R. F., Bratslavsky, E., Muraven, M., & Tice, D. M. (1998). Ego depletion: Is the active self a limited resource? *Journal of Personality and Social Psychology*, *74*(5), 1252–1265.

Besculides, M., & Laraque, F. (2004). Unintended pregnancy among the urban poor. *Journal of Urban Health*, *81*(3), 340–348.

Blum, L. M. (1999). *At the breast: Ideologies of breastfeeding and motherhood in the contemporary United States*. Boston, MA: Beacon Press.

Boyas, J. F. (2013). Correlates of health literacy among Latinos in Arkansas. *Social Work in Public Health*, *28*, 32–43.

Bridges, K. M. (2012). Pregnancy, medicaid, state regulation, and legal subjection. *Journal of Poverty*, *16*, 323–352.

Buckles, K., & Kolka, S. (2014). Prenatal investments, breastfeeding, and birth order. *Social Science & Medicine*, *118*, 66–70. doi:10.1016/j.socscimed.2014.07.055.

Colen, C. G., & Ramey, D. M. (2014). Is breast truly best? Estimating the effects of breastfeeding on long-term child health and wellbeing in the United States using sibling comparisons. *Social Science & Medicine*, *109*, 55–65.

Cooklin, A. R., Rowe, H. J., & Fisher, J. R. W. (2012). Paid parental leave supports breastfeeding and mother–infant relationship: A prospective investigation of maternal postpartum employment. *Australian and New Zealand Journal of Public Health, 36*(3), 249–256. doi:10.1111/j.1753-6405.2012.00846.x

D'Angelo, D. V., Gilbert, B. C., Rochat, R. W., Santelli, J. S., & Herold, J. M. (2004). Differences between mistimed and unwanted pregnancies among women who have live births. *Perspectives on Sexual and Reproductive Health, 36*(5), 192–197. Retrieved from https://www.guttmacher.org/pubs/journals/3619204.html

Dehlendorf, C., Rodriguez, M. I., Levy, K., Borrero, S., & Steinauer, J. (2010). Disparities in family planning. *American Journal of Obstetrics and Gynecology, 202*(3), 214–220. doi:10.1016/j.ajog.2009.08.022.

Dodgson, J. E. (2012). Racism, race, and disparities in breastfeeding. In P. H. Smith, B. Hausman, & M. Labbok (Eds.), *Beyond health, beyond choice: Breastfeeding constraints and realities* (pp. 74–83). New Brunswick, NJ: Rutgers University Press.

Donovan, P. (1995). Physical violence toward pregnant women is more likely to occur when pregnancy was unintended. *Family Planning Perspectives, 27*(5), 222–223.

Dumas, A., Robataille, J., & Jette, S. L. (2014). Lifestyle as a choice of necessity: Young women, health and obesity. *Social Theory & Health, 12*(2), 138–158.

Dye, T. D., Wojtowycz, M. A., Aubry, R. H., Quade, J., & Kilburn, H. (1997). Unintended pregnancy and breast-feeding behavior. *American Journal of Public Health, 87*(10), 1709–1711. Retrieved from http://www.ncbi.nlm.nih.gov/pmc/articles/PMC1381142/pdf/amjph00509-0135.pdf

Evenhouse, E., & Reilly, S. (2005). Improved estimates of the benefits of breastfeeding using sibling comparisons to reduce selection bias. *HSR: Health Services Research, 40*(6), 1781–1802.

Gibson-Davis, C. M., & Brooks-Gunn, J. (2007). The association of couples' relationship status and quality with breastfeeding initiation. *Journal of Marriage and Family, 29*, 1107–1117.

Guttmacher Institute. (2015, February). Unintended pregnancy in the United States. Retrieved from http://www.guttmacher.org/pubs/FB-Unintended-Pregnancy-US.html

Hausman, B. L. (2012). Feminism and breastfeeding: Rhetoric, ideology, and the material realities of women's lives. In P. H. Smith, B. Hausman, & M. Labbok (Eds.), *Beyond health, beyond choice: Breastfeeding constraints and realities* (pp. 15–24). New Brunswick, NJ: Rutgers University Press.

Hausman, B. L., Smith, P. H., & Labbok, M. (2012). Introduction: Breastfeeding constraints and realities. In P. H. Smith, B. Hausman, & M. Labbok (Eds.), *Beyond health, beyond choice: Breastfeeding constraints and realities* (pp. 1–11). New Brunswick, NJ: Rutgers University Press.

Heikkilä, K., Sacker, A., Kelly, Y., Renfrew, M. J., & Quigley, M. A. (2011). Breast feeding and child behaviour in the millennium cohort study. *Archives of Disease in Childhood, 96*(7), 635–642. doi:10.1136/adc.2010.201970.

Hromi-Fiedler, A., & Pérez-Escamilla, R. (2006). Unintended pregnancies are associated with less likelihood of prolonged breast-feeding: An analysis of 18 demographic and health surveys. *Public Health Nutrition, 9*(3), 306–312. Retrieved from http://journals.cambridge.org/download.php?file=%2FPHN%2FPHN9_03%2FS1368980006000577a.pdf&code=b111054a3a84b2f690aecae20ceafeb1

Hummer, R. A., Hack, K. A., & Raley, R. K. (2004). Retrospective reports of pregnancy wantedness and child well-being in the United States. *Journal of Family Issues, 25*(3), 404–428.

Jacknowitz, A. (2008). The role of workplace characteristics in breastfeeding practices. *Women & Health, 47*(2), 87–111. doi:10.1080/03630240802092357.

Jacobson, J. L. (1993). Women's health: The price of poverty. In M. Koblinsky, J. Timyan, & J. Gay (Eds.), *The health of women: A global perspective* (pp. 3–31). Boulder, CO: Westview Press.

Johnston, M. L., & Esposito, N. (2007). Barriers and facilitators for breastfeeding among working women in the United States. *Journal of Obstetric, Gynecologic, & Neonatal Nursing, 36*(1), 9–20.

Joyce, T., Kaestner, R., & Korenman, S. (2000). The stability of pregnancy intentions and pregnancy-related maternal behaviors. *Maternal & Child Health Journal*, *4*(3), 171–178. Retrieved from http://www.ncbi.nlm.nih.gov/pubmed/11097504.

Kendalla, C., Afable-Munsuzb, A., Speizerc, I., Averya, A., Schmidta, N., & Santellid, J. (2005). Understanding pregnancy in a population of inner-city women in New Orleans – Results of qualitative research. *Social Science & Medicine*, *60*, 297–311.

Kidd, C., Palmeri, H., & Aslin, R. N. (2013). Rational snacking: Young children's decision-making on the marshmallow task is moderated by beliefs about environmental reliability. *Cognition*, *126*(1), 109–114.

Kimbro, R. T. (2006). On-the-job moms: Work and breastfeeding initiation and duration for a sample of low-income women. *Maternal and Child Health Journal*, *10*(1), 19–26. doi:10.1007/s10995-005-0058-7.

Kimbro, R. T., Lynch, S. M., & McLanahan, S. (2008). The influence of acculturation on breast-feeding initiation and duration for Mexican–Americans. *Population Research and Policy Review*, *27*(2), 183–199. doi:10.1007/s11113-007-9059-0.

Kogan, M. D., Singh, G. K., Dee, D. L., Belanoff, C., & Grummer-Strawh, L. M. (2008). Multivariate analysis of state variation in breastfeeding rates in the United States. *American Journal of Public Health*, *98*(10), 1872–1880. doi:10.2105/AJPH.2007.127118.

Kost, K., Landry, D. J., & Darroch, J. E. (1998). The effects of pregnancy planning status On birth outcomes and infant care. *Family Planning Perspectives*, *30*(5), 223–230. Retrieved from http://www.ncbi.nlm.nih.gov/pubmed/9782045.

Kost, K., & Lindberg, L. (2015). Pregnancy intentions, maternal behaviors, and infant health: Investigating relationships with new measures and propensity score analysis. *Demography*, *52*(1), 83–111. doi:10.1007/s13524-014-0359-9.

Kramer, M. S., Matush, L., Vanilovich, I., Platt, R. W., Bogdanovich, N., Sevkovskaya, Z., ... Shapiro, S. (2009). A randomized breast-feeding promotion intervention did not reduce child obesity in Belarus. *Journal of Nutrition*, *129*, 1S–5S.

Lee, H. J., Elo, I. T., McCollum, K. F., & Culhane, J. F. (2009). Racial/ethnic differences in breast-feeding initiation and duration among low-income inner-city mothers. *Social Science Quarterly*, *90*(5), 1251–1271.

Link, B. G., & Phelan, J. C. (1995). Social conditions as fundamental causes of disease. *Journal of Health and Social Behavior*, *35*(Extra Issue), 80–94.

Lubold, A. M., & Roth, L. M. (2012). The impact of workplace practices on breastfeeding experiences and disparities among women. In P. H. Smith, B. Hausman, & M. Labbok (Eds.), *Beyond health, beyond choice: Breastfeeding constraints and realities* (pp. 157–166). New Brunswick, NJ: Rutgers University Press.

Lucas, J. C., & McCarter-Spaulding, D. (2012). Working out work: Race, employment, and public policy. In P. H. Smith, B. Hausman, & M. Labbok (Eds.), *Beyond health, beyond choice: Breastfeeding constraints and realities* (pp. 144–156). New Brunswick, NJ: Rutgers University Press.

Marsiglio, W., & Mott, F. L. (1988). Does wanting to become pregnant with a first child affect subsequent maternal behaviors and infant birth weight? *Journal of Marriage and Family*, *50*(4), 1023–1036.

Mauldon, J., Foster, D. G., & Roberts, S. C. M. (2015). Effect of abortion vs. carrying to term on a woman's relationship with the man involved in the pregnancy. *Perspectives on Sexual and Reproductive Health*, *47*(1), 1–8. doi:10.1363/47e2315.

Maxson, P., & Miranda, M. L. (2011). Pregnancy intention, demographic differences, and psychosocial health. *Journal of Women's Health*, *20*(8), 1215–1223. doi:10.1089/jwh.2010.2379.

Mulford, C. (2012). 'Are we there yet?' Breastfeeding as a gauge of carework by mothers. In P. H. Smith, B. Hausman, & M. Labbok (Eds.), *Beyond health, beyond choice: Breastfeeding constraints and realities* (pp. 123–132). New Brunswick, NJ: Rutgers University Press.

Murtagh, L., & Moulton, A. D. (2011). Working mothers, breastfeeding, and the law. *American Journal of Public Health*, *101*(2), 217–223. doi:10.2105/AJPH.2009.185280.

National Center for Chronic Disease Prevention and Health Promotion. (2014). Breastfeeding report card. Retrieved from http://www.cdc.gov/breastfeeding/pdf/2014breastfeedingreport-card.pdf

National Center for Health Statistics. (2015, 6/22/2015). National survey of family growth. Retrieved from http://www.cdc.gov/nchs/nsfg.htm

Peters, E., Wehkamp, K.-H., Felderbaum, R. E., Krüger, D., & Linder, R. (2006). Breastfeeding duration is determined by only a few factors. *The European Journal of Public Health*, *16*(2), 162–167.

Phelan, J. C., Link, B. G., & Tehranifar, P. (2010). Social conditions as fundamental causes of health inequalities: Theory, evidence, and policy implications. *Journal of Health and Social Behavior*, *51*(S), S28–S40.

Pulley, L., Klerman, L. V., Tang, H., & Baker, B. A. (2002). The extent of pregnancy mistiming and its association with maternal characteristics and behaviors and pregnancy outcomes. *Perspectives on Sexual and Reproductive Health*, *34*(4), 206–211. Retrieved from http://www.ncbi.nlm.nih.gov/pubmed/12214911.

Rippeyoung, P. L. F. (2013). Can Breastfeeding Solve Inequality? The relative mediating impact of breastfeeding and home environment on poverty gaps in Canadian child cognitive skills. *Canadian Journal of Sociology*, *38*(1), 65–85.

Rippeyoung, P. L. F., & Noonanb, M. C. (2012a). Breastfeeding and the gendering of infant care. In P. H. Smith, B. Hausman, & M. Labbok (Eds.), *Beyond health, beyond choice: Breastfeeding constraints and realities* (pp. 133–143). New Brunswick, NJ: Rutgers University Press.

Rippeyoung, P. L. F., & Noonanb, M. C. (2012b). Is breastfeeding truly cost free? Income consequences of breastfeeding for women. *American Sociological Review*, *77*(2), 244–267.

Roberts, S. C. M., Biggs, M. A., Chibber, K. S., Gould, H., Rocca, C., & Foster, D. G. (2014). Risk of violence from the man involved in the pregnancy after receiving or being denied an abortion. *BMC Medicine*, *12*, 144–150.

Rudzik, A. E. F. (2012). The experience and determinants of first-time breast-feeding duration among low-income women from Sao Paulo, Brazil. *Current Anthropology*, *53*(1), 108–117.

Ruowei, L., Darling, N., Maurice, E., Barker, L., & Grummer-Strawn, L. M. (2005). Breastfeeding rates in the United States by characteristics of the child, mother, or family: The 2002 National Immunization Survey. *Pediatrics*, *115*(1), e31–e37. doi:10.1002/prot.20244.

Ruspini, E. (2001). The study of women's deprivation: How to reveal the gender dimension of poverty. *International Journal of Social Research Methodology*, *4*(2), 101–118.

Seipel, M. M. O., & Shafer, K. (2013). The effect of prenatal and postnatal care on childhood obesity. *Social Work*, *58*(3), 241–252. Retrieved from http://www.ncbi.nlm.nih.gov/pubmed/24032305.

Shah, A. K., Mullainathan, S., & Shafir, E. (2012). Some consequences of having too little. *Science*, *338*, 682–685.

Smith, J. P., McIntyre, E., Craig, L., Javanparast, S., Strazdins, L., & Mortensen, K. (2013). Workplace support, breastfeeding and health. *Family Matters*, *93*, 58–73.

Stein, Z., & Kuhn, L. (2009). Breast feeding: A time to craft new policies. *Journal of Public Health Policy*, *30*(3), 300–310. doi:10.1057/jphp.2009.23.

Taylor, J. S., & Cabral, H. (2002). Are women with an unintended pregnancy less likely to breastfeed? *Journal of Family Practice*, *51*(5), 431–436. Retrieved from http://www.ncbi.nlm.nih.gov/pubmed/12019050.

Taylor, J. S., Risica, P. M., Geller, L., Kirtania, U., & Cabral, H. (2006). Duration of breastfeeding among first-time mothers in the United States: Results of a national survey. *Acta Paediatrica*, *95*(8), 980–984. doi:10.1080/08035250600750064.

Whaiey, S. E., Koleilat, M., Whaiey, M., Gomez, J., Meehan, K., & Saluja, K. (2012). Impact of policy changes on infant feeding decisions among low-income women participating in the special supplemental nutrition program for women, infants, and children. *American Journal of Public Health*, *102*(12), 2269–2273.

Wolf, J. B. (2007). Is breast really best? Risk and total motherhood in the national breastfeeding awareness campaign. *Journal of Health Politics, Policy and Law*, *32*(4), 595–636.

Woloshin, S., Schwartz, L. M., & Welch, H. G. (2008). The risk of death by age, sex, and smoking status in the United States: Putting health risks in context. *Journal of the National Cancer Institute*, *100*(12), 845–853. doi:10.1093/jnci/djn124.

World Health Organization. (2015). The World Health Organization's infant feeding recommendation. Retrieved from http://www.who.int/nutrition/topics/infantfeeding_recommendation/en/

TAKING INSURANCE IN ABORTION CARE: POLICY, PRACTICES, AND THE ROLE OF POVERTY

Katrina Kimport and Brenly Rowland

ABSTRACT

Most women seeking abortion pay out-of-pocket for care, partly due to legal restrictions on insurance coverage. These costs can constitute a hardship for many women. Advocates have sought to ensure insurance coverage for abortion, but we do not know whether the intermediaries between policy and patient – abortion-providing facilities – are able and willing to accept insurance.

We interviewed 22 abortion facility administrators, representing 64 clinical sites in 21 states that varied in their legal allowance of public and private insurance coverage for abortion, about their facility's insurance practices, and experiences.

Respondents described challenges in accepting public and/or private insurance that included, but were not limited to, legal regulations. When public insurance broadly covered abortion, its low reimbursement failed to cover the costs of care. Because of the predominance of low income patients in abortion care, this caused financial challenges for facilities, leading one in a state that allows broad coverage to nonetheless decline public insurance. Accepting private insurance carried its own risks, including nonpayment because costs fell within patients' deductibles. Respondents described work-arounds to protect their facility from nonpayment and enable patients to use their private insurance.

Health and Health Care Concerns among Women and Racial and Ethnic Minorities
Research in the Sociology of Health Care, Volume 35, 39–57

ISSN: 0275-4959/doi:10.1108/S0275-495920170000035003

The structure of insurance and the population of abortion patients mean that changes at the political level may not translate into changes in individual women's experience of paying for abortion.

This research illustrates how legal regulations, insurer practices, and the socioeconomics of the patient population matter for abortion-providing facilities' decision-making about accepting insurance.

Keywords: Abortion; insurance; Medicaid; poverty

INTRODUCTION

On July 8, 2015, U.S. Congressional Representative Barbara Lee introduced the Equal Access to Abortion Coverage in Health Insurance Act, known as the EACH Woman Act. The act would require public and private insurance providers to cover abortion care. Although unlikely to come up for a vote, let alone be passed, while the antiabortion Republican party holds the majority of seats in Congress, the act represents the latest foray in decades of political contestation over insurance coverage for abortion. In 1976, with the Hyde Amendment, Congress voted to exclude abortion care from the services federal funds contributed to public health insurance (known as Medicaid) can cover, save for abortion for reasons of rape or incest, or when the pregnant woman's life is in danger. The Hyde amendment has been regularly reapproved over the years, and 33 states and the District of Columbia have mirrored that language to similarly restrict the use of state funds contributed to public insurance for abortion (Guttmacher Institute, 2017b). Even with Hyde still firmly in place, in 2009, controversy over insurance coverage for abortion led to delays in the approval and implementation of the Affordable Care Act (Gold, 2010). To placate antiabortion members of congress, the act includes special rules regarding abortion services, including requiring separate, opt-in funds for abortion coverage for plans offered through the newly established health exchanges (Cohen, 2010; Schaler-Haynes, Chesnokova, Cox, & Feinstein, 2011) and allowing states to ban private insurance plans from covering abortion (Rosenbaum, 2011).

As these policy fights have played out, abortion remains one of the most common medical procedures in the United States, with one in three women obtaining abortion care in her lifetime (Jones & Kavanaugh, 2011). Currently, most women obtaining abortions pay out-of-pocket, even those eligible for insurance coverage (Jones, Upadhyay, & Weitz, 2013). Among insured women, regardless of type of insurance, only about one-third receive coverage for their abortions (Bessett, Gorski, Jinadasa, Ostrow, & Peterson, 2011; Roberts, Gould, Kimport, Weitz, & Foster, 2014). Many women with private insurance plans fail to use their coverage for reasons including because they assume abortion is not a covered service (Cockrill & Weitz, 2010; Van Bebber, Phillips, Weitz, Gould, & Stewart, 2006) and because they were given incorrect information regarding their plan's policies on covering abortions (Jones et al., 2013). Staff confusion and/or obfuscation regarding insurance coverage for abortion are not restricted to private insurers. Dennis, Blanchard, and Córdova (2011) found that Medicaid representatives in states that permit the use of state funds to cover abortion care were sometimes reluctant to give information about abortion services and often discouraged callers from seeking coverage at all.

The costs women bear to obtain abortion care are not insignificant (Van Bebber et al., 2006). In 2009, the median cost of a first trimester abortion, which constitute nearly 90% of all procedures (Pazol et al., 2011), was $470 and cost ranged as high as $629 (Jones & Kooistra, 2011). Women additionally face costs related to travel, lost work time, and childcare for existing children. Roberts et al. (2014) found, for example, that half of the women in their sample spent more than one-third of their monthly income to cover the costs associated with their abortion, potentially foregoing rent, utilities, and even food. Cost sometimes becomes a complete barrier to abortion: Cook, Parnell, Moore, and Pagnini (1999) estimate that lack of public funding for abortion contributes to as many as one-third of women who would choose abortion instead carrying their pregnancies to term due to their inability to afford abortion services. Scholars have used these findings to argue for the importance of public insurance coverage for abortion (Dennis, Manski, & Blanchard, 2015).

However, while the literature has examined the structure of insurance policies around abortion care and how women actually pay for care, little work has honed in on a third aspect of the insurance and payment for abortion services equation: the role of the facility. As an intermediary between patients and insurers, providers play a key role in securing insurance coverage for abortion care, but we know little about how they navigate this task. Research has shown that the actions of individual providers and facilities matter for securing Medicaid coverage for individual, eligible abortions (Dennis & Blanchard, 2013; Dennis et al., 2011), but also that more than half of Medicaid-eligible cases are not reimbursed (Kacanek, Dennis, Miller, & Blanchard, 2010). If providers do not accept insurance, or experience the obstacles to accepting insurance as prohibitive, changes in public policy such as the EACH Woman Act will not impact women's experience of paying for care.

The stakes are high. Abortion care is gendered care: women (and a very small number of transmen) get abortions. Policies and practices related to care are thus inherently gendered and can further – or potentially contest – gender inequality. Additionally, 42% of abortion patients report household incomes below the federal poverty line (Jones & Kavanaugh, 2011) meaning that insurance practices have a notable impact on economically vulnerable populations, with abortion decisions impacting not only the woman herself but also other people in her life (Dennis, Manski, & Blanchard, 2014). Abortion patients are also disproportionately women of color (Jones & Kavanaugh, 2011), meaning that obstacles to care created by insurance coverage policies and practices have disproportionate impact on populations that are already socially marginalized (Dehlendorf, Harris, & Weitz, 2013).

Here, we investigate facilities' practices around accepting public and private insurance for abortion care under a variety of regulatory settings, including broad allowance and broad prohibition of abortion coverage. We find that legal allowance and prohibition mattered to facilities' deciding to accept insurance, as did public insurance's reimbursement rates and the structure of private insurers. We further identify how the predominance of low income women in the patient population produces difficulties unique to abortion care that can make the costs of accepting insurance outweigh any benefits. Our findings illustrate how legal regulations and insurer practices *as well as* the socioeconomics of the patient population matter for abortion-providing facilities' decision-making about accepting insurance.

METHODS

To examine the insurance policies and practices of facilities that provide abortions, we conducted key informant interviews with staff members at abortion-providing facilities who had familiarity with billing practices and policies. Because target respondents would have extensive experience in the administrative aspects of abortion provision, with some having insight into insurance practices and decisions for more than one clinical site and/or across multiple regulatory settings, we considered them key informants. As part of a separate study, we worked with the National Abortion Federation (NAF), a professional association of abortion providers in the United States that includes both individual people and facilities, to identify member facilities that would be interested in participating in research about abortion and insurance. Because not all abortion providing facilities are NAF members, we also drew on professional contacts to identify administrators at non-NAF facilities who might be willing to participate in this study.

Anticipating that state policies might impact facility insurance practices, we sorted facilities based on the state laws regarding public and private insurance coverage for abortion of the state(s) they were located in. Facilities fell into three categories: they were located in states with (1) public and private insurance coverage broadly allowed; (2) private insurance coverage broadly allowed but public insurance coverage broadly restricted (i.e., limited to the exceptions to the Hyde amendment: rape, incest, or life endangerment); or (3) private insurance coverage restricted (e.g., prohibiting abortion coverage in plans available through the state health exchange) and public insurance coverage broadly restricted. There are no states that fit the fourth scenario of this cross tab of broad public insurance and restricted private insurance coverage.

Next, the second author emailed the administrative contact at up to five facilities in each category, purposively chosen for geographic diversity. The email described the study as an investigation into facility policies and practices related to accepting insurance coverage for abortion and requested a phone interview with whomever at the facility would be most knowledgeable on this topic (with additional inclusion criteria that prospective participants be over 18 and English-speaking). We sent two follow-up emails, at 1 week and 2 weeks after the initial email. If we did not hear from someone at that facility, we emailed the administrative contact at another facility located in a state with the same public and private insurance allowance profile.

Between October 2015 and February 2016, we conducted 22 in-depth phone interviews. At the end of each interview, respondents were asked to invite others they thought could speak to our research questions to contact us about the study. This recruitment strategy yielded 15 interviews from direct email and seven interviews through snowball referral. Interviews were conducted by phone at a time convenient to the respondent. Most took place during business hours, while the respondent was at work. Respondents verbally consented to participate in the study and were offered a $35 gift card to compensate them for their time. We collected but did not retain contact information to mail the gift cards.

Interviews were semistructured, allowing respondents to introduce new ideas. They included questions about the respondent's facility's current policies and practices regarding accepting public and private insurance, the history of these practices, and the various pros and cons of current and past practices. Additionally, we collected basic demographic information about respondents and their facilities. Interviews were audio recorded and transcribed. They ranged in length from about 20 minutes (owing to the demands of the respondent's work schedule) to an hour, averaging just under 40 minutes. All study protocols were approved by the institutional review board at the authors' institution.

Sample Characteristics

Of the 22 key informants, all but one were women, most were white, and most held a 4-year college or advanced degree (Table 1). They ranged in age from 32 to 68. Four respondents had worked at their facility for fewer than 5 years, while the remaining 17 reported 5 years or more at the same facility, including one respondent with 27 years at her facility.

Respondents represented 16 different facilities. Eight of the facilities operated a single clinical site that exclusively or predominantly provided abortion care. Five facilities operated multiple clinical sites, ranging from two to 36, that similarly specialized in abortion care. Outpatient clinics like these account for just under half of all the abortion-providing facilities in the United States, and

Table 1. Respondent Characteristics.

Characteristics	Respondents ($n = 22$)
Age (in years)	
30–39	9
40–49	6
50–59	3
60–69	3
Declined to provide	1
Race/ethnicity	
Asian	1
Black	3
Latina	1
Multiracial (Black and Native American)	1
White	15
Declined to provide	1
Highest educational attainment	
High school	1
Technical degree or some college	3
4-year college degree	5
Advanced degree	9
Declined to provide	4

provide 94% of all abortions performed annually (Jones & Jerman, 2014). The four remaining facilities represented in our sample were hospitals that offered a broad range of care. Hospitals account for 35% of the abortion providers in the United States, but just 4% of abortions performed annually (Jones & Jerman, 2014). These 16 facilities represented a total of 64 clinical sites located in 21 US states, including in all four general regions of the country: seven in the Midwest, eight in the northeast, nine in the south, and 40 in the west (most of these sites in the west were part of a single multisite facility). It is important to note that this regional distribution is not representative of the geographical distribution of providers (Jones & Jerman, 2014). This sample over-represents clinics in the west and under-represents providers in the northeast and south.

Analysis

Both authors read all transcripts in full. Because our focal unit of analysis is individual clinical sites rather than the respondent, the second author wrote a summary of the insurance policies, including reported challenges to and debates about, for each of the facilities represented in our sample. Then, both authors examined the summaries for patterns and trends in insurance acceptance policy. We identified three broad areas relevant to insurance acceptance policies: prework to accept insurance, variation in law and coverage, and the stakes of accepting insurance. Using these general topics as sensitizing concepts (Charmaz, 2006), the first author developed an initial codebook of broad topics and concepts, which the second author used to code three transcripts, simultaneously identifying new codes and possibly redundant codes. The first author independently coded the same transcripts and compared results. Although coding was generally consistent, there were areas of disagreement, which the authors discussed and resolved. With the revised codebook, the second author coded the remainder of the transcripts.

Next, we exported the excerpts for each topic and concept code and, using modified grounded theory (Charmaz, 2006), identified emergent patterns relevant to these more general codes. Each author performed the subcoding for about half the initial codes, discussing findings regularly. We considered coding complete when no new subcodes emerged.

RESULTS

In our interviews, respondents reported that accepting insurance, both public and private, took a great deal of staff time and effort, including research, physician credentialing, and the actual work of billing insurers. Taking insurance, in other words, was work – sometimes a lot of work. That accepting insurance requires staff work, both one-time activities and ongoing tasks, is not unique to abortion care. Nonetheless, respondents identified several ways in which accepting insurance for abortion care was uniquely complicated and costly. For some facilities, accepting insurance was so complicated and costly in terms of staff time and resources that they chose not to accept insurance all together.

Identifying Insurers

In order for facilities to take insurance, they had to first identify available insurers. The patchwork of state laws restricting Medicaid and private insurance coverage of abortion made this complicated for many facilities. We start with respondents' accounts of identifying Medicaid insurers.

In 33 states and the District of Columbia, state law broadly prohibits Medicaid coverage of abortion, with a few exceptions (e.g., pregnancy as the result of rape). On one level, it would seem that these bans would simplify facilities' experience of deciding whether to accept public insurance: they simply could not and would not. This was the case for several respondents, who

Table 2. Site Practices on Public Insurance.

State Law Regarding Public Insurance Coverage for Abortion	Site Accepts Public Insurance	Site Does Not Accept Public Insurance
Prohibits broadly ($n = 22$)	1[a]	21
Allows broadly ($n = 42$)	40	2

[a]This site accepted public insurance from patients who were residents of a neighboring state that allows public insurance coverage of abortion.

explained their facility's policy of not accepting Medicaid as rooted in a state law prohibition. In our sample, 21 clinical sites declined to accept public insurance because of legal restrictions on the use of Medicaid for abortion care (Table 2). The Director of Operations at a single site facility in the northeast was blunt in explaining why they do not accept Medicaid: "state Medicaid doesn't cover abortion services. So, you know, we don't obviously bill them, because they don't cover." Like many of the other sites in our sample that declined to accept Medicaid, her clinic developed their policy in response to the legal ban on public insurance coverage.

In theory, though, these laws included exceptions that allowed patients to use Medicaid for abortion care – usually for cases of rape, incest, and the life of the pregnant woman. In practice, however, facilities reported difficulty securing Medicaid coverage for these few exceptions allowed by the law. A physician at a single site facility in the west explained:

> Even in cases of rape, incest, or health of the mother, it [Medicaid coverage] is extremely rare. I just did kind of a research project […] to try to find out if they ever pay. We found 25 cases in 5 years where they paid, and they were hospital cases and the [abortion] pill. There were no abortion providers [like my facility] that provided those abortions, in other words.

As the physician explained, Medicaid did not cover abortions provided in facilities like hers, further cementing her facility's decision not to accept Medicaid.

The Billing Coordinator at a multisite facility with clinics throughout the United States faced a different challenge in regards to securing Medicaid reimbursement for exceptional cases that the law allows coverage for. She explained that, although one of the states where they had a clinical site explicitly allowed for Medicaid insurance coverage of abortions deemed "medically necessary," it had a parallel law that prohibited any physician who performs abortions from being credentialed by Medicaid. This created a legal paradox: without a credentialed physician, the site could not submit claims to Medicaid, even for abortions Medicaid is supposed to cover.

Not all states, however, made it difficult – or legally impossible – to bill Medicaid for abortion care, even when they had a law on the books limiting Medicaid coverage to certain circumstances. In some states, despite an ostensible ban on Medicaid coverage of most abortions, Medicaid staff interpreted allowable exceptions broadly. For example, a clinic director from a multisite facility in the south and west described how one of the states where her facility had a clinical site allowed Medicaid coverage for abortion if continuing the pregnancy could impact the woman's mental health. She continued, "I don't know if you have kids, but, yes, of course they have a mental impact on you." She reported that her facility was able to regularly and successfully bill Medicaid for abortion care under that portion of the law. Thus, what could appear to be a ban on Medicaid coverage of abortion, save for specific circumstances, did not, in practice, greatly restrict the application of Medicaid funds for abortion.

Similarly, a clinic situated in a state that banned the use of Medicaid for abortion for its residents might still get reimbursed by Medicaid for care provided to patients who reside in another state. The Director of a single site facility in the Midwest noted that her facility is located near the state border, so it sees many patients from a neighboring state that allows Medicaid coverage of abortion. The facility is contracted with all the neighboring state's Medicaid plans and has even coordinated with their Department of Health Services to expedite claim submission and processing, enabling them to take public insurance for patients who are residents of that state.

Still, as respondents explained, coverage for abortion care in states where Medicaid is broadly permitted to cover abortions was rarely straightforward either. A Billing Coordinator, whose facility had clinical sites in three states where Medicaid broadly covers abortion care, explained that these states had both standard Medicaid and Medicaid Managed Care Organizations (MCOs). In some states, MCOs will not pay for abortion care, but, as the Billing Coordinator explained, "They pay for what they call the 'nonabortion charges,' which is your office visit, your ultrasound, and your lab work." Similarly, a Director of Family Planning described how many of the patients at her northeast facility come from a state with multiple Medicaid providers, only some of which cover abortion, although state law allows Medicaid coverage of abortion: "there's some that will cover it, some that will not. So, that also adds a layer of complexity." A Counseling Manager explained that the state where her facility is located has several versions of Medicaid, all of which pay for abortion care, but they each reimburse for abortion care differently, which the facility has to attend to in its budgeting. As these idiosyncrasies illustrate, taking Medicaid in a state that broadly allows public insurance coverage of abortion was not necessarily easy.

On the private insurance front, respondents reported that many plans simply did not include abortion as a covered benefit. Twenty-five states currently ban private insurers on the state health exchanges from covering abortion in most instances (Guttmacher Institute, 2017a). Ten of these states, moreover, ban all private insurers from covering abortion in most instances (Guttmacher Institute, 2017a). For some facilities, this simplified their insurance policies regarding private insurers since such insurers were banned from covering abortion services. In our sample, seven clinical sites were located in states where

Table 3. Site Practices on Private Insurance.

State Law Regarding Private Insurance Coverage for Abortion	Site Accepts Private Insurance	Site Does Not Accept Private Insurance
Prohibits broadly ($n = 7$)	2[a]	6
Restricts some ($n = 8$)	5	3
Allows broadly ($n = 49$)	47	2

[a]These clinics accepted private insurance when the insurers covered abortion care, usually because the insurance company was based out-of-state and not subject to the state ban.

private insurers were broadly prohibited from covering abortion care (Table 3). An additional eight clinical sites operated in states that restricted some forms of private insurance (e.g., plans purchased on the state-run health exchange).

As with Medicaid, however, there were oddities that made the private insurance experience complicated. As the Director of a single site facility in the Midwest explained, state prohibitions on covering abortion generally apply to insurance companies based in her Midwestern state, but patients may have their insurance with companies based out-of-state. Although the state her facility is in "has a law that says abortion cannot be paid for," they have been successful billing private insurers as an out-of-network provider:

> We have many women who have policies through [an insurer] which is based out of [state]. We have billed those folks' insurance for their abortion, and there have been payments.

This facility was not alone in identifying and acting on this quirk in how state laws applied to private insurers; one other respondent described handling similar cases.

The Costs of Accepting Public Insurance

In our sample, 42 clinical sites operated in states that broadly allow public insurance coverage of abortion (Table 2). As respondents explained, however, while the existence of public insurance coverage of abortion care was necessary for a facility to decide to accept insurance, it was not sufficient; other factors went into their facilities' calculus of whether or not to accept Medicaid. Indeed, two of the clinical sites in our sample (one that operated as a standalone clinic and one that was part of a multisite facility) that were not subject to a state prohibition on using public insurance funds for abortion did not accept Medicaid (Table 2). Although the other 40 sites located in states where Medicaid broadly allowed coverage for abortion did accept public insurance, respondents nonetheless described tension around this practice. The interviews highlight how fraught the decision to take Medicaid can be, even in the absence of a ban on abortion coverage.

Chief among these tensions around accepting public insurance, respondents reported, was its low reimbursement rate for abortion. Despite reports from early providers of abortion care that money was a motivator to become a provider (Goldstein, 1984), our respondents reported that contemporary abortion care is poorly reimbursed. The specific dollar amount Medicaid reimburses for abortion varies by state, but interviewees universally described it as very low. From a business perspective, taking Medicaid did not always make financial sense; it did not cover the costs to the facility of providing care. As a Counseling Manager explained about her facility in the west, the Medicaid reimbursement "doesn't even come close to the expenditures for a service." The Director of a single site facility in the Midwest which recently raised its prices, described how they lost money when they took Medicaid: "[Even before raising our prices,] we were probably writing off about half of the fee [for aspiration procedures]. And then, for the medication [abortion], it was probably two-thirds. The reimbursement is awful." Reimbursement rates were also generally stagnant even as costs went up. The Senior Project Director at a multisite facility with sites in the east and south noted that:

> We're probably still getting the same amount that we got when I started 13 years ago. And, you know, our prices are ever increasing, in terms of staffing and physicians and just the cost of doing business.

Other respondents described their difficulty with Medicaid's reimbursement specifically for abortion at later gestations. Although the abortion procedure – and its associated costs – is different for later versus earlier gestations, most Medicaids offer only a single reimbursement rate for abortion. The Clinic Director at a multisite facility with clinics in the south and west explained, "they allow [reimbursement of] a certain dollar amount for that [abortion billing] code, and so it doesn't matter if she's 2 weeks or 20 weeks," even though her facility's costs were substantially different at those gestations.

Additionally, several respondents pointed out that Medicaid was slow to reimburse facilities, and consistently slower than private insurers. Respondents reported average times to payment by Medicaid that ranged from 90 to 120 days, along with experiences of payment taking far longer, including one case where payment took 2 years and other cases where the respondent described ultimately giving up on receiving payment all together.

Accepting Medicaid for any health service, with its notoriously low reimbursements and delays in payment, is a challenge for many medical practices, but it poses an especially acute problem in abortion care because of the patient mix. In the United States, abortion patients are disproportionately low income or poor. Jones and Kavanaugh (2011) found that 68.9% of abortion patients report family incomes of less than 200% of the federal poverty level. This means that many, if not most, abortion patients qualify for Medicaid, which is available to residents at or below 100% of the federal poverty level in all states and, in states that expanded Medicaid as part of the 2010 Affordable Care Act, to residents at or below 138% of the federal poverty level. Thus, for abortion-providing facilities, accepting public insurance meant being underpaid and experiencing substantial delays in reimbursement for the majority of their patients.

The Director of Operations at a multisite facility with clinics in the south, Midwest, and west explained how the predominance of low income patients had become a financial issue in keeping her facility open: "60% of our patients overall are insurance patients and 60% of those are Medicaid patients. That becomes, financially, quite a critical issue for us [because Medicaid's reimbursement is so low]." She was not alone. Across the interviews, respondents described the challenge of serving a high number of Medicaid patients, given Medicaid's low and often slow reimbursement, to their ability to cover costs and continue to provide care. As the Billing Coordinator from a multisite facility with sites throughout the United States summed up, taking Medicaid posed a dilemma wherein clinics had to choose between their need to cover costs and their desire to provide abortion services to women who seek care:

> From a business perspective, it doesn't make sense to take Medicaid. It just doesn't. I mean, you lose money every time you see patients. But when you look at the majority of people in some of these places, you would be turning a lot of people away.

The difficulties posed by this disproportionately poor patient population were compounded by the landscape of abortion provision. The majority of abortion care in the United States (63%) is provided by outpatient, standalone facilities that primarily or exclusively provide abortion care (Jones & Jerman, 2014). Facilities like these do not offer other services that may attract a different mix of patients with different insurers and, instead, are especially vulnerable to Medicaids' low and delayed reimbursement.

The Costs of Accepting Private Insurance

Respondents' accounts of working with private insurers did not include the same pitfalls of low and delayed reimbursement that characterized Medicaid, but that did not mean accepting private insurance was without problems. Working with private insurers entailed different challenges. For most of the facilities in our sample that operated in states that allowed private insurance coverage of abortion, the benefits of accepting private insurance outweighed any costs. However, some facilities decided otherwise and chose not to accept private insurance despite no state-level restriction on private insurance coverage of abortion. Specifically, one hospital and one single site facility in states with no restrictions on private insurance coverage of abortion and one hospital and three single site facilities located in states that restricted abortion coverage in plans on the health exchange judged the costs prohibitive and declined to accept private insurance for abortion care (Table 3).

Broadly, the biggest difficulty in taking private insurance was determining whether private insurers would actually pay for the abortion care their clients received. This difficulty manifested in several ways. For one, facilities often had trouble initially determining a patient's eligibility for insurance coverage, sometimes because of the technical language of an individual plan. The Senior Project Director at a facility with clinical sites in the south and northeast explained, for example, that policies might cover abortion, but with restrictions: "we make sure that there's no medical necessity kind of clause on it [a patient's private insurance plan], because they can also say, 'Oh, a termination is covered but only medical necessity,' and each one of them can have their own definition of what 'medical necessity' is." She also described complications in determining coverage depending on who was the named insured on a given plan. She said:

> Sometimes there'll be coverage for the policyholder but not for the dependent, specific to abortion. And so, for instance, like, a dad's policy might not cover his daughter's abortion, or his wife's.

As these examples illustrate, for clinics whose patients used a variety of insurers and plans, keeping track of whether, when, and for whom abortion was a covered service was complicated.

Respondents further reported that private insurer representatives did not always give accurate information about coverage to facility staff members. This was not necessarily because of hostility to abortion but, more mundanely, usually owed to the bureaucracy of private insurance. The Director of a single site facility in the Midwest gave an example:

> We would call their insurance company and see if it [abortion] was a covered service, and the insurance company would say "yes, and it's a 100 percent," and, you know, all this stuff. Well, that's just a quote of benefits; that's not a guarantee. And so, we would have these women come in, and they would not pay anything but their copay. We would bill the insurance, and then the insurance would in fact not pay 100 percent.

When her facility would follow-up, the insurer would reiterate that they gave a quote, not a guarantee. As this respondent further explained, "It wasn't that they were lying to us or misleading us. You know, and they were very clear on the phone about, you know: 'This is not a guarantee of payment; it's just a quote of benefits.' " The upshot for her facility, however, was that it did not get paid for the care it provided.

Even once facility staff had confirmed a patient was eligible for abortion coverage, that did not guarantee payment. Abortion care, with an average cost of $470 in 2009 for a first trimester procedure (Jones & Kooistra, 2011), could fall within a patient's deductible. This meant that, although abortion was a covered benefit, the patient might still be responsible for the full amount of the procedure. As the Director of Operations at a single site facility in the northeast explained, in cases like these when a facility charged the patient only a co-pay in anticipation of reimbursement from private insurers, they risked not being paid at all:

> We ran into tons of cases where, yes, abortion was a covered service [by a private insurer], but [the cost] went to deductible, or the [patient's] coinsurance was huge.[...] A lot of times we ended up getting burned where, you know, the insurance ended up saying that the patient portion was higher than what they had originally quoted us. And then, when we billed the client [afterwards], we had a lot of cases where women no longer have the incentive to pay us, now that they were no longer pregnant.

Several other respondents similarly explained how high deductibles meant that they could not always depend on payment for patients with private insurance.

Respondents also described running up against policies in the insurance system that were incompatible with abortion care. For instance, a physician from a single site facility in the west identified a complication in securing reimbursement for medication abortion: according to the protocol approved by the Food and Drug Administration, the drug used in medication abortions must be given to the patient by a clinician; it cannot be dispensed by a pharmacist. One private insurer, by the physician's account, however, refused to reimburse for pills given at the facility, citing their expectation that pills should be dispensed at a pharmacy: "they didn't understand why a patient had to get the pill here and not at a pharmacy. They wouldn't pay for it. It was huge. I fought and fought. I think about year eight I finally just gave up." Although the insurer considered abortion a covered benefit, it simultaneously enforced policies that made it impossible to reimburse for legally dispensed medication abortion. In this way, although abortion was covered on the books for this insurer, patients could not actually use this benefit in practice.

Faced with the uncertainty of reimbursement from private insurance, regardless of what a patient's policy specified on paper, some facilities developed a work-around to enable patients to use their insurance while also ensuring against providing free care: require upfront payment, bill insurance, and reimburse the patient for her upfront costs if and when the insurer paid. This approach is not uncommon across the health care field for services provided by an out-of-network provider but typically is not allowed when a facility has contracted with an insurer. Nonetheless, facilities like a Director of Operations' single site clinic in the northeast regularly did so. As she related, insurers initially pushed back:

> I actually had gotten a couple of calls from [private insurers] asking why we were requiring payment upfront for a covered service. You know, in our contracts, you're supposed to bill the insurance and then bill the client any patient portion. And so, once I explained the situation, [that we were finding] it would all go to deductible, and then the client's incentive to pay wasn't as strong as it is on the front end. [...] And they were like, "Oh, that makes sense."

Insurers recognized that abortion clinics were in a unique billing position. This work-around of requiring upfront payment enabled facilities to serve privately insured patients without the risk of inadvertently providing free care.

As with accepting Medicaid, the demographics of abortion patients figured into facilities' decision-making regarding accepting private insurance, too. The Associate Medical Director at a single site clinic in the Midwest pointed out that so few of her facility's patients had private insurance that covered abortion that it did not make sense for them to contract with any private insurers. Similarly, a Counseling Manager explained that part of the reason why her facility in the west declined to accept insurance, despite no legal prohibitions on doing so, related to the patient population it served: only about 10% of its patients had private insurance. Still, although the Counseling Manager's facility did not do the work-around of billing insurance and reimbursing patients, they did encourage patients with private insurance to submit their bills themselves for reimbursement. Other respondents reported similar practices of encouraging patients to submit claims directly to their insurer. A physician at a single site facility in the west reported that some patients were successful in pursuing direct reimbursement: "I've had a few patients get reimbursed." In other words, patients with private insurance coverage could still get reimbursed for abortion care, even without the participation of the facility.

DISCUSSION

With evidence that women obtaining abortions have difficulty paying for their care out-of-pocket (Jones et al., 2013; Roberts et al., 2014), advocates have begun to push to mandate public and private insurance coverage for abortion. Our interviews suggest, however, that eliminating legal restrictions may not be enough to remove the financial burdens of paying for abortion from women themselves. While the complexity of legal allowances and prohibitions on abortion coverage by both public and private insurers impacted respondents' facilities' decision-making around accepting abortion, other factors also mattered. Indeed, according to our respondents, taking insurance in abortion care is not always good business. They explained that, with Medicaid, facilities could expect low and sometimes nonexistent reimbursement. Meanwhile, with private insurance, facilities risked nonreimbursement because the costs of care fell within the patient's deductible. Thus, even with a law requiring Medicaid and private insurance coverage of abortion, facilities might not receive enough in paid claims to cover the costs of providing care. Facilities might reasonably conclude that they cannot afford to take insurance and keep their doors open.

Central to understanding this possible outcome is recognition of the composition of the population of abortion patients. Certainly, there are challenges for any facility in accepting insurance, but our interviews show that the challenges are particularly acute for abortion providers because of the predominance of poor and low income patients – who qualify for Medicaid – and the dearth of private insurance patients. With this patient mix, abortion care provision is not lucrative – indeed, respondents reported regularly losing money on care to Medicaid recipients. It bears noting that the abortion patient population was not always this way: women seeking abortion in the initial decades after the 1973 *Roe v. Wade* decision were usually white and affluent (Jones, Kost, Singh, Henshaw, & Finer, 2009), seeking to avoid derailing educational and/or occupational plans (Freedman & Weitz, 2012). Contemporary abortion patients, in contrast, are predominantly low income and disproportionately women of color (Jones & Kavanaugh, 2011) who want to avoid further financial hardship (Biggs, Gould, & Foster, 2013).

Scholars have sourced this shift in the population of abortion patients to disparities in the rates of unintended pregnancy (Dehlendorf et al., 2013), with low income women and women of color more likely to experience an unintended pregnancy than white and affluent women (Finer & Zolna, 2011). Further, scholars have argued that disparities in rates of unintended pregnancy are themselves the product of unequal access to comprehensive sex education and effective contraception that is patterned by race and class (Dehlendorf et al., 2013). The predominance of low income women in abortion care – and the attendant financial strain that poses for abortion-providing facilities – in other words, is partly a result of a broader pattern of health inequalities.

The answer to whether removing restrictions on abortion coverage would substantially change the provision of abortion care is also impacted by the existing landscape of abortion providers. It is reasonable to expect that the changes in the regulatory environment over the decades since *Roe* have induced changes in the characteristics of abortion providers. Although the types of providers have not substantially changed over time (i.e., outpatient clinics continue to provide most of the abortion care in the United States, Jones & Jerman, 2014), it is likely that the increasing regulation has affected the mix of motivations to provide. Providers motivated by an ideological commitment to abortion access may weather the increasing regulation of care to the detriment of their financial circumstances, but entrepreneurial providers like those Goldstein (1984) studied in the early years of legal abortion may find it is no longer a desirable business opportunity. This complexity and regulatory environment may also operate as a barrier to new providers entering the field, in parallel to institutional structures (Freedman, 2010) and interpersonal interactions (Kimport, Weitz, & Freedman, 2016) that serve to marginalize abortion provision in medicine.

Supporting this hypothesis that contemporary abortion providers are more often ideologically motivated to provide care than spurred by a profit interest, we note that even as our respondents detailed the hardships to their facility of accepting insurance, most continued to do so when legally able. Implicit in their accounts of creating work-arounds for patients to use private insurance and stretching their budgets in order to accept Medicaid was their commitment to preserving access to abortion, even at the expense of the financial health of their facility. Our convenience sampling methodology means we cannot know how commonly facilities opt to accept insurance despite financial penalties for doing so. Future research should investigate how widespread these practices are.

Future research should also examine the overlap between the shift in the patient population seeking abortion toward more vulnerable groups and the increase in regulation of insurance (and other aspects of abortion care). Does the fact that abortion patients are disproportionately low income and of color – i.e., socially vulnerable populations – invite or enable regulation in a way that services predominantly accessed by more privileged populations would not?

Ultimately, our study identifies how legal policy, insurer practices, and the patient population matter for clinics' calculus as to whether to accept insurance for abortion care. By focusing on the actions of clinics themselves, we address a gap in the literature on insurance for abortion care, examining the practices of the intermediary between patients and insurance companies. To best meet the health care needs of women, particularly low income women, who most commonly pay for abortion care out-of-pocket (Jones et al., 2013; Roberts et al., 2014), we need to attend not only to how abortion is legally regulated but also what it means for abortion provision that its patient population is uniquely characterized by poverty.

ACKNOWLEDGMENTS

The authors would like to thank Amanda Dennis for her comments on an early draft. Funding support for the data collection and analysis came from the National Health Law Program.

REFERENCES

Bessett, D., Gorski, K., Jinadasa, D., Ostrow, M., & Peterson, M. J. (2011). Out of time and out of pocket: Experiences of women seeking state-subsidized insurance for abortion care in Massachusetts. *Women's Health Issues*, *21*(3S), S21–S25.

Biggs, M. A., Gould, H., & Foster, D. G. (2013). Understanding why women seek abortions in the US. *BMC Women's Health*, *13*(1), 29–42.

Charmaz, K. (2006). *Constructing grounded theory*. London: Sage.

Cockrill, K., & Weitz, T. A. (2010). Abortion patients' perceptions of abortion regulation. *Women's Health Issues*, *20*, 12–19.

Cohen, S. A. (2010). Insurance coverage of abortion: The battle to date and the battle to come. *Guttmacher Policy Review*, *13*(4), 2–6.

Cook, P. J., Parnell, A. M., Moore, M. J., & Pagnini, D. (1999). The effects of short-term variation in abortion funding on pregnancy outcomes. *Journal of Health Economics*, *18*(2), 241–257.

Dehlendorf, C., Harris, L. H., & Weitz, T. A. (2013). Disparities in abortion rates: A public health approach. *American Journal of Public Health*, *103*(10), 1772–1779.

Dennis, A., & Blanchard, K. (2013). Abortion providers' experiences with Medicaid abortion coverage policies: A qualitative multistate study. *Health Services Research*, *48*(1), 236–252.

Dennis, A., Blanchard, K., & Córdova, D. (2011). Strategies for securing funding for abortion under the Hyde Amendment: A multistate study of abortion providers' experiences managing Medicaid. *American Journal of Public Health*, *101*(11), 2124–2129.

Dennis, A., Manski, R., & Blanchard, K. (2014). Does Medicaid coverage matter?: A qualitative multi-state study of abortion affordability for low-income women. *Journal of Health Care for the Poor and Underserved*, *25*(4), 1571–1585.

Dennis, A., Manski, R., & Blanchard, K. (2015). A qualitative exploration of low-income women's experiences accessing abortion in Massachusetts. *Women's Health Issues*, *25*(5), 463–469.

Finer, L. B., & Zolna, M. R. (2011). Unintended pregnancy in the United States: Incidence and disparities, 2006. *Contraception*, *84*(5), 478–485.

Freedman, L. R. (2010). *Willing and unable: doctors' constraints in abortion care*. Nashville, TN: Vanderbilt University Press.

Freedman, L. R., & Weitz, T. A. (2012). The politics of motherhood meets the politics of poverty. *Contemporary Sociology*, *41*(1), 36–42.

Gold, R. B. (2010). Insurance coverage and abortion incidence: Information and misinformation. *Guttmacher Policy Review*, *13*(4), 7–10.

Goldstein, M. S. (1984). Abortion as a medical career choice: Entrepreneurs, community physicians, and others. *Journal of Health and Social Behavior*, 211–229.

Guttmacher Institute. (2017a). Restricting insurance coverage of abortion. Retrieved from https://www.guttmacher.org/state-policy/explore/restricting-insurance-coverage-abortion

Guttmacher Institute. (2017b). State funding of abortion under medicaid. Retrieved from https://www.guttmacher.org/state-policy/explore/state-funding-abortion-under-medicaid

Jones, R. K., & Jerman, J. (2014). Abortion incidence and service availability in the United States, 2011. *Perspectives on Sexual and Reproductive Health*, *46*(1), 3–14.

Jones, R. K., & Kavanaugh, M. L. (2011). Changes in abortion rates between 2000 and 2008 and lifetime incidence of abortion. *Obstetrics and Gynecology*, *117*(6), 1358–1366.

Jones, R. K., & Kooistra, K. (2011). Abortion incidence and access to services in the United States, 2008. *Perspectives on Sexual and Reproductive Health*, *43*(1), 41–50.

Jones, R. K., Kost, K., Singh, S., Henshaw, S. K., & Finer, L. B. (2009). Trends in abortion in the United States. *Clinical Obstetrics and Gynecology*, *52*(2), 119–129.

Jones, R. K., Upadhyay, U. D., & Weitz, T. A. (2013). At what cost? Payment for abortion care by US women. *Women's Health Issues*, *23*(3), e173–e178.

Kacanek, D., Dennis, A., Miller, K., & Blanchard, K. (2010). Medicaid funding for abortion: Providers' experiences with cases involving rape, incest and life endangerment. *Perspectives on Sexual and Reproductive Health*, *42*(2), 79–86.

Kimport, K., Weitz, T., & Freedman, L. R. (2016). The stratified legitimacy of abortion. *Journal of Health and Social Behavior*, *57*(4), 503–516.

Pazol, K., Zane, S. B., Parker, W. Y., Hall, L. R., Berg, C., & Cook, D. A. (2011). Abortion surveillance: United States, 2008. *Morbidity and Mortality Weekly Report*, *60*(15), 1–44.

Roberts, S., Gould, H., Kimport, K., Weitz, T. A., & Foster, D. G. (2014). Out-of-pocket costs and insurance coverage for abortion in the United States. *Women's Health Issues*, *24*(2), e211–e218.

Rosenbaum, S. (2011). The Patient Protection and Affordable Care Act: Implications for public health policy and practice. *Public Health Reports*, 130–135.

Schaler-Haynes, M., Chesnokova, A., Cox, C., & Feinstein, M. (2011). Abortion coverage and health reform: Restrictions and options for exchange-based insurance markets. *The University of Pennsylvania Journal of Law and Social Change*, *15*, 323.

Van Bebber, S. L., Phillips, K. A., Weitz, T. A., Gould, H., & Stewart, F. (2006). Patient costs for medication abortion: Results from a study of five clinical practices. *Women's Health Issues*, *16*(1), 4–13.

THE PATIENT–HEALTHCARE WORKER RELATIONSHIP: HOW DOES IT AFFECT PATIENT VIEWS TOWARDS VACCINATION DURING PREGNANCY?☆

Rose Jane Wilson, Tracey Chantler, Shelley Lees, Pauline Paterson and Heidi Larson

ABSTRACT

Relational autonomy proposes that persons are socially embedded, with decisions being made within social relationships. Through this theoretical lens, this article explores how the healthcare professional–patient relationship can affect pregnant women's decisions to accept pertussis and influenza vaccines.

Hackney was chosen as the study site as it has very low vaccine uptake rates. In-depth interviews were conducted with 40 pregnant and recently pregnant women, as well as 10 healthcare professionals. Interviews explored experiences of the UK's National Health Service (NHS) health care and views towards vaccination in pregnancy. An observation of a consultation between

☆All authors are based at the London School of Hygiene and Tropical Medicine (LSHTM)

Health and Health Care Concerns among Women and Racial and Ethnic Minorities
Research in the Sociology of Health Care, Volume 35, 59–77

ISSN: 0275-4959/doi:10.1108/S0275-495920170000035004

a pregnant patient and her General Practitioners (GPs) was also conducted in order to understand how the vaccination discussion takes place.

The findings of this study indicate that advice from friends and family can greatly influence a pregnant woman's vaccination decisions. The patient's social context, including influences on her decisions, must be understood by healthcare professionals, so that discussions about concerns can take place. If close relationships with patients are formed, healthcare professional advice is more likely to be trusted. With support from healthcare professionals, patients feel competent, empowered to make the right decision for them, and are more likely to vaccinate.

This research will help to inform contextualised policies aimed at increasing vaccination acceptance and reducing inequality in access to vaccination during pregnancy in Hackney.

To the author's knowledge, this chapter is the first to apply the theory of relational autonomy to views towards maternal vaccination and decision making. It provides valuable insights into how healthcare professionals' interactions with their pregnant patients can influence vaccination acceptance. The chapter contains advice on how both healthcare professionals and policy-makers can include mothers in vaccine decision-making processes in more personalised ways, by adopting a dialogue that appreciates and understands the social processes around vaccination concerns.

Keywords: Maternal vaccination; relational autonomy; healthcare worker; pertussis; influenza

INTRODUCTION

Pertussis and influenza are preventable diseases with potentially severe consequences for newborn infants and in the case of influenza, for pregnant women. Infants under the age of 6 months are vulnerable to transmission of pertussis and influenza infection from others, especially their mothers (Mcintyre & Wood, 2009). Influenza immunisation was first recommended for all pregnant women in 2009 (Dlugacz et al., 2012) and due to a pertussis (whooping cough) outbreak in 2012, which caused 14 infant deaths, the UK Department of Health temporarily introduced pertussis vaccination for all pregnant women (Flory, 2012).

A systematic literature review of 155 articles relating to acceptance of vaccines, provided during pregnancy, showed that little research has been conducted into how pregnant patients' social context and relationships with others, especially their healthcare workers (HCWs), affects vaccination acceptance

(Wilson, Paterson, Jarrett, & Larson, 2015). In this chapter, I (RW) explore, in relation to the theory of relational autonomy, how the patient–HCW relationship can affect general trust in HCW advice, and thus vaccination, which could affect vaccine acceptance during pregnancy. I also explore other influences on vaccine decision making and how these should be taken into account in patient–HCW encounters. I start my chapter by analysing the various social influences on pregnant women's vaccination decisions. I then explore the influence of trust in government, the NHS and healthcare professionals on vaccination acceptance, and how vaccination acceptance is shaped by communities' historical and socio-political contexts. I illustrate this point through narratives of Black British Caribbean women interviewed. Finally, I analyse how empowerment, in a way that is related to theories of relational autonomy, can help in the vaccine decision-making process. These are particularly important issues in today's chaotic care environment, with changes to organisational structures, time limitations, staff shortages, mandatory overtime and lack of continuity, where it is sometimes difficult to practice in a manner that fosters partnership or provides support to patients (Ritchie, Ritchie, & Ritchie, 1997).

Relational autonomy is a feminist formulation of autonomy which presents a different way of thinking about autonomy that is relational rather than individualistic (Walter & Friedman Ross, 2014), accepting that persons are socially embedded, with their identities being formed within social relationships and shaped by intersecting social determinants such as race, class, gender and ethnicity (Mackenzie & Stoljar, 2000). This approach opposes the current emphasis on the individual's ability to access and acquire skills, where patients who do not conform to this model are alluded to as apathetic and ignorant, needful of persuasion to change their behaviour, resistant to change and 'hard to reach' (Leach & Fairhead, 2007). Rather, relational autonomy understands that dialogue, especially with HCWs, which involves advice-giving, is not an affront to individual autonomy, but allows individual autonomy to flourish (Walter & Friedman Ross, 2014).

All names used in this chapter are pseudonyms.

FIELDWORK AND INTERPRETIVE APPROACH

The borough of Hackney, London was chosen as it has one of the lowest vaccine coverage rates among pregnant women in England, with influenza vaccine coverage rates at 31.3% (Public Health England, 2016) and pertussis coverage rates at 27.4% (Byrne, 2015). Hackney is also very ethnically and socially diverse. According to the 2011 Census, just over a third (36%) of respondents in Hackney described themselves as White British. The remaining population consists of Black and minority ethnic groups, with the largest group Other White 16.3%, followed by Black African 11.4% and Black Caribbean people

7.8%. Hackney has the largest group of Charedi Jewish people in Europe, which represents about 7.4% of the borough's overall population. At least 4.5% of the Hackney population is Turkish. Other significant communities in Hackney include Chinese, Vietnamese and Eastern Europeans especially Polish, Western Europeans particularly Spanish and French people, Australasians and residents from North and Latin America (LB Hackney Policy Team, 2016). Hackney is an area of growing economic opportunity; however, this growth sits alongside significant deprivation, with persistent inequalities and child poverty, unemployment and welfare dependency in some areas (LB Hackney Policy Team, 2016).

Participants were recruited from nine parent-toddler groups across Hackney, which were free to attend; four community centres/migrant support groups, three general practitioners (GP) practices with median vaccination uptake rates and a diverse patient population (according to Public Health England (PHE) data) and two community antenatal clinics.

Semi-structured interviews were conducted between December 2016 and June 2017, with 40 pregnant women and women who had given birth in the past year at the commencement of the fieldwork, as well as 10 HCWs. Where necessary, an interpreter attended the interviews. In addition, one consultation between a pregnant patient and her GP was video recorded. The video recording acted as an ethnographic observation method which allowed the exploration of interactions between HCWs and pregnant women. It must be noted, however, that the Hawthorne effect (Mayo, 1949) may have occurred with this method, as the GP being video recorded knew that the study was looking at vaccine discussions and so would have been more likely to bring it up in the consultation.

Pregnant and recently pregnant participants interviewed were between ages 18 and 41 and were from a wide variety of backgrounds. Fifteen out of forty participants described themselves as White British, five were Black British Caribbean, two were Black British, two Chinese, two German, two Nigerian, two Orthodox Jewish, two Turkish, one was Australian, one British Brazilian, one Italian, one Lithuanian, one Norwegian, one Pakistani British, one Somalian and one was South African. Sixteen participants had not undergone higher education, nine had a bachelor's degree and fifteen had a master's degree. The participant who took part in the video recording of the consultation was age 34, White British and employed. Healthcare professionals interviewed were all female and between age 23 and 62. Five were White British, two were Black British Caribbean, two were British Indian and one was Black British. Six participants were GPs, two were midwives and two were practice nurses.

Data was analysed using a thematic analysis approach. Thematic analysis is often utilised when research is used in policy, and thus must be accessible to those outside of academia (Braun & Clarke, 2014). Thematic analysis was used in this study as a 'contextualist' method, characterised by theories of constructionism and critical realism, which acknowledge the ways individuals make meaning of their experience, and, in turn, the ways the broader social context impinges on those meanings, while retaining focus on the limits of 'reality' (there is no singular, objective, universal truth, waiting to be uncovered through the application of 'the scientific method. Instead, there is a multiplicity of interrelated, subjective and often oppositional understandings) (Taylor & Ussher, 2001). Therefore, thematic analysis conducted within a constructionist framework does not seek to focus on motivation or individual psychologies, but instead, to theorise the socio-cultural contexts, and structural conditions, that enable individual accounts (Braun & Clarke, 2014). Using thematic analysis, themes within the interviews and video recording were identified and analysed in rich detail. A detailed and nuanced account of one particular theme within the data (Patient–HCW interaction) was conducted, which relates to a specific question and area of interest within the data: how relational autonomy affects acceptance of vaccines.

IMPACT OF SOCIAL INFLUENCES ON VACCINATION DECISIONS

I spent a lot of time in participant's homes and at their local cafés, chatting over tea and crying babies, about their experiences using the healthcare system during pregnancy and their views towards vaccination. In this section, I will explore in-depth, the various social influences on patient's decisions, and the importance of HCWs to understand these influences and build their own relationships with patients.

When asked who made decisions about their health, all 40 women interviewed immediately and proudly said 'me'. However, later on in the interview, when asked if there was anyone or anywhere they would typically go to for advice regarding their health or specifically, vaccination, all participants mentioned a friend or family member, as well as, or rather than her GP. While these answers seem to contradict each other, relational autonomy suggests that, due to the nature of 'society' and the idea that no-one is completely individual or untouched by others, one can engage with others in important health decisions and value their input, while still feeling autonomous. This is especially true if those engaging in the conversation are trusted friends, family members or healthcare providers. According to Walter and Friedman Ross (2014), discussion of challenging decisions with various social contacts in fact increases feelings of autonomy as it allows an in-depth exploration of the issue and thus empowers the individual to make the 'right' decision for them (Walter & Friedman Ross, 2014).

Participants often had very close relationships with female family members such as sisters who already had children, mother-in-laws, mothers and aunts. It seemed that the participants were not looking for actual information from these contacts, as they would with a HCW, instead they wanted personal interaction and to feel comfortable and cared for.

> My mother-in-law she could tell me quite a lot... she's had a lot of kids... My mum's only had one...and my mum seems to know a lot, probably because she's looked after kids in the past...It doesn't mean because you've only had one you don't know, so no matter what, I go to my mum. (Beth, age 22)

This participant had support from her mother, mother-in-law and partner in making her vaccination decision. She also had a good relationship with her midwife and said that all of her friends had been vaccinated. Possibly as a result of these trusted influences, who had positive attitudes towards vaccination, the participant also trusted vaccination.

This desire for personal interaction was also seen in the participants' wide use of Internet forums, especially Mumsnet and Netmums, often before seeking advice from their GP. Many participants said they used such forums but at the same time were quick to criticise incorrect information and the opinions of other users who are *all going a bit potty* (mother, age 34). These forums and other Internet sites provided an extension to mothers' 'real life' social networks, enabling them to discuss or just read about other people's opinions towards pregnancy issues and vaccination. These Internet forums often became personified as a best friend, even if it was acknowledged that this relationship was not always healthy.

> Within my pregnancy, that internet became my best friend, and it gave me information I didn't really want to know, but it wasn't actually... the right information. So, I was always told not to always believe everything that's on Google, because it's not 100% accurate...so you never know if it's the truth. (Lucy, age 27)

The media has often portrayed mothers' opinions as driven by emotion, and fathers' opinions influenced by 'scientific evidence' (Leach & Fairhead, 2007). However, participants in my study often laughed and employed a rather patronising attitude towards her male partner's understanding of vaccination and pregnancy, and illustrated that they themselves were in control of their body.

> My partner doesn't factor in... I read, when I was pregnant... an article... this man is, like... 'when my wife was pregnant, I discovered all the things she couldn't eat, so I had to cook her a special meal every night...' I'd have murdered him if he'd said anything like this... I know some people feel like it's their [partner's] baby. But, I don't...When it's inside me, it's my baby. (Rita, age 27)

Women therefore tended not to seek advice from male partners as much as from their female friends and family members, thus sometimes excluding male partners from the vaccine decision-making process. Through extended time spent between HCWs and pregnant patients over the course of the pregnancy, in-depth discussions could be facilitated, which could enable HCWs to understand these influences and the patient's background and social context more broadly, thus identifying any specific vaccination concerns.

UNDERSTANDING THE IMPORTANCE OF TRUST IN THE GOVERNMENT, THE NHS AND THE HEALTHCARE WORKER

You're putting your whole trust in these people... to make sure that you come through the other end perfectly fine. (Mother, age 27)

'Trust' in this sense can be defined as an acceptance of decisions without questioning the rationale behind them (Löfstedt, 2005). However, my research demonstrated that notions of trust and distrust are complex. Distrust in government motivation to vaccinate was evident when participants expressed that *vaccination is only pushed so that healthcare workers do not go off sick* (mother, age 34), and *to stop hospital admissions in order to save money* (mother, age 34). This distrust became palpable in the use of metaphors by participants when speaking about vaccination. Metaphors are important because they are influenced by wider socio-political discourses in society and are unconsciously drawn on as ways of thinking that have always been, and continue to be acceptable to the groups with which individuals identify, when perceived risks are encountered. When such events are objectified, groups favour the symbols and/or metaphors compatible with in-group values (Joffe, 2003). In analysing vaccine anxieties, we must therefore understand how parents conceptualise the bodily processes involved in keeping healthy and how, in their context, they consider vaccines. This involves understanding the concepts and metaphors parents use and how their framings integrate bodily, social and political reflection (Leach & Fairhead, 2007).

Three participants in my study used the term 'guinea-pig' to describe how they felt with regard to being offered vaccines. As well as using this metaphor, one Black British Caribbean mother stated that in accepting vaccination, you are taking 'a Russian Roulette chance' that your baby would be affected (Shiloh, age 19). In my study, the use of metaphors arose when participants felt strongly against vaccination. Use of powerful metaphors (i.e. guinea-pig, Russian Roulette chance), especially by Black British Caribbean mothers, which have connotations of forced experimentation and violence, as well as participants' recalling stories from family members who, when arriving in the UK, became ill from vaccines, could be linked to distrust in the UK government and the NHS. This is plausible when acknowledging past British–Caribbean colonialism, as well as the relatively recent post-colonial experimentation with the contraceptive pill on Caribbean women *with Caribbean women acting as guinea-pigs of one of the most revolutionary drugs in the history of medicine* (Oudshoorn, 2002).

Of the five self-described Black British Caribbean women interviewed, none had accepted the influenza vaccine and only two had (hesitantly) accepted the pertussis vaccine during pregnancy. One Black British Caribbean midwife interviewed (who was against vaccination in pregnancy herself) mentioned that more Afro-Caribbean women than White women decline vaccination due to distrust of what's in vaccination, as it is 'something that the government are putting in people' (Midwife Renee, age 41). This sentiment was evident in an interview with a British Caribbean mother, who said,

> I read a lot of things of, about the way the, um, vaccines effect people and affect different cultures differently. Different races and things like that. And that concerned me. (Tessa, age 27)

Implicit distrust in vaccination goes deeper than fears of vaccines themselves and are indicative of the socio-political context in which vaccines and those they are intended for are situated (Leach & Fairhead, 2007). In the early 20th century, many vaccine anxieties reflected the fears and concerns of institutions of the colonial state (White, 2005). Colonial control over African societies and bodies deeply entwined with the establishment of public health regimes including immunisation (White, 2005). Post-independence, vaccine anxieties have arisen at particular times and places in ways that reflect shifts in local–national state politics, the political economy of neoliberal reforms and the relationships between states, citizens and global institutions (Leach & Fairhead, 2007). However, Western researchers have been criticised for investigating women's experiences without considering the impact of colonial legacy, power and social inequalities in the woman-healthcare institution relationship (Kumar, 2013). Here I analyse the ways Black British Caribbean mothers in my study drew connections between vaccines and wider historical and political issues, and how they represent them in ways that make sense given their everyday experiences (Leach & Fairhead, 2007).

Shiloh and Jane are both young, single, unemployed Black British Caribbean mothers, educated up to high-school level respectively. Below are some examples of their interactions with midwives, GPs and social services.

> I was signed on to Social Services...It was like they was just watching me, every move I was making with them...they was looking to see... if you're doing everything right... so it just felt not right... because of my past [domestic violence by ex-partner] and my ex-partner, he came there [hospital] for the first time... because we both thought that was right... all of us... going to these appointments. And soon as I went there with him... they [hospital staff] called Social Services to say I came here with him....and then through that it just felt I had to go the clinic by myself after that. (Shiloh, age 19)

> I was told, if you don't... *make* the child get all their injections that... they can... bring up, like, my background... see if I had a social worker, and social worker can get onto my case because... it's like I'm not protecting the child... that's what I was told by one of my midwives... she's the one that closed my case, after I told her, 'yes, [my daughter] will get all her, um, injections', and she has... these injections are new to me, so for me to just say, yeah,

> I'm going to give it to [my daughter], it's something that I was kind of being forced to do, without ...thinking about it ... and the same GP...she told me that you need to... and I-I felt intimidated, and I feeled under pressure because she was telling me that... these are the things that can happen if you don't get the child [vaccinated].... (Jane, age 24)

Here, the threat given by the midwife and GP that the state will be involved, in the form of Jane having a social worker 'on her case' if she did not vaccinate her child, was akin to blackmail and led Jane to feeling forced to vaccinate her child without having a chance to consider or discuss it.

Parents with little resources are less able to demand services, less likely to view providers as contributing advice rather than dictating behaviours and are more likely to be reported to state agencies or social workers than privileged parents. Privileged parents do not have to worry so much about these issues and so have more choice in their decisions. They also receive more respect from providers as potential partners in their care (Reich, 2016).

As mentioned above, perceived risks are often constructed through elements of group attachment and the experiences of these groups and themselves, in terms of both the narratives they are exposed to and past misfortunes. These elements do not distort a 'real risk' but are the 'reality' in the minds of those who consider the risks (Joffe, 2003). Shiloh said her mother and aunt advised her against vaccination because 'when [her aunt] first came to the country 21 years ago...when she did take the flu jab, she constantly got sick' (Shiloh, age 19). Two other Black British Caribbean mothers also relayed family members' experience and advice about the flu vaccine,

Samantha:	I've never had the flu vaccine, but I've had loads of friends, family have it, and it's always negative things. Like even my granddad, they call him for flu vaccines... and he's always grumbling afterwards of like feeling a bit like weak with the flu, and it's kind of like why would I have that if, if I've seen other people go through that? No... especially in a pregnancy as well. You already feel tired and weak.
RW:	... you said you, you, um, ask your mum if you're not sure what to do. Did you discuss vaccination with her?
Samantha:	Yeah... she said 'no, don't have it'... She's more like... natural health person, like not to do with medicated stuff... so she's... against that kind of stuff anyway.
RW:	And... do you think... what she said influenced your decision?
Samantha:	I had already made my decision, but... when you talk to her and she's... saying all of this kind of... add[s] to all the things you already thought of (Samantha, age 28).
Jane:	They [healthcare professionals] asked me if I wanted the flu jabs. Um, I told them no, not after my aunty was ill, and my cousin was ill... my aunty advised me not to get the flu jab
RW:	You said you had a discussion with your-your aunt about it... do you think... because she advised not to get it... you were influenced by her?
Jane:	Yeah... None of my family's got it. None of my family members mentioned anything about it... now, we're Jamaicans, we've got friends, we've got more relatives that's Jamaicans, I've heard it through... So, obviously... if I was [pregnant now], I would get it done because... I've heard it several times now.

RW:	Okay... and, how much do you trust the advice given on vaccination by the doctor or midwife.
Jane:	I would ask the doctor how she got it done... I would have to see in personal writing that they have had this done... and how many people since this new thing has come out, has actually got the actual injection... And how much people's been sick from it... so I know if I should ...I just think it's just silly... My dad got the flu the other day... and he had to go to the doctors, and they had to give him some strong medicine... he didn't get the flu jab... I just think it's ridiculous, because anybody can get a flu...So, I don't think that will cure the flu (Jane, age 24).

The above narratives show that distrust in the UK government, the NHS and vaccines are passed down through generations, with family members being very clear that they are against vaccination, thus greatly influencing other family members' decisions to vaccinate. Rather than trust and engage with healthcare professionals around this issue, these participants preferred to listen to family advice and the advice of those within their community. This is evident with Jane's comment above: now that she has heard of the vaccine from Jamaican friends and family, she would accept it if she was pregnant again. This is unsurprising given the perceived disapproval of those who do not vaccinate, by some HCW, who sometimes put so much pressure on mothers to vaccinate, that they feel they cannot discuss the decision with their HCW. For example, when Samantha's GP recommended the vaccines, she said that she gave the impression that she would think about receiving them, but had already decided not to accept the vaccines (Samantha, age 28).

Distrust in the government, and therefore the NHS (as a government-funded service), can translate into distrust in healthcare professionals. Again, this matter is nuanced. Some participants reported an extremely positive experience with their GP, nurse or midwife. One particular participant said that her midwife was very supportive and became her friend, always asking the participant how she was and what she had been up to, making her feel welcome and comfortable. This participant also trusted HCW advice on vaccination *100%* (Beth, age 22) and believed that there are no disadvantages to vaccination or side effects. Although this participant had a negative birth experience, she still trusted the NHS, due to her positive antenatal experience and close relationship with her midwife.

These sentiments contrast greatly with the experience of Shiloh, age 19 (who used the guinea-pig metaphor), who felt that while she was pregnant, she was not a main priority. Apart from having family support, she was isolated; she could not go to antenatal classes as she was moving house and she did not know about parenting classes, even though she would have liked to attend some. Shiloh felt neglected and expressed lack of empathy from her HCW. This sentiment of neglect during her pregnancy and the birth ran through Shiloh's entire interview. She felt alone unless her family was with her and defending her; *My mum, my sister was at work... I didn't have no one there until my auntie [said]... 'she's in pain can't you give her a bit more... paracetamol?'* (Shiloh, age 19). Shiloh reported that she and her mother made decisions about her health. She had a great deal of trust in her mother and aunt's advice, which tended to be against vaccination; her mother had *found out that a lot of these vaccinations do mess you up during pregnancy* (Shiloh, age 19). Additionally, Shiloh's's aunt had told her that when she arrived in the country 21 years ago, she had received the influenza vaccine and now constantly got sick. She needed to clarify that the sickness started when she arrived in the country, resonating with the sentiments of distrust in the UK government. The higher level of trust in advice from family over that of HCWs was also evident when she attributed the survival of her son to her mother and aunt;

> They didn't concentrate on my pregnancy, all they were worried about [was]... your baby has a lot of hair...and my auntie was like ... 'can't you see that the coil is wrapped around his neck? ... get the coil off his neck...' if it wasn't for my aunt and my mum... he wouldn't be here. (Shiloh, age 19)

When asked if enough information was provided during her pregnancy, Shiloh expressed, *I was just working off my own mind...I... had no help from doctors... I had to learn by myself* (Shiloh, age 19). This fear of neglect extended to the current state of the NHS and possible funding cuts; *Midwifes, are getting paid less...and it's going to mess up the NHS... it will go back to where people are having their kids at home themselves...where they're giving birth to their own child* (Shiloh, age 19). Shiloh did not vaccinate during pregnancy and reported no trust in HCW advice on vaccination.

Ten participants had family members who were HCWs, from whom they tended to ask advice. One participant asked her grandfather (a retired doctor) and her step-mother (a paediatrician) for advice. When asking her grandfather about the influenza vaccination during pregnancy, he responded; '*You're not allowed to medicate pregnant women and especially vaccines... Don't get anything because there is no research how it will affect an unborn child, it needs to be studied for 20/30 years to know... if there is any effect... don't become a guinea-pig*' (Aldona, age 29, quoting her grandfather). Here again the powerful 'guinea-pig' metaphor is used. Not only is this advice coming from a trusted family member but a family member who is also a HCW. These people tended to be trusted more than non-related HCWs.

> I would've trusted my sister [who is a midwife] more for honest advice because ...they'd [HCW] be promoting all the... injections... and I've read lots of stories of children being really unwell after having them... a doctor, a nurse wouldn't tell you that, they'd say, 'Oh no of course you have to have that'. (Anna, age 34)

Trust in friends and family was strong even if that person did not know the answer to a question. When talking about the leader of a parent-toddler group, one participant said;

> She's got three kids of her own, so... with her experience ... I felt comfortable with her advice ... It was very reassuring; I didn't feel patronised by her... If she's not sure, she's not sure, but most of the time, when she is sure, it sounds... convincible... so... I can understand what she's saying and I can relate to it. (Lucy, age 27)

From the point of view of the participant, if an advisor was honest, it did not matter if they did not have all the answers. It did not matter that the woman running the toddler group was not a medic; she listened and was not patronising, she had three children of her own and so could empathise. On the other hand, when a HCW did not have a close relationship with a participant (one participant had been introduced to her midwives as 'Midwife 1 and Midwife 2'), the patient could be very scathing. When talking about a midwife who checked for an answer on her phone, the participant called her *uneducated* and *sly* (Lucy, age 27). However, according to another participant, when a midwife did admit to not knowing, it was appreciated and they were trusted; *My midwife concentrated on my needs... I can ask her anything. Any sort of problems... she always says 'I don't know but I can see into it' and she'll get back to me...within that hour* (Shiloh, age 19). Often, however, questions were not answered and no re-assurance provided. Any chances of a trusting relationship were further eroded in some cases by midwives being rude to the patients; *Midwives were rather rude... and not so compassionate... not so sympathetic... that affected... my whole experience of my labour* (Mahsa, age 31). *I asked something, it was... patronising... the attitude... how they came across with the answer – it was, like, mm, was I meant to ask you that?* (Lucy, age 27). Often, however, there was no chance for a relationship to be built. One of the main factors affecting the patient-HCW relationships and patient's experience of care was midwife continuity; *If you had that same midwife... or if there was someone who knew you I think it would make quite a difference because you could at least trust what they had to say... at least trust one person when people are telling* [you] *different things* (Julia, age 38). One participant expressed the want for a HCW to take time to discuss her concerns and ask her what she was comfortable with *so that they can actually understand you as a person* (Lucy, age 27). Often, if advice came from a trusted source, even if this person was 'unqualified' in the subject matter, individuals were likely to follow their advice. If a person offering advice was highly qualified but did not have a close relationship with the person asking, or if they had a patronising attitude, their advice was sometimes disqualified and distrusted.

EMPOWERMENT

According to Kabeer (1999), empowerment is the process by which individuals acquire an ability to make strategic life choices. The ability to exercise choice incorporates three interrelated dimensions: resources (with regard to vaccination, this would include access to healthcare and vaccination); agency (processes of discussion, negotiation and decision making); and achievements (well-being outcomes) (Kabeer, 1999). Empowerment is essential for relational autonomy but is only possible when one can trust their HCW and the advice they provide. Parents' perceptions about their agency in the vaccination decision have often been neglected as possible drivers of their vaccination behaviour (Fadda, Depping, & Schulz, 2015).

In a study on the measles-mumps-rubella (MMR) vaccine decision, Fadda, Galimberti, Carraro, and Schulz (2016) found that the majority of parents reported feeling competent and, consequently, autonomous when they could obtain vaccination-related information and guidance from an expert whom they could trust (Fadda et al., 2016). These sentiments were reflected in my study: if patients trusted HCW advice, they were more empowered to make the decision that was right for them, with support from their HCW.

> My midwife... was really, really good, bubbly, had a laugh, my partner would come there and she would make my partner feel shy...and no one makes him feel like that and I felt like I took control with her... I discuss it with her but I make all the decisions. (Beth, age 22)

Participants were clear that they did not want to be left to make vaccine decisions alone. Pertussis and (if it is flu season) influenza vaccines should be recommended at the pregnant patient's 16-week check with her GP, and then at antenatal appointments with her midwife. However, when and how (and sometimes if) these discussions happen, vary by GP practice and individual HCWs. One of the HCWs interviewed said that the discussion about vaccination is *a tick box discussion rather than one we invite* and another said the discussion is just *part of going through all the things that are needed* (Dr. Amber, age 29). This approach left some participants feeling unclear about their options and even neglected by their HCW, and distrustful of the whole healthcare system. One participant described a traumatic experience at the hospital. She was given conflicting advice and asked to make decisions herself. Her response was; '*I'm not the doctor, I don't know what's best for me and the baby... no-one knows what they're doing in here*' (Ava, age 26). Mothers often had to decide whether or not to vaccinate with no advice from their HCW provided. As a result, some questioned the importance of the vaccines. This is concerning considering that Fadda et al. (2016) found that confidence in vaccine decisions is related to the perceived importance of this decision (Fadda et al., 2016).

> My midwife she laughed at it [vaccination], she said well it's up to what you want to do... No one's stopping you... just do what you want to do... I called him [GP] and he said he

> was fine with it as well... [not having vaccines]. They just say 'we're not here to force you, it's just your decision'. (Shiloh, age 19)

> I think you have to go with your instinct... if you feel like... you're not getting the right information, then you won't go for it [vaccination]... needs to be a lot more... one to one... communication... especially with pregnant women... there needs to be... more... understanding between one another... 'I've understood what you're saying, and what you're saying to me doesn't make me feel like I have to go to somewhere else to get another opinion' ... to make someone feel like they have to do their own investigation... it's like being at school... this is different. This is to do with an unborn... human. (Lucy, age 27)

One component of patient-centred care is whether HCWs explicitly solicit questions about vaccination. One participant stated that while HCWs were in general very pro-vaccine, there was no scope for discussion (Idda, age 27). Sometimes participants needed re-assurance, which also tended to be missing from the vaccine conversation.

> It's almost taken as a given that if they tell you about it [vaccination]... you'll just do it... as opposed to proactively looking to reassure you, if you haven't specifically asked. So if I had questions... 'What are the known side effects?' ... and I'm confident enough to ask that... it's not like they were...withholding anything, but they won't proactively volunteer the information. (Isobel, age 40)

In cases like this, the implicit message given to patients who turn to HCWs for advice is that the patient is on their own, and should be able to think clearly about the decision. There is an assumption that being autonomous means being self-reliant and rational. The consequence of this is that the burden of making a decision is carried exclusively by the pregnant patient (Wendler & Rid, 2011). Further to this, there was sometimes the assumption that some information was being withheld, reflecting sentiments of other participants of distrust in the government and its organisations.

When discussing the influenza vaccine, one participant stated that she felt 'down' because she did not receive the vaccine during pregnancy. This patient also mentioned that HCWs *did not care* (Haleefa, age 27). If an in-depth discussion with a trusted HCW had taken place, which accounted for the patient's personal emotions and needs, she may have felt more competent and thus empowered to make the right decision for her. She would be more likely to have felt satisfied and confident with her decision without experiencing feelings of guilt after the decision was made.

An empowered decision could also prevent the phenomenon of 'omission bias', the concept of favouring potentially harmful omissions over less harmful acts. The phenomenon arises because it is often perceived that one is more responsible for the consequences of one's actions than for the consequences of one's inactions, and so the former would cause more blame and regret (Asch, 1994). For example, Shiloh, age 19, stated that if something went wrong with her pregnancy after receiving vaccination, she would be annoyed with herself. A decision to vaccinate which is shared with a HCW could lesson these fears of blame and regret.

The way in which the topic of vaccination is initiated is important because it can significantly affect the nature and extent of patients' responses (Opel et al., 2012). A video recording of a 16-week check consultation between a GP and her pregnant patient in this study showed that the GP had an open, participatory approach to the vaccine discussion. From the start, the GP built a relationship with the patient: she smiled at the baby scan and said; *It doesn't matter how many times I see this, I still think it's amazing... its phenomenal.* The GP then clearly outlined what will happen in the consultation and, initiating the vaccine discussion by saying that they would *have a little chat about vaccines and things like that. Is that kind of what you were expecting?* The patient expressed how nice it felt to receive the call about the consultation and to be looked after. The GP told the patient she could stop her if she had any questions. She said she would touch on the pertussis vaccine and asked if the patient knew much about the infection and the vaccine. The patient told the GP the story of having whooping cough as a child and being given fish fingers. The GP and patient were able to laugh about this as an idea for a cure. The GP explained why the vaccine was introduced, the dangers of an infant contracting pertussis and when and by whom it would be administered. She asserted that it is rare to have any side effects from the vaccine, reassuring the patient that *we keep an eye on you when we give it... but it's incredibly rare to have any kind of allergic reaction...you should be perfect; you won't notice anything.* The patient was able to ask questions during this discussion which were answered confidently and at the end of the discussion, expressed, *that makes perfect sense to me.* The GP finished the consultation by asking about the patient's mood, if she had a supportive partner, and telling her that she seemed clued up.

From the perspective of the participant, the GP personalised the consultation and showed caring for the individual with true delight in the baby scan, and asking about her emotional needs. She was able to make the patient feel comfortable and at ease by sharing a joke. The question format (i.e. *have you heard of pertussis?*) and the assurance that the patient could ask questions allowed patient participation in the vaccination decision process (Opel et al., 2012). Any concerns could be discussed and the patient was re-assured. The result of this was that the patient felt cared for and confident in the vaccine recommendation.

CONCLUSIONS

Patients face many influences on their decisions to vaccinate including family, friends, health professionals, religious institutions and government agencies, as well as their personal characteristics (Ells, Hunt, & Chambers-Evans, 2011). Often pregnant women are greatly influenced by trusted female family members to whom they have approached for advice. The advice given has great influence on a pregnant woman's decision to vaccinate. Social conditions and relationships can even shape available choices for patients (Ells et al., 2011). It is important therefore that HCWs understand these influences, as well as the wider social context in which their patient is situated. If HCWs know who these influencers are, they are more able to talk through any concerns brought about by them with the patient (possibly by debunking myths and reassuring confused patients after receiving conflicting advice). The HCW may also then notice that partners are not being engaged in the conversation, as was observed in this study, thus affecting their ability to provide advice and support. HCWs could then engage such family members in discussions about the vaccination decision, unburdening the pregnant patient from making health decisions on her own. This approach would incorporate a broader conception of the patient's needs in context (Walter & Friedman Ross, 2014), while engaging in a dialogue about how vaccines make sense in people's lives and thus engendering a feeling of understanding and trust between the HCW and patient. For this understanding to arise (which entails in-depth discussion of a very personal nature, sometimes including patient's family members), pregnant patients must trust their HCWs.

While some participants in this study had a close relationship with their HCW, in many cases, good patient–HCW relationships and understanding of the patient's social context was lacking and so distrust in HCWs and vaccination was not surprising. A relational autonomy approach requires the same one or two HCWs to spend time with their patient during her pregnancy, to understand the contextual features of her identity and experience, including key relationships with others, and the role the patient wishes herself and others to play. These features of a relational autonomy approach help the HCW to understand the patient as a whole, and foster a relationship of collaboration between patient and health professional, as well as address any circumstances that hinder patient autonomy (Ells et al., 2011).

The role of the HCW therefore is not only to provide information but also to build a trusting, close relationship with their patient, ensuring she feels comfortable, taken care of, and in control. In this way, HCWs can be key in patient's empowerment in the vaccination decision. They should be willing to address parents' questions and concerns and recognise how their interactions and relationships with patients can either enable or impair empowerment. Misconceived assumptions about what empowerment means might be a contributing factor to vaccine hesitancy (Fadda et al., 2016). It must be understood that patients can at the same time be compliant with the HCW recommendation, but claim the decision as their own as it was guided by a trusted source with whom they have a good relationship (Kukla, 2005). In fact, patients feel more in control of their decision when it is recommended by a trusted medical professional (Mendick, Young, Holcombe, & Salmon, 2010). Thus, to feel empowered does not necessarily mean patients must make decisions on their own. Having the ability to negotiate the extent to which one is involved in decision making is key; it is a wholly context-specific decision (Jackson,

Cheater, & Reid, 2008). These features of relational autonomy lead not only to greater patient satisfaction, less symptom burden, and lower rates of referral (Little et al., 2001) but could also increase levels of trust in vaccination and thus create higher rates of vaccination acceptance.

Those who do not accept prescribed vaccination schedules should be seen neither as ignorant nor as resisting in a negative sense. Such assumptions lead to flawed and ineffective policy prescriptions (Poltorak, Leach, Fairhead, & Cassell, 2005). Such parents are often following positive, informed strategies geared to their health, which understand vaccination in personalised ways. The current popularity of individualist thinking makes the 'one size fits all' vaccine programme and the discourse of herd immunity seem impersonal, without much scope for patient inclusion in the decision-making process. Therefore, individualised care may create a more positive experience of healthcare (Reich, 2016). If policy-makers and health professionals are to engage effectively with mothers, one-way information delivery needs to be replaced with dialogue that appreciates and understands the social processes around vaccination concerns (Poltorak et al., 2005). Health professionals should move away from implicit expectations of compliance, incorporating definitions of science and evidence to include a wider variety of views (Leach & Fairhead, 2007). This would open it up to public critique and thus create a more democratised health care system.

ACKNOWLEDGEMENTS

I would like to acknowledge the Brocher Foundation in Geneva for hosting me and giving me the time and space to analyse and write up my research. I am also extremely grateful to Dr. Sophie Zadeh for introducing me to the theory of relational autonomy.

This research was funded by the National Institute for Health Research Health Protection Research Unit (NIHR HPRU) in Immunisation at LSHTM, in partnership with Public Health England (PHE). The views expressed are those of the authors and not necessarily those of the NHS, the NIHR, the Department of Health or of Public Health England.

REFERENCES

Asch, D. A. (1994). Omission bias and pertussis vaccination. *Medical Decision Making*, *14*, 118–123.

Braun, V., & Clarke, V. (2014). What can thematic analysis offer health and wellbeing researchers? *International Journal of Qualitative Studies on Health and Well-being*, *9*, 26152.

Byrne, L. (30th June 2015). RE: Registered Patient GP practice data. Prenatal pertussis Immunisation Vaccine Uptake Monitoring Programme England Apr 2015 to Mar 2016. Type to WILSON R.

Dlugacz, Y., Fleischer, A., Torroella Carney, M., Copperman, N., Ahmed, I., & Ross, Z. (2012). 2009 H1N1 vaccination by pregnant women during the 2009-10 H1N1 influenza pandemic. *Obstetrics*, *206*, 339.e1–339.e8.

Ells, C., Hunt, M. R., & Chambers-Evans, J. (2011). Relational autonomy as an essential component of patient-centered care. *International Journal of Feminist Approaches to Bioethics*, *4*, 79–101.

Fadda, M., Depping, M. K., & Schulz, P. J. (2015). Addressing issues of vaccination literacy and psychological empowerment in the measles-mumps-rubella (MMR) vaccination decision-making: A qualitative study. *BMC Public Health*, *14*, 836.

Fadda, M., Galimberti, E., Carraro, V., & Schulz, P. J. (2016). What are parents' perspectives on psychological empowerment in the MMR vaccination decision? A focus group study. *BMJ Open*, *6*(4), e010773.

Flory, D. (2012). *Commissioning the pertussis (whooping cough) vaccination programme for pregnant women*. Retrieved from https://www.gov.uk/government/uploads/system/uploads/attachment_data/file/212948/David-Flory-PERTUSSIS-27-09-2012.pdf. Accessed 15 September 2014.

Jackson, C., Cheater, F. M., & Reid, I. (2008). A systematic review of decision support needs of parents making child health decisions. *Health Expect*, *11*, 232–251.

Joffe, H. (2003). Risk: From perception to social representation. *British Journal of Social Psychology*, *42*, 55–73.

Kabeer, N. (1999). Resources, agency, achievements: Reflections on the measurement of women's empowerment. *Development and Change*, *30*, 435.

Kukla, R. (2005). Conscientious autonomy: Displacing decisions in health care. *Hastings Center Report*, *35*, 34–44.

Kumar, R. (2013). How are women's experiences of childbirth represented in the Literature? A critical review of qualitative health research set in the global South. *Women's Health Urban Life*, *12*, 19–38.

LB Hackney Policy Team (2016). A profile of Hackney, its people and place *[Online]*. London: LB Hackney Policy Team. Retrieved from http://hackney.gov.uk/Assets/Documents/Hackney-Profile.pdf

Leach, M., & Fairhead, J. (2007). *Vaccine anxieties: Global science, child health and society*. London: Earthscan.

Little, P., Everitt, H., Williamson, I., Warner, G., Moore, M., Gould, C., & Payne, S. (2001). Observational study of effect of patient centeredness and positive approach on outcomes of general practice consultations. *BMJ*, *323*(7318), 908–911.

Löfstedt, R. E. (2005). *Risk management in post-trust societies*. New York, NY: Palgrave Macmillan.

Mackenzie, C., & Stoljar, N. (2000). *Relational autonomy: Feminist perspective on autonomy, agency, and the social self*. New York, NY: Oxford University Press.

Mayo, E. (1949). *Hawthorne and the Western Electric Company, the social problems of an industrial civilisation*. Harvard, MA: Routledge.

Mcintyre, P., & Wood, N. (2009). Pertussis in early infancy: Disease burden and preventive strategies. *Current Opinion in Infectious Diseases*, *22*, 215–223.

Mendick, N., Young, B., Holcombe, C., & Salmon, P. (2010). The ethics of responsibility and ownership in decision-making about treatment for breast cancer: Triangulation of consultation with patient and surgeon perspectives. *Social Science & Medicine*, *70*, 1904–1911.

Opel, D. J., Robinson, J. D., Heritage, J., Korfiatis, C., Taylor, J. A., & Mangione-Smith, R. (2012). Characterizing providers' immunization communication practices during health supervision visits with vaccine-hesitant parents: A pilot study. *Vaccine*, *30*, 1269–1275.

Oudshoorn, N. (2002). Drugs for healthy people: The culture of testing hormonal contraceptives for women and men. In: G. M. Van Heteren & E. M. Tansey (Eds.), *Biographies of remedies: Drugs, medicines, and contraceptives in Dutch and Anglo American healing cultures*. Amsterdam: Rodopi.

Poltorak, M., Leach, M., Fairhead, J., & Cassell, J. (2005). 'MMR talk' and vaccination choices: An ethnographic study in Brighton. *Social Science & Medicine*, *61*, 709–719.

Public Health England (2016). *Seasonal influenza vaccine uptake amongst GP Patients in England: Provisional monthly data for 1 September 2015 to 31 January 2016 [Online]*. England: Public Health England. Retrieved from https://www.gov.uk/government/uploads/system/uploads/attachment_data/file/503124/January_2016_Seasonal_flu_GP_patients_01Sept_31Jan.pdf. Accessed 20 August 2016.

Reich, J. (2016). *Calling the shots: Why parents reject vaccines*. New York, NY: New York University Press.

Ritchie, B., Ritchie, B., & Ritchie, J. (1997). Nurses' practices and perceptions of family-centered care. *Journal of Pediatric Nursing*, *12*, 214–222.

Taylor, G. W., & Ussher, J. M. (2001). Making sense of S&M: A discourse analytic account. *Sexualities*, *4*, 293–314.

Walter, J. K., & Friedman Ross, L. (2014). Relational autonomy: Moving beyond the limits of isolated individualism. *Pediatrics*, *133*, 16–23.

Wendler, D., & Rid, A. (2011). Systematic review: The effect on surrogates of making treatment decisions for others. *Annals of Internal Medicine*, *154*, 336–346.

White, L. (2005). The needle and the state: Immunizatio nand innoculation in Africa. Or, the practice of un-national sovreignty. *Locating the field: The ethnocgraphy of biomedical research in Africa*. Kilifi, Kenya.

Wilson, R. J., Paterson, P., Jarrett, C., & Larson, H. J. (2015). Understanding factors influencing vaccination acceptance during pregnancy globally: A literature review. *Vaccine*, *33*, 6420–6429.

AN EXAMINATION OF STATE-LEVEL MANDATES FOR INSURANCE COVERAGE ON HEALTH-SEEKING BEHAVIORS FOR INFERTILITY

Nicole Maki Weller

ABSTRACT

Health-seeking behaviors (HSB) for infertility are influenced my multiple factors. The Behavioral Model of Health Services Utilization states that enabling resources and predisposing factors are essential in predicting HSB, and this study examined the relationship between state-level mandates that insurance providers cover infertility service on the rates of HSB for infertility among a nationally representative sample of women.

This study used data from the National Survey of Family Growth, identified 15 states with state-level mandates as enabling resources, and used sociodemographic characteristics as predisposing resources. Using discrete-time event-history analyses, and retrospective accounts of infertility HSB, these variables were examined to determine if residing in a state with state-level insurance mandates would increase the likelihood of HSB for infertility.

Results indicated an impact of state-level mandates on HSB for infertility. Specifically, the rates of HSB for infertility were higher among women residing in states with state-level mandates.

Health and Health Care Concerns among Women and Racial and Ethnic Minorities
Research in the Sociology of Health Care, Volume 35, 79–95

ISSN: 0275-4959/doi:10.1108/S0275-495920170000035005

A limitation in this research stems from a data restriction that forced identifying a place-of-residence before or after 2000. To overcome this, multiple analyses, and a nested model comparison were tested to measure the effect of state-level mandates on HSB.

The comparative analysis of the rates of HSB for women residing in states with state-level mandates has not been considered before, and the results provide further detail into the infertility experience for women and their partners.

Keywords: Health-seeking behaviors; infertility; insurance coverage; state-level mandates

INTRODUCTION

Health-seeking behaviors (HSB) for infertility are influenced by multiple social and individual factors such as socioeconomic status, age, health history, and access to health insurance coverage (Pescosolido, 1992; Schoen, Astone, Kim, Nathanson, & Fields, 1999; Stephen and Chandra, 2006). One of the largest obstacles to seeking help for infertility is the cost of treatment (Bitler & Schmidt, 2006; Schmidt, 2007). Less invasive procedures for infertility, like hormone therapy, can cost between $500 to $3000 dollars per cycle; tubal surgeries can total upwards of $10,000; in vitro fertilization (IVF) averages $12,500 per procedure; and the total cost of just one, medically assisted live birth will cost an average of $44,000 (Smith et al., 2010). In addition to the financial obstacles associated with HSB for infertility, there is debate on the actual total number of women experiencing infertility when rates are determined by the number of women engaging in HSB for infertility is the measure of assessment. This stems from the understanding that the percentage of women who actually seek treatment for infertility are not representative of the number of women who are actually experiencing any infertility complications (Guzick & Swan, 2006; Johnson & Fledderjohann, 2012). With these two obstacles in consideration, this research examined if there was a relationship between residing in a state with state-level insurance mandates to cover/offer-to-cover infertility services on the rates of HSB for infertility among all women – with particular attention given to the marginalized populations of women that are not typically represented in the percentages of women seeking infertility treatment.

It is important to examine the contextual effects of state-level insurance mandates on HSB for infertility for three reasons. First, the number of women who engage in any HSB for infertility is disproportionately fewer than the actual number of women who report any lifetime infertility. Furthermore, the sociodemographics of women who are seeking treatment overwhelmingly represent women from higher socioeconomic status groups (i.e., highly educated, employed, and higher incomes) (Greil & McQuillan, 2010). By comparing the rates of HSB when insurance coverage is available, it will shed some light on the sociodemographic differences in HSB for infertility by identifying one measure, (insurance coverage) that may contribute to these differences. Second, as the proportion of women who delay childbearing until later or older maternal ages increases, in part due to changing social dynamics, it can be presumed that the rates of women experiencing any lifetime infertility will also increase. This logic stems from the physiological realties that an increased risk for infertility comes with advanced maternal age. Therefore, examining the effects of state-level insurance mandates on HSB for infertility can specify how a measure that extends beyond the personal control of the individual (i.e., not getting older, or improving socioeconomic status) may influence HSB. The third and final reason takes into consideration the changing social and political policies regarding options covered by health insurance programs. Ongoing debates as to what should be included in health insurance coverage, specific to reproductive health, currently focuses on birth control methods. However, with the high costs of infertility services and treatments, it is necessary to explore any potential influence that access to insurance coverage may have on the rates of HSB for infertility (Bitler & Schmidt, 2006). Therefore, this study set out to identify if there were observable differences in the rates of HSB for infertility when state-level mandates for insurance to cover/offer-to-cover infertility services was considered.

BEHAVIORAL MODEL OF HEALTH SERVICE UTILIZATION

According to the Behavioral Model of Health Services Utilization (Behavioral Model), health-seeking behaviors for all health needs are influenced by predisposing factors, enabling resources, internal factors, and external factors (Andersen, 1968, 1995; Bradley et al., 2002). Predisposing factors include sociodemographic characteristics, social status, and health beliefs (Andersen, 1968, 1995; Bradley et al., 2002). Enabling resources include individual, family, and community resources as well as social networks, access to health insurance, having a regular health care professional, and/or, having access to a health care facility (Andersen, 1968, 1995; Bradley et al., 2002). Over time the Behavioral Model developed to include internal factors (i.e., exercise, diet, and health history) and external factors (i.e., the economic environment), to predict HSB for general health conditions (Andersen, 1968, 1995; Bradley et al., 2002). According to the Behavioral Model, the likelihood of an individual seeking treatment is dependent upon the interaction of predisposing factors, enabling resources, and internal and external factors (Andersen, 1968, 1995; Bradley et al., 2002). Using the Behavioral Model as a theoretical guide, this study proposed that residing in a state with state-level insurance mandates is an enabling resource that allows women greater access to infertility treatments and services. Furthermore, predisposing factors observed among women residing within these states, such as their socioeconomic status, subsequently influences their rates of HSB for infertility. Applying Behavioral Model theory to this research supports the assertion that there is an impact on the rates of HSB for infertility among women residing in a state with state-level mandates that insurance providers cover/offer-to-cover infertility services (enabling resource), and that this is further impacted by the unique sociodemographic differences (predisposing factors) of these women.

STATE-LEVEL INSURANCE MANDATES

Health-seeking behaviors for general health conditions are influenced by an interaction of enabling resources and external factors. Enabling resources include access to health insurance, but more specifically, insurance plans that cover infertility treatments. External factors that influence HSB for general health conditions include the availability and costs of the services. In the case of insurance mandates and infertility, residing in a state with state-level mandates for insurance coverage could alleviate some of the high costs associated with infertility treatments, ultimately increasing the availability and accessibility of treatment options. Previous research has shown that states with state-level insurance mandates to cover/offer-to-cover infertility services have unique HSB trends as compared to states without any mandates (Bitler & Schmidt, 2006). For example, states with mandated coverage of IVF have the highest reported rates of IVF usage and the highest medically prescribed rates of IVF treatment for infertility (Bitler & Schmidt, 2006). Other studies have observed that the rates of twin births to women aged 35 or older are highest in states with infertility insurance mandates (Bitler & Schmidt, 2006). The higher rates of twin births in these states may be explained in part by the fact that access to infertility treatments, like IVF, may increase the risks for multiple births, but it remains a unique trend among states with these mandates.

In response to the increasing expense of infertility treatments as well as changing socio-reproductive trends, 15 states have issued state-level insurance mandates. While state-mandated policies vary across each state, the mandates essentially require group-health insurance companies to include coverage for infertility treatment in every policy, or, offer the option of purchasing a policy that would cover infertility treatment. There are exceptions to this rule with some states making allowances for health maintenance organizations (HMOs). Table 1 lists the 15 states that either mandate coverage for infertility services or mandate an option to purchase coverage for infertility services.

Table 1. States that Mandate Insurance Programs Cover, or Offer-to-Cover Infertility Services.

	Year Mandate Enacted	Mandate to Cover Infertility Insurance	Mandate to Offer Coverage
Arkansas	1987	Cover	
California	1989		Offer
Connecticut	1987	Cover	
Hawaii	1991	Cover	
Illinois	1991		Offer
Louisiana	2001		Offer
Maryland	1985	Cover	
Massachusetts	1987	Cover	
Montana	1987	Cover	
New Jersey	2001	Cover	
New York	1990	Cover	
Ohio	1991	Cover	
Rhode Island	1989	Cover	
Texas	1987		Offer
West Virginia	1977	Cover	

Source: Retrieved from RESOLVE (http://www.resolve.org) and accessed on January 30, 2017.

INFERTILITY

Infertility in the United States is quite common with data from the National Survey of Family Growth (NSFG) and the National Survey of Fertility Barriers (NSFB) estimating that over 7 million men and women of reproductive age, at least 51.3% of women aged 25–45, have experienced infertility at some point in their lives (Greil, McQuillan, & Slauson-Blevins, 2011; Chandra & Stephen, 2010). Studying the changing trends of infertility is important for multiple reasons, such as providing insight into the social construction of health and illness, and providing insight into the sociocultural disparities that exists in the American health care system. An additional aspect of infertility that is relevant to sociological studies on health outcomes is the idea that with increasing public knowledge about infertility and treatment options, there will be an increase in the number of individuals that seek advice and treatment for infertility. This in turn influences the number of physicians and health care providers that provide these services as well as influencing how health care insurance programs provide coverage for these types of services.

An additional consideration regarding the importance of studying infertility health-seeking behaviors stems from the fact these behaviors, like all health-seeking behaviors, are overwhelmingly determined by socioeconomic status. Access to prenatal services, infertility services and treatments, or even insurance plans covering reproductive health is influenced by socioeconomic status in the US marginalized populations of women in the US society and culture are systematically isolated from reproductive health resources that would alleviate fertility barriers (Bell, 2009; Nachtigall et al., 2005). Popular perception of the educated, affluent, and non-Hispanic white women struggling with infertility is vastly different from the perception of the under-educated, poor, minority women who cannot stop having babies (Bell, 2009; Nachtigall et al., 2005). The impact of social construction of infertility on HSB is observed in the racial/ethnic differences of who actually seeks treatment for infertility, even though rates of infertility are often higher for nonwhite women (Bitler & Schmidt, 2006; Macaluso et al., 2010).

Examining and identifying social determinants that influence the rates of HSB for infertility not only benefits women and their partners coping with infertility, but may also provide a better understanding of how the limitations regarding access to any health care service, can be observed across the broader US population. While previous studies have shown that changing social environments and prior reproductive health outcomes have significant impacts on the HSB for women experiencing infertility, no previous research has considered the contextual relationship between state-level effects on individual health behaviors among women experiencing infertility (Kelly-Weeder & O'Connor, 2006; Martinez, Daniels, & Chandra, 2012).

HYPOTHESIS

Borrowing from the Behavioral Model of Health Services Utilization, this study proposed that HSB for infertility was more likely observed among women residing in states with state-level mandates for insurance providers to cover/offer-to-cover infertility treatments, when compared to women residing in states without these mandates. This expectation stems from three assumptions regarding HSB and infertility. First, treatment for infertility is very costly which impedes some women from pursuing treatment. However, if a woman is residing in a state with state-level mandates that insurance providers cover/offer-to-cover infertility treatments, this could alleviate some of the financial burdens of treatment; ultimately increasing the rates of HSB for infertility. In this regard, state-level mandates act as an enabling resource that increases the likelihood of utilization. At a minimum, women residing in states with state-level insurance mandates may explore the options surrounding infertility treatments even if they opt out of pursuing treatment.

Second, external factors such as increased public awareness of infertility treatment options may be associated with living in a state with state-level mandates (Bitler & Schmidt, 2006; Bunting & Boivin, 2007; Schmidt, 2007). For example, women residing in these states may have greater access to information delivered by their medical and/or insurance providers that their infertility needs could be serviced as part of the state-level mandates. Similarly, there are numerous social networks for women experiencing infertility. For women residing in states with state-level mandates, these social networks could disseminate information regarding treatment options that are available as part of these mandates.

The final assumption is that belonging to an insurance group that will cover/offer-to-cover infertility treatments, may increase the availability of a network of physicians that are experts in the field of infertility. It may be that within the professional network of physicians there is shared knowledge or information about what services are provided by certain health care professionals, therefore making referrals based on services needed and the type of insurance coverage included more feasible.

Therefore, the overarching hypothesis for this study was that residing in a state with state-level mandates that insurance providers cover/offer-to-cover infertility treatments will increase the rates of HSB for infertility for women. Moreover, the rates of HSB for infertility will be higher among all sociodemographic groups of women residing in states with state-level insurance mandates; demonstrating that enabling resources, like access to insurance, may be more influential on HSB for infertility than predisposing factors.

DATA AND METHODOLOGY

Retrospective data from female respondents that were interviewed in the 2006–2010 National Survey of Family Growth (NSFG) survey were examined to test the hypothesis that residing in a state with state-level insurance mandates would increase the rates of HSB for infertility. The female respondent's state-of-residence was determined using variables that asked the respondent if they had been living in the same state since 2000, then merging those variables with data from a contextual file that indicated which state the respondent was residing in at that time. All 50 US states, including Washington D.C., were included in the state variables. Respondents were observed as living in only one of the 50 US states. Since the NSFG only interviews civil, noninstitutionalized members of the US population, consideration for military personnel stationed over-seas with a permanent US address, was not an issue.

Admittedly, there were methodological constraints using variables that asked about state-of-residence using 2000 as a point-in-time reference. However, this research employed two unique statistical analyses to overcome this issue. The first set of analyses was informed by recent data from the US Census, which states over 55% of women of reproductive age (18–44) reside in the same state of birth (Ren, 2011). Therefore, the first set of analyses only measures the rates of HSB for female respondents reporting any HSB since 2000 onward, based on the fact that the respondent indicated they have lived in the same state since 2000 and any state-level effects would be present only from that time onward. The second set of analyses stems from data presented by the Pew Research Center which suggests adults that are moving with frequency are likely to be younger and unmarried. This demographic characteristic is in contrast to the typical sociodemographics of women actively trying to get pregnant (Cohn and Morin, 2010). Therefore, the second assumption informing the analysis is that female respondents who are moving with frequency are not actively trying to get pregnant, and as such, are not actively engaging in HSB for infertility. Consequently, this subset of women would not be greatly impacted by state-level mandates regarding infertility services. For these reasons, the second set of analyses measured HSB for infertility for all female respondents as one large cohort, not removing any cases based on the variable regarding year of residence since 2000. Further discussion on the justification of this methodological approach will be discussed later in this chapter. In both sets of analyses, the main predictor of HSB for infertility was residing in a state with state-level mandates that insurance providers cover/offer-to-cover infertility treatments. At the time of this study, there were 15 states with these state-level mandates for coverage, which were presented in Table 1.

For this research, all 15 states with the state-level mandates were combined into one group in an effort to focus only on the influence of the mandates, rather than on the unique, individual state-level effects that could influence HSB for infertility, above and beyond the insurance mandates. Respondents were coded 1 if they lived in any of these 15 states, or 0 if they lived in a state without any state-level mandates. Finally, to examine if the enabling resources of state-level mandates for insurance coverage of infertility treatments could be more influential than predisposing factors of sociodemographic marginalization, additional variables were considered including race/ethnicity, socioeconomic status, and maternal age. These variables were included in the analyses because they are frequently cited determinants of HSB for health in general, but infertility specifically.

ANALYTIC STRATEGY

Event-history discrete-time hazard models were used to estimate the rates of HSB for infertility. The NSFG measures health-seeking behaviors for infertility based on responses to questions about experience seeking help to get pregnant, or help to prevent a miscarriage, at a monthly level. Therefore, HSB for infertility were conceptualized as discrete-time units, rather than continuous time and person-months. Although using person-months for the unit of analysis increases the sample size substantially, discrete-time methods are appropriate for these analyses for two reasons. The first is that discrete-time methods do not deflate the standard errors and subsequent tests for statistical significance are provided (Allison, 1982). Second, the probability of HSB for infertility within a given month is so small that the estimates provided through discrete-time methods would be very similar to estimates given from continuous methods (Axinn & Barber, 2001). Logistic regression models were used to predict if HSB for infertility did or did not occur for each respondent during the period of observation using residence in a state with state-level mandates as the primary predictor, and sociodemographic characteristics as the secondary predictor.

$$\mathrm{Ln}[p/(1-p) = \alpha + \sum(\beta k)(Xk)$$

In this formula, p is the monthly probability of HSB for infertility and $p/(1-p)$ is the monthly odds of HSB occurring. In the logit model, coefficients indicate the log-odds of HSB for infertility for a one unit change in the explanatory variables. Coefficients from the models are presented as exponentiated log-odds, or odds ratios. This allows for interpretation of the coefficients as the monthly odds of HSB for infertility. Odds ratios greater than 1 indicate a positive effect, odds ratios less than 1 indicate a negative effect, and odds ratios equal to one indicate no effect.

Four separate models were analyzed in this study. The first model examined the impact of selected sociodemographic measures on the rates of HSB for infertility. The second model built on the first model to examine selected sociodemographic variables as well as a measure for residing in a state with state-level insurance mandates. The third model maintained the measures of selected sociodemographic variables, and the measure of residing in a state with state-level insurance mandates, but added a new measure of residing in the same state since 2000. The fourth and final model was a nested comparison model testing the goodness-of-fit of the measure for residing in the same state since 2000.

RESULTS

Selected descriptive statistics from Table 2 indicate that 37% of female respondents lived in one of the 15 states with state-level mandates; 74% lived in the same state since 2000; and 11% had ever engaged in HSB for infertility. The sociodemographics of the 11,210 respondents surveyed was representative of US population demographics where 52% of the sample was non-Hispanic white; 21% was non-Hispanic black; 22% was Hispanic; with 5% self-identifying as some other race/ethnicity. In addition, 51% of the sample had at least a

Table 2. Means and Standard Deviations for $N = 11{,}210$ female respondents.

	Mean	Std. Dev.	Min.	Max.
Ever use infertility services	0.11	0.31	0	1
Parity status (at time of interview)				
Nulliparous	0.42	0.49	0	1
Parous	0.58	0.49	0	1
Educational attainment				
No high school degree/GED	0.35	0.48	0	1
High school degree	0.51	0.50	0	1
Bachelor's degree	0.12	0.33	0	1
Graduate degree (MA or PhD)	0.02	0.13	0	1
Employment status				
Full- or part-time employment	0.63	0.48	0	1
Unemployed/working unpaid labor	0.37	0.29	0	1
Cumulative years of employment				
Full- or part-time years of employment	13.4	2.71	1	20
Relationship type				
Married	0.35	0.17	0	1
Cohabiting	0.18	0.25	0	1
Single	0.47	0.23	0	1
Relationship duration				
0 to 1 years	0.11	0.12	0	1
1 to 3 years	0.39	0.15	0	1
3 to 5 years	0.28	0.11	0	1
5 or more years	0.22	0.12	0	1
Age cohorts				
Age 15–19	0.33	0.47	0	1
Age 20–24	0.27	0.44	0	1
Age 25–29	0.19	0.39	0	1
Age 30–34	0.12	0.33	0	1
Age 35–39	0.07	0.25	0	1
Age 40–45	0.02	0.15	0	1
Race/ethnicity				
Non-Hispanic White	0.52	0.50	0	1
Non-Hispanic Black	0.21	0.41	0	1
Hispanic	0.22	0.41	0	1
Non-Hispanic other	0.05	0.23	0	1
Childhood sociodemographics				
Biological parents married at birth	0.78	0.42	0	1
Mother's education				

Table 2. (*Continued*)

	Mean	Std. Dev.	Min.	Max.
No high school diploma/GED	0.25	0.44	0	1
High school diploma/GED	0.32	0.47	0	1
Two years of college	0.24	0.42	0	1
Bachelor's degree	0.19	0.39	0	1
Mother worked full or part time	0.72	0.45	0	1
Mother's age at first baby				
Age 19 or younger	0.37	0.48	0	1
Age 20–24	0.37	0.48	0	1
Age 25–30	0.18	0.38	0	1
Age 30 or older	0.08	0.27	0	1

Source: National Survey of Family Growth, 2006–2010 Continuous Data File.

high school degree (12% had a bachelor's degree or higher) and the cumulative years of employment at the time of survey was 13.4 years.

Table 3 presents the results from analyses conducted to measure the effects of various selected sociodemographic variables; residing in a state with state-level mandates that insurance cover/offer-to-cover infertility services; and residing in the same state since 2000 on the rates of HSB for infertility.

The results from Model 1 largely support national sociodemographic trends regarding HSB for infertility. For example, results show that non-Hispanic white women are more likely to engage in HSB for infertility compared to non-Hispanic black and Hispanic women. Likewise, women with more advanced educational degrees and with more years of employment are also more likely to engage in HSB for infertility compared to their counterparts with less education and less employment experience. In the following sections, the outcomes from Model 2, Model 3, and Model 4 are presented which highlight the rates of HSB for infertility among women when various sociodemographic characteristics and the main predictor of state-level mandates was examined.

Model 2 of Table 3 presents the results from the analyses looking at the impact of residing in a state with state-level mandates for insurance coverage on the rates of HSB for infertility. To begin, the findings indicate that rates of HSB for infertility among respondents living in a state with state-level mandates are 38% higher than female respondents who did not reside in a state with state-level mandates. Similarly, the rates of HSB among women residing in a state with state-level mandates, are higher for non-Hispanic white women compared to Hispanic and non-Hispanic black women, and they are higher still among women with higher levels of education and employment experience

Table 3. Effects of Residing in a State a with State-Level Mandates that Insurance Providers Cover/Offer-to-Cover Infertility Services, on Rates of HSB for Infertility.

Model	1	2	3
State-Level Mandates for Insurance Coverage			
Reside in state with coverage/offer-to-cover	–	1.38*	1.32*
Reside in the same state since 2000	–	–	1.14*
Time-Varying Control Measures			
High School Degree (GED Equivalent)	1.82*	1.83*	1.79*
Bachelor's Degree	3.06*	3.09*	2.99*
Graduate Degree (Masters or PhD)	6.09*	6.01*	6.03*
Working full time for at least 6 months	2.37*	2.35*	2.29*
Cumulative years of full-time employment	0.88*	0.88*	0.92*
Married	4.38*	4.42*	4.61*
Cohabiting	1.85	1.79	1.74
Time-Invariant Control Measures (from childhood)			
Age Cohorts			
20–24	2.77**	2.80**	2.84**
25–29	4.97**	5.03**	5.07**
30–34	7.16**	7.23**	7.24**
35–39	4.85**	4.91**	4.97**
40–45	2.98*	3.06*	3.10*
Race/ethnicity			
Non-Hispanic Black	0.70*	0.70*	0.69*
Hispanic	0.94*	0.98*	0.94*
Non-Hispanic other	0.75*	0.76*	0.76*
Biological parents married at birth	0.78	0.79	0.74
Mother's education & employment status			
Mother's highest degree was high school	1.13	1.09	1.11
Mother's highest degree 2 years college	1.10	1.12	1.09
Mother's highest degree was BA	1.13	1.11	1.11
Mother worked full or part time	0.88	0.87	0.89
Mother's Age at First Baby			
Age 20–24	0.81	0.81	0.80
Age 25–29	0.79	0.78	0.78
Age 30 or older	0.40	0.40	0.39
Person-months	1,096,796	1,096,796	1,096,796

Coefficients are odds ratios, with z-ratios in parentheses.
$^{*}p < 0.05$, $^{**}p < 0.01$, $^{***}p < 0.001$.

compared to women with lower levels of education and employment experience.

The results from Model 3 in Table 3 present the rates of HSB for infertility when residing in a state with state-level mandates was examined with a measure of living in the same state since 2000. In this model, the rates of HSB for infertility are 32% higher for women who lived in a state with state-level mandates that insurance providers cover/offer-to-cover infertility treatments, and it was 14% higher among women who had lived in the same state since 2000, compared to respondents who did not live in a state with state-level mandates. With regard to the sociodemographic differences on the rates of HSB for infertility, results from Model 3 resemble those observed in Model 1 and Model 2. For example, non-Hispanic white women residing in a state with state-level mandates for insurance coverage of infertility treatments are more likely to engage in HSB compared to their non-Hispanic black and Hispanic counterparts. Hispanic respondents were 6% less likely to engage in HSB for infertility, and non-Hispanic black respondents were 31% less likely to engage in HSB for infertility.

In the fourth and final model (not shown), a likelihood ratio (*lr*) test was used in a nested model comparison of female respondents who had lived in the same state since 2000, to all female respondents regardless if they have lived in the same state since 2000. This test was conducted to determine if the variable for residing in the same state since 2000 was a better fit for predicting HSB for infertility when compared against the rates of HSB for infertility among women who had not lived in the same state since 2000. The purpose of this final model was to determine if there was a significant difference on the rates of HSB for infertility, when the year-of-reference variable was considered. The likelihood ratio test statistic was 25.14 and was statistically insignificant ($p < 0.05$) indicating a statistically significant difference among the rates of HSB of infertility among women who have lived in the same state since 2000 compared to all women who had not lived in the same state since 2000. This supports the results presented in Model 3 were only women who have lived in the same state since 2000 are analyzed, and their rates of HSB for infertility are statistically significantly higher among the women who reside in states with state-level insurance mandates.

CONCLUSION

This study set out to examine the relationship between various enabling and predisposing factors that influence health-seeking behaviors for infertility. Specifically, the study examined if HSB for infertility would be influenced by residing in a state with state-level mandates that insurance provider's cover/offer-to-cover infertility services. Similarly, the study examined if residing in a state with these state-level mandates would produce significant outcomes on the rates of HSB for a subset of the population that is typically marginalized from accessing infertility services and treatments. This is an important question to ask partly in response to the growing rates of infertility currently in the United States, due to projected population structure changes that contribute to delayed childbearing until more advanced maternal ages, and in part due to shifting federal programs surrounding health care coverage at the macro-level. This second point highlights the potential for state-level insurance mandates to cover/offer-to-cover infertility services may be renegotiated and removed as part of shifting federal laws on health care coverage. By exploring this contextual relationship on the HSB for infertility, this research highlighted the social importance of maintaining state-level insurance mandates for women and their partners seeking infertility treatment.

Prior to the discussion on the results from this research, it is necessary to address a challenge of the study that impacted the overall analytical procedures. This challenge stemmed from the limiting construction of the point-in-time measure with regard to residing in the same state since 2000. This is largely a limitation of using secondary, precoded data. This presented problems in making broad interpretations of HSB for infertility because there was no systematic collection of residence data prior to 2000. However, results from the models testing the effects of residing in a state with state-level mandates and residing in the same state since 2000 were shown to be a statistically better fit and demonstrated that among female respondents in these categories, the rates of HSB for infertility were higher when compared to their counterparts. Furthermore, the unique aspect of this particular research inquiry regarding state-level mandates is highlighted by the lack of any previous research into this area. Therefore, approaching an analysis of these measures in unique and creative ways provides the groundwork for future research into this particular area. The proceeding discussion addresses the unique contributions of this research, above and beyond the limitation of the point-in-time reference.

The overall findings from each of the analytical models examined, indicated that among women experiencing infertility, those who resided in a state with state-level mandates for insurance coverage of infertility services had higher rates of HSB for infertility compared to their counterparts living in states without any state-level mandates. This can be explained in part by the perception that state-level insurance mandates act as an enabling resources. For example, medical and health care providers located in states with state-level mandates may be more knowledgeable of coverage options and providers who are covered under various insurance programs. This knowledge benefits women and their partners experiencing infertility and needing to seek services and treatments from specialists for their fertility needs. Likewise, residing in a state with state-level mandates may increase the rates of HSB for infertility because it increases the chances of external factors promoting HSB for infertility. For example, it is possible that the benefits of residing in a state with state-level mandates extend beyond knowledgeable physicians and health care providers, and can be observed among social network groups that provide tremendous support to women and their partners experiencing infertility. In this regard, the external factors present themselves when a woman seeks information from her peers and she is directed to health care providers that participate in the state-level mandates and provide various treatments. Finally, there may be additional state-level characteristics that were not measured in this study, that are present among these states that simultaneously contribute to higher rates of HSB for infertility. For example, population demographics such as higher rates of educated, employed, and health-conscious workforce that would be more likely to engage in HSB for any health care need.

Previous research on the broader topic of HSB for infertility consistently highlight that select groups of women are limited in their access to services and treatments for infertility. This stems from historical stratification from receiving fair and equitable health care services, from social misconceptions that racial/ethnic minorities are not experiencing infertility, but rather are hyper fertile, and finally from the social reality that infertility treatments are costly and there is tremendous socioeconomic inequality in our society preventing some women and their partners from seeking treatment. Results from this study suggest that one potential solution to this social inequity in HSB for infertility may be state-level mandates for insurance coverage. In each of the models tested in this study, the rates of HSB for infertility were higher among women residing in states with state-level insurance mandates regardless of their race/ethnicity and socioeconomic status. In this regard, the state-level mandates as enabling resources may be more influential on HSB for infertility than are predisposing factors.

One final point of discussion that was not tested in the analytical models of this research, but is nevertheless important to the study of infertility, is the influence of fertility intentions HSB. This research did not test fertility expectations specifically but rather made the assumption that any women actively seeking infertility services was motivated in part by her fertility intentions. An additional component specific to infertility behaviors that goes beyond the scope of this research is consideration to a cost/benefit analysis of fertility intentions and subsequent HSB behaviors. For example, our understanding of HSB for infertility would be enhanced if we could interpret the overall gains of residing in a state with state-level mandates in HSB for infertility. Women who reside in states without these mandates will no doubt seek treatments and services for their infertility. Future considerations should examine at what point, or level of financial investment, will residing in state with state-level mandates produce higher rates of HSB for infertility compared to states without mandates.

Future research goals exploring the relationship between state-level mandates and HSB for infertility should focus on exploring data that can provide improved time-ordering information regarding state-of-residence and any infertility related HSB. A second research option would be to consider additional contextual effects on the rates of HSB. For example, exploring poverty levels, immigration flows, economic and wealth distributions, and even historical political associations of a state would provide further insight into how contextual effects have various outcomes on the rates of HSB. Finally, this research would be improved if there was a better understanding of how fertility intentions and desires may supersede any financial and contextual restrictions in terms of HSB. Put another way, future research should consider if there is a tipping point for women and their partners seeking infertility assistance when fertility intentions are no longer guiding the HSB, but rather, the restrictive and personal costs associated with prolonged infertility treatment influences HSB.

The greatest contributing factor of this research to the existing research on infertility is the comparative analysis of the rates of HSB for women residing in states with progressive state-level mandates to cover/offer-to-cover infertility services – an analysis that has not previously been considered. In addition to the comparative analysis of this research, testing the effects of select sociodemographics variables supports existing research on fertility and infertility by building upon existing studies linking education, employment, and relationship status to various outcomes of HSB, by highlighting innovative approaches to studying the effects of maternal age or lifetime diagnosis of STI in HSB, and by proposing that rates of HSB for infertility extend beyond the individual level and can be observed at macro-levels.

The findings from this research have overall implications for social science researchers interested in the changing social impacts on fertility trends, for medical and mental health professionals that interact and work with women and couples coping with infertility, and in public health policies in developing greater public awareness of the risks factors not only associated with infertility, but the health-seeking behaviors for infertility. More specifically, this research and the findings from the substantive research questions further promote the idea that the infertility experience is significantly different for women of all sociodemographic backgrounds, but also, it is significantly different based on various contextual effects.

REFERENCES

Allison, P. D. (1982). Discrete-time methods for the analysis of event histories. *Sociological Methodology*, *13*, 61–98.

Andersen, R. A. (1968). *A behavioral model of families' use of health services*. Chicago, IL: University of Chicago Center for Health Administration Studies.

Andersen, R. A. (1995). Revisiting the behavioral model and access to medical care: Does it matter? *Journal of Health and Social Behavior*, *36*(1), 1–10.

Axinn, W. G., & Barber, J. S. (2001). Mass education and fertility transition. *American Sociological Review*, *66*(4), 481–505.

Bell, A. V. (2009). It's way out of my league. *Gender & Society*, *23*(5), 688.

Bitler, M., & Schmidt, L. (2006). Health disparities and infertility: Impacts of state-level insurance mandates. *Fertility and Sterility*, *85*(4), 858–865.

Bradley, E. H., McGraw, S. A., Curry, L., Buckser, A., King, K. L., Kasl, S. V., & Andersen, R. (2002). Revisiting the andersen model: The role of psychosocial factors in long-term care use. *Health Services Research*, *37*(5), 1221–1242.

Bunting, L., & Boivin, J. (2007). Decision-making about seeking medical advice in an internet sample of women trying to get pregnant. *Human Reproduction*, *22*(6), 1662–1668.

Cohn, D. V., & Morin, R. (2010). *American mobility: Who moves? Who stays put? Where's home?* (December 2008). Washington, DC: Pew Research Center. Retrieved from http://www.pew-socialtrends.org/files/2010/10/Movers-and-Stayers.pdf, Accessed on June 2017.

Chandra, A., & Stephen, E. H. (2010). Infertility service use among us women: 1995 and 2002. *Fertility and Sterility*, *93*(3), 725–736.

Greil, A., McQuillan, J., & Slauson-Blevins, K. (2011). The social construction of infertility. *Sociology Compass*, *5*, 736–746.

Greil, A. L., & McQuillan, J. (2010). Trying times: Medicalization, intent, and ambiguity in the definition of infertility. *Medical Anthropology Quarterly*, *24*(2), 137–156.

Guzick, D. S., & Swan, S. (2006). The decline of infertility: Apparent or real? *Fertility and Sterility*, *86*(3), 524–526.

Johnson, K. M., & Fledderjohann, J. (2012). Revisiting "her" infertility: Medicalized embodiment, self-identification and distress. *Social Science & Medicine*, *75*(5), 883–891.

Kelly-Weeder, S., & O'Connor, A. (2006). Modifiable risk factors for impaired fertility in women: What nurse practitioners need to know. *Journal of the American Academy of Nurse Practitioners*, *18*(6), 268–276.

Macaluso, M., Wright-Schnapp, T. J., Chandra, A., Johnson, R., Satterwhite, C. L., Pulver, A., … Pollack, L. A. (2010). A public health focus on infertility prevention, detection, and management. *Fertility and Sterility*, *93*(1), 1–16.

Martinez, G. M., Daniels, K., & Chandra, A. (2012). Fertility of men and women aged 15–44 years in the United States: National Survey of Family Growth, 2006–2010. National health statistics reports no. 51. Hyattsville, MN: National Center for Health Statistics.

Nachtigall, R. D., Castrillo, M., Shah, N., Turner, D., Harrington, J., & Jackson, R. (2005). The challenge of providing infertility services to a low-income immigrant latino population. *Fertility and Sterility*, *92*(1), 116–123.

Pescosolido, B. (1992). Beyond rational choice: the social dynamics of how people seek help. *American Journal of Sociology*, *97*, 1096–1138.

Ping, R. (2011). Lifetime mobility in the United States: 2010. Survey. *US Census Bureau*. American Community Survey Briefs, Issued November 2011.

Schmidt, L. (2007). Effects of infertility insurance mandates on fertility. *Journal of Health Economics*, *26*(3), 431–446.

Schoen, R., Astone, M. A., Kim, Y. J., Nathanson, C. A., & Fields, J. M. (1999). Do fertility intentions affect fertility behavior? *Journal of Marriage and Family*, *61*(3), 790–799.

Smith, J. F., Eisenberg, M. L., Millstein, S. G., Nachtigall, R. D., Shindel, A. W., Wing, H., … Katz, P. P. (2010). The use of complementary and alternative fertility treatment in couples seeking fertility care: Data from a prospective cohort in the united states. *Fertility and Sterility*, *93*(7), 2169–2174.

Stephen, E. H., & Chandra, A. (2006). Infertility service use among us women: 1995–2002. *Fertility and Sterility*, *93*(3), 725–736.

PART III
HEALTH CARE PRACTITIONERS AND HEALTH AND HEALTH CARE

BEARING THE BURDEN OF CARE: EMOTIONAL BURNOUT AMONG MATERNITY SUPPORT WORKERS

Miriam Naiman-Sessions, Megan M. Henley and Louise Marie Roth

ABSTRACT

This research examines effects on emotional burnout among "maternity support workers" (MSWs) that support women in labor (labor and delivery (L&D) nurses and doulas). The emotional intensity of maternity support work is likely to contribute to emotional distress, compassion fatigue, and burnout.

This study uses data from the Maternity Support Survey (MSS) to analyze emotional burnout among 807 L&D nurses and 1,226 doulas in the United States and Canada. Multivariate OLS regression models examine the effects of work–family conflict, overwork, emotional intelligence, witnessing unethical mistreatment of women in labor, and practice characteristics on emotional burnout among these MSWs. We measure emotional burnout using the Professional Quality of Life (PROQOL) Emotional Burnout subscale.

Work–family conflict, feelings of overwork, witnessing a higher frequency of unethical mistreatment, and working in a hospital with a larger percentage of cesarean deliveries are associated with higher levels of burnout among MSWs. Higher emotional intelligence is associated with lower levels of burnout, and the availability of hospital wellness programs is associated with less burnout among L&D nurses.

Health and Health Care Concerns among Women and Racial and Ethnic Minorities
Research in the Sociology of Health Care, Volume 35, 99–125

ISSN: 0275-4959/doi:10.1108/S0275-495920170000035006

While the MSS obtained a large number of responses, its recruitment methods produced a nonrandom sample and made it impossible to calculate a response rate. As a result, responses may not be generalizable to all L&D nurses and doulas in the United States and Canada.

This research reveals that MSWs attitudes about medical procedures such as cesarean sections and induction are tied to their experiences of emotional burnout. It also demonstrates a link between witnessing mistreatment of laboring women and burnout, so that traumatic incidents have negative emotional consequences for MSWs. The findings have implications for secondary trauma and compassion fatigue, and for the quality of maternity care.

Keywords: Emotional burnout; compassion fatigue; maternity support; secondary trauma

INTRODUCTION

Helping occupations are a growing field of workers that nurture the physical, emotional, and social well-being of others. Within this field, helping professionals face significant emotional, physical, and spiritual demands as they confront human suffering and meet the needs of society's most vulnerable members. Workers in helping occupations provide care and compassion in a society that often devalues it. As a result, these workers face elevated risks of emotional burnout and compassion fatigue, presenting important problems for the retention of care workers and for quality of care.

In the field of helping occupations, we define workers that support women in labor as "maternity support workers" (MSWs). MSWs offer women information, emotional, and/or physical support, and advocacy during pregnancy, childbirth, and postpartum (Morton & Clift, 2014; Roth et al., 2014). MSWs are present for life-changing events, and the intensity of maternity support work is likely to contribute to high levels of emotional burnout and compassion fatigue. Within maternity support work, labor and delivery (L&D) nurses provide support, monitor labor progress, and administer medications, while doulas provide continuous support to laboring women but do not provide medical services or advice. L&D nurses and doulas have different organizational positions and relation to medical procedures, which may influence their attitudes toward birth and consequently their susceptibility to emotional burnout. However, existing research has not considered contributors to burnout in a maternity care setting. How do MSWs manage the emotional intensity of their work? What influences the level of emotional burnout among MSWs? Also, given their different positions within the medical establishment, how do the factors that influence burnout differ for these two groups of MSWs?

Many MSWs do this work because they have a desire to care for others or strong beliefs about the importance of birth in women's and families' lives (Eley, Eley, Bertello, & Rogers-Clark, 2012; Morton & Clift, 2014). Those beliefs may be based on their own life experiences, their experiences supporting women with traumatic birth experiences, and/or their views of common medical practices in hospital birth. This study contributes to the literature on emotional burnout among care workers by analyzing the effects of experience-based attitudes toward birth, views of common obstetric practices, and frequency of witnessing unethical mistreatment. We use data from the Maternity Support Survey (MSS) to analyze emotional burnout among L&D nurses and doulas in the United States and Canada. The MSS contains data on the characteristics and attitudes of L&D nurses, childbirth educators, and doulas, although this analysis focuses on L&D nurses and doulas who physically support pregnant women during labor and birth. It includes measures of experiential knowledge, attitudes toward common medical practices, and the frequency of witnessing traumatic events, all of which may influence burnout for MSWs.

MSWs

Research shows that labor support is associated with improved birth outcomes, less reliance on pain medication, shorter labor, fewer cesarean sections and assisted vaginal deliveries using vacuum or forceps, greater satisfaction with the birth experience, and lower rates of postpartum depression (Deitrick & Draves, 2008; Flamm, Berwick, & Kabcenell, 1998; Hodnett, Gates, Hoymeyr, & Sakala, 2013; Klaus, Kennell & Klaus [1993] 2012; Kozhimannil et al., 2016; Mander, 2001; Manning-Orenstein, 1998; McGrath & Kennell, 2008; Simkin, 1991). However, research has yet to examine how the emotional labor that MSWs perform influences the emotional well-being of the workers themselves (Ekström, Guttke, Lenz, & Wahn, 2011; Liva, Hall, Klein, & Wong, 2012; Monari, Di Mario, Facchinetti, & Basevi, 2008; Morton & Clift, 2014; Reime et al., 2004; Sandelowski, 1984).

MSWs have limited influence in the medical model of hospital birth, where obstetricians have authority over other workers (Simonds, Rothman, & Norman, 2007). Over 99% of births in the United States and Canada occur in hospitals and hospital births involve high rates of medical procedures, including continuous electronic fetal monitoring (CEFM), the use of intravenous medication (Pitocin) to stimulate labor, and cesarean delivery. Changes in the healthcare system, like shorter hospital stays, an increased reliance on technology, and decreased staff ratios, have also led to a dehumanization of the birth process in hospital settings (Goldberg, 2002). L&D nurses increasingly monitor multiple laboring women from a nursing station outside the L&D room and have limited opportunities to support women one-on-one (Payant, Davies,

Graham, Peterson, & Clinch, 2008). This creates a conflict between values that emphasize birth as an important life experience and the realities of hospital birth. Hospital practices may also have different effects on burnout for L&D nurses and doulas because nurses are integrated into the hospital system and their job involves implementing medical protocols. In contrast, doulas often enter maternity support work because they are committed to a midwifery model of care and a woman's right to make informed choices about her healthcare (Morton & Clift, 2014). As a result, these two maternity support roles are likely to hold different views of common hospital procedures, which may influence their levels of emotional burnout and compassion fatigue.

EMOTIONAL BURNOUT AND MATERNITY SUPPORT WORK

Emotion work refers to individuals' efforts to manage their own and others' feelings and emotional expressions (Hochschild, 1979). Emotion management can involve the suppression and evocation of emotion through cognitive, bodily, or expressive processes, like deliberate changes in thoughts, control of physical symptoms, or changes in gestures (Hochschild, 1979). The term emotional labor applies when this work is commodified and performed in service and caring occupations (Cancian & Oliker, 2000; Hochschild, 1983). These occupations are often susceptible to emotional burnout and compassion fatigue.

Emotional burnout is a state of physical and emotional depletion that results from excessive job and/or personal demands and continuous stress (Lee & Ashforth, 1990; Maslach, 2003; Maslach & Jackson, 1981). Burnout often occurs gradually, as a long-term result of working in draining situations. Emotional burnout can be hard to treat because of the way it builds over time (Pines & Aronson, 1988). Compassion fatigue is a related condition that occurs due to a "state of tension and preoccupation with the cumulative impact of caring" (Figley, 1983: 10). Those who work in care occupations, like nursing, are susceptible to compassion fatigue because caring and empathy are core values of these type of work (Figley, 1983; Melvin, 2012). Compassion fatigue can lead to feelings of isolation, fear, and anxiety, which can have serious consequences for care workers and their patients (Figley, 2002; Larsen, Stamm, & Davis, 2002). It can also occur after isolated incidences of trauma and in this respect is similar to secondary traumatic stress, which occurs when care workers experience sudden incidences of extreme distress, leading to feelings of fear, anxiety, and isolation that can have lasting effects on them (Beck & Gable, 2012; Figley, 1995, 2002; Killian, 2008).

Emotional burnout and compassion fatigue can encourage absenteeism and turnover among care workers and can lead to the loss of one's capacity to care for others (Figley, 2002; Maslach, 2003). As a result, care workers may give impersonal care as they attempt to distance themselves from their patients (Beckstead, 2002; Maslach, 2003; Miller, Stiff, & Ellis, 1988; Smith & Kleinman, 1989). Previous research has found that care workers who receive support from colleagues, report a satisfying work–life balance, and have higher levels of education are best equipped to combat emotional burnout and compassion fatigue (Beck & Gable, 2012; Perry, Toffner, Merrick, & Dalton, 2011; Townsend & Campbell, 2009). However, some influences on burnout are structural: deep-seated workplace policies and organizational culture frequently contribute to burnout, and this is especially difficult to treat (Pines & Aronson, 1988). Organizations can also underestimate the negative impact of emotional burnout and compassion fatigue on their workers and the care that they provide.

Many studies of emotional burnout focus on nurses as a prime example of care work and previous research has found that nurses have high rates of emotional burnout (Beckstead, 2002; Melvin, 2012; Miller et al., 1988; Pines & Aronson, 1988). Young nurses burn out faster and are less likely to engage in techniques to manage their emotions than more experienced nurses, who may develop strategies over time that shield them from burnout (Beckstead, 2002; Erickson & Grove, 2007; Smith, 1992). However, existing studies do not focus specifically on maternity support work, where L&D nurses traditionally performed the tasks that involve the most emotional labor – making women feel cared about and appearing calm and confident (Corbett & Callister, 2000). Now, L&D nurses spend only about 10% of their time providing direct support to laboring women and maternity care involves increasing use of technology (Davis-Floyd, 2003; McNiven, Hodnett, & O'Brien-Pallas, 1992). This is partly due to staffing and organizational constraints in the nursing profession, but it is aggravated by the fact that emotional labor is not highly valued (Davies & Hodnett, 2002; Huynh, Alderson, & Thompson, 2008). Hence, while the general public and new nursing students often perceive nursing as a profession that fills a care deficit left by physicians, L&D nurses face contradictory expectations as a traditional caring occupation that is undergoing processes of depersonalization. Over time, this can contribute to emotional overextension and exhaustion (Maslach, 2003).

The counterpoint to this maternity support role is doulas, whose specific mandate is to fill the care deficit and counteract depersonalization in the medical model of birth by providing one-on-one continuous support during labor. Research on the effectiveness of doula support has shown that doula-assisted births have fewer medical interventions, greater maternal satisfaction, and better infant outcomes (Hodnett et al., 2013; Kennell, Klaus, McGrath, Robertson, & Hinkley, 1991; Kozhimannil et al., 2016; Langer, Campero, Garcia, & Reynoso, 1998). Doulas are in a unique position because they support laboring women both within and outside the hospital setting. However, because doulas typically occupy no formal position within the medical establishment, they must walk a fine line between challenging the medicalized birth model and accommodating it (Henley, 2015). Surveys suggest that doulas' biggest challenge in hospital settings is the lack of respect they receive from other healthcare professionals (Lantz, Low, Kane, Varkey, & Watson, 2005). Coupled with an emphasis on emotional aspects of the birth experience, this can contribute to burnout among doulas, whose culture emphasizes caring and commitment (DONA International, 2014). Thus, tensions with the medical model of birth may undermine the emotional needs of these MSWs.

BURNOUT: MITIGATING AND AGGRAVATING FACTORS

In this chapter, we focus on individual and organizational circumstances that affect the likelihood of emotional burnout and compassion fatigue among these MSWs, including work–family conflict; feeling overworked; emotional intelligence; positive and negative personal birth experiences; views on epidural analgesia, induction, and cesarean delivery; frequency of witnessing unethical mistreatment; percentage of births that MSWs attend that involve cesarean delivery; and presence of a hospital wellness program. This study makes unique contributions to the empirical literature by considering the effects of views of common medical procedures and witnessing mistreatment as factors that influence emotional resilience or susceptibility to burnout.

Work–Family Conflict

Family relations can serve an important role in one's mental, emotional, and physical well-being and family support can buffer emotional resilience (Carr & Springer, 2010). This is one reason that marriage can decrease vulnerability to burnout, although work and family commitments also pose emotional and time demands that can lead to work–family conflict (Killian, 2008; Peeters, Montgomery, Bakker, & Schaufeli, 2005). Work–family conflict increases the likelihood of emotional burnout, and the significant demands of care work can increase work–family conflict (Hochschild, 1979, 1983; Killian, 2008).

Overwork

Another important influence on emotional burnout is work overload. Long hours and excessive job demands can increase compassion fatigue in care occupations (Shirom, Nirel, & Vinokur, 2010). Among MSWs, nurses are in high demand, work long shifts, and face pressures to provide personalized care to multiple patients at a time while balancing patient care with other tasks (Beckstead, 2002; Maslach, 2003; Shirom et al., 2010). This can be overwhelming, leaving L&D nurses depleted and unable to give as much as they would like. In contrast, doulas do not work long regular shifts, but they often attend long labors and can become overloaded if they attend more than one or two births per month. Perceptions of overwork among MSWs can aggravate problems of compassion fatigue and contribute to emotional burnout.

Emotional Intelligence

Previous research has found that emotional intelligence (EI) can serve as a protective factor against burnout (Mikolajczak, Menil, & Luminet, 2007). Nurses view EI, especially in the form of the ability to recognize and regulate emotions in oneself and others, as an important personal skill (Graham, Logan, Davies, & Nimrod, 2004; Huynh et al., 2008). Those considered "good" nurses by their peers can regulate their emotions, hiding their reactions and cultivating professional distance and detachment when necessary (Lawler, 2006). Doula training programs teach doulas how to regulate their own emotions and help others manage feelings of panic and anxiety. Thus, emotional regulation is an important skill for MSWs to master. MSWs with high EI may also have better protection against burnout (Mikolajczak et al., 2007).

Positive and Negative Birth Experiences

While previous research on emotional burnout among care workers has highlighted the importance of work–family conflict, overwork, and EI, it has paid less attention to the effects of personal experiences and beliefs on workers' emotional reactions to their work. For both L&D nurses and doulas, personal experiences can inspire empathy and compassion, and many MSWs (especially doulas) enter their field because they had positive experiences with their own births and they want to help others to have similar experiences (Henley, 2016). On the other hand, nurses and doulas who have had negative experiences with their own births may enter maternity support as a way to prevent other women from having a similar experience (Henley, 2016). This creates an emotional risk, because caring for women who have adverse events or suffer mistreatment may trigger secondary traumatic stress for MSWs who have had a negative personal birth experience, putting them at risk for depressive and post-traumatic stress symptoms that negatively influence their capacity to care for others (Olde, van der Hart, Kleber, & van Son, 2006; Zaers, Waschke, & Ehlert, 2008). Thus, while positive experiences may play an important role in the decision to enter care work, negative experiences may influence the ability to provide effective care (Henley, 2016; Roth et al., 2014). In this chapter, we look specifically at how both positive and negative birth experiences affect burnout among L&D nurses and doulas.

Views of Common Medical Procedures

Previous research on emotional burnout has largely ignored the possibility that workers may hold negative views of common organizational practices in their work environment, and that this could increase their likelihood of burnout. For example, many MSWs (especially doulas but also some L&D nurses) have negative views of obstetrical procedures like induction, epidural analgesia, and cesarean section and advocate for low-intervention approaches to childbirth. However, most MSWs support labor in hospital environments where L&D is medically managed, most labors involve CEFM and epidural analgesia, and induction is common. Moreover, L&D nurses must implement medical protocols as part of a hospital team, regardless of their own views. Consequently, they may find it easier to effectively care for women in labor when they hold positive views of obstetric interventions. In contrast, doulas do not engage in medical procedures, but they do witness them. When hospital practices contradict their views and their clients' birth plans, it can be emotionally deflating. Thus, we expect MSWs with more negative views of medical procedures to have higher levels of burnout.

Unethical Mistreatment

Mistreatment is unfortunately common in obstetric practice and there has been growing recognition of the high frequency with which women experience unethical mistreatment and emotional trauma while giving birth (Anonymous, 2015; Laine, Taichman, & laCombe, 2015; Roth, Henley, Seacrist, Torres, & Morton, 2016; Schiller, 2015). Mistreatment can come in various forms, including providers making demeaning remarks, ignoring women's requests, and engaging in procedures against the woman's wishes. MSWs witness these experiences, which may produce secondary trauma and compassion fatigue (Roth et al., 2016). Thus, traumatic incidents can have negative emotional consequences for both patients and the support people who care for them. The more frequently care workers observe this type of mistreatment, the more one expects them to experience emotional burnout.

Cesarean Sections

The medical model of birth involves a "cascade of interventions," in which each successive intervention incrementally increases the probability of a cesarean delivery. In 2011, 32.8% of births in the United States and 27.0% of births in Canada involved cesarean delivery, which is associated with substantial increases in maternal mortality and morbidity (CIHI, 2012; Liu et al., 2007;

Martin, Hamilton, Ventura, Osterman, & Mathews, 2013). Quality initiatives aim to reduce the primary cesarean rate, and birth advocates view technology and surgery as a significant contributor to worsening maternal outcomes (Morris, 2013). Most MSWs have negative attitudes toward cesarean deliveries, viewing them as an overused procedure with negative consequences for women's physical and emotional well-being. However, MSWs support many laboring women who have cesarean deliveries. Given their negative views of cesareans, one expects MSWs who attend a larger percentage of cesarean deliveries to suffer from more emotional burnout.

Hospital Wellness Programs

Finally, a crucial component in a study of emotional burnout involves organizational policies and programs that contribute to burnout susceptibility (Pines & Aronson, 1988). For example, the availability of a Hospital Wellness Program may reduce emotional burnout among L&D nurses who have access to wellness services. Programs focused on reducing stress and emotional burnout can include discussions of risk factors specific to care providers, development of personalized wellness plans, instruction in relaxation techniques, development of a supportive peer environment, and/or normalizing the experience of work-related emotional burnout (Medland, Howard-Ruben, & Whitaker, 2004; Zadeh, Gamba, Hudson, & Wiener, 2012). Prior research suggests that programs addressing psychosocial wellness can reduce emotional burnout and increase retention (Kravits, McAllister-Black, Grant, & Kirk, 2010; Medland et al., 2004; Zadeh et al., 2012). (We analyze this for nurses only, because doulas often work in various locations and are not organizational employees.)

Hypotheses

Based on the literature review and theoretical framework, we tested eight hypotheses about L&D nurses' and doulas' experiences with emotional burnout. First, MSWs who experience more work/family conflict will have higher levels of emotional burnout (H_1). Second, MSWs who perceive themselves to be overloaded will have higher levels of emotional burnout (H_2). Third, MSWs with greater emotional regulation will have lower levels of emotional burnout (H_3). Fourth, MSWs whose positive birth experiences influenced their birth views will have lower levels of emotional burnout (H_{4A}), while those whose negative birth experiences shaped their birth views will have higher levels of emotional burnout (H_{4B}). Fifth, MSWs with more negative views of obstetrical procedures will have higher levels of emotional burnout (H_5). MSWs who witness unethical mistreatment more frequently will also have higher levels of emotional burnout (H_6), and MSWs who attend a higher proportion of cesarean deliveries will have higher levels of burnout (H_7). Finally, nurses with access to a hospital-based wellness program will experience lower levels of burnout (H_8).

DATA AND METHODS

Data for this study come from the MSS, a cross-sectional online survey of L&D nurses, doulas, and childbirth educators in the United States and Canada. For this analysis, we excluded respondents who worked exclusively as childbirth educators, because they were unlikely to provide active labor support. The survey recruited participants between November 2012 and March 2013 through each occupation's professional associations. The organizations for nurses were the Association of Women's Health, Obstetric and Neonatal Nurses (AWHONN) and the Canadian Nurses Association (CNA). The doula organizations were DONA International, Health Connect One, toLABOR (formerly ALACE), CAPPA Canada, and Doula C.A.R.E. (Canada). The professional organizations emailed their current members a recruitment letter via email with a link to the survey, followed by up to two reminders. The research team also publicized the survey to other MSWs via social media (Facebook, Twitter, and maternity blogs) and email networks. The survey collected no personal identifiers, and the Institutional Review Board at the primary investigator's University determined the study to be exempt.

The survey contained questions about demographic characteristics, training and credentials in the maternity support field, sources of information/knowledge about birth, financial rewards of maternity support work, childbirth and breastfeeding experience, attitudes toward common labor practices and breastfeeding, attitudes toward other maternity support roles, work experiences including witnessing mistreatment, work satisfaction and burnout, hospital characteristics, understandings of informed consent, experiences with and knowledge of quality improvement initiatives, and questions specific to each maternity support role. A total of 3,325 respondents started the survey and 2,781 completed it, for a completion rate of 83.6%. Because of the recruitment methods, we cannot ascertain how many potential respondents were in the sampling frame and consequently cannot calculate an accurate response rate. After we excluded cases with missing values on relevant variables, 1,996 respondents remained (807 L&D nurses and 1,226 doulas). Some respondents held multiple maternity support roles, so the number of nurses plus the number of doulas totals more than 1,996.

Dependent Variable

The dependent variable for this analysis is the Professional Quality of Life (PROQOL) Emotional Burnout subscale. The Emotional Burnout subscale consists of 10 questions with responses on a Likert scale (1 = never to 5 = very often). Table 1 presents the PROQOL emotional burnout subscale items with their means and standard deviations. The internal consistency reliability of the emotional burnout subscale was strong for the whole sample ($\alpha = 0.76$) and within roles (nurses $\alpha = 0.79$, doulas $\alpha = 0.72$). Prior studies using this tool report a similar internal consistency reliability ($\alpha = 0.75$) (Stamm, 2010).

Independent Variables

Demographic characteristics included age, race, household income, level of education, and marital status. Over 99.5% of respondents identified as female. Regions included Canada and the Northeastern, Midwestern, Southern, and Western Census regions in the United States (West = reference). We tried to include both age and years in nursing in the models for nurses, but could not because of multicollinearity. To maintain consistency across nurse and doula models, we used age in both models and excluded years in nursing.

Table 1. Descriptive Statistics for Professional Quality of Life (PROQOL) Emotional Burnout Subscale Items.

	All Mean (SD)	Nurses Mean (SD)	Doulas Mean (SD)
I am happy[a]	4.40 (0.64)	4.30 (0.68)	4.46*** (0.61)
I feel connected to others[a]	4.39 (0.66)	4.26 (0.68)	4.49*** (0.63)
I am not as productive at work because I am losing sleep over traumatic experiences of a woman I cared for	1.74 (0.73)	1.78 (0.71)	1.72** (0.74)
I feel trapped by my job in maternity care	1.56 (0.88)	1.82 (1.00)	1.40*** (0.74)
I have beliefs that sustain me[a]	4.41 (0.79)	4.31 (0.83)	4.48*** (0.76)
I am the person I always wanted to be[a]	4.05 (0.75)	3.98 (0.76)	4.11** (0.75)
I feel worn out because of my work in maternity care	2.52 (1.03)	2.77 (1.09)	2.35*** (0.96)
I am a very caring person[a]	4.61 (0.57)	4.57 (0.59)	4.64* (0.54)
I feel "bogged down" by the system	3.10 (1.12)	3.38 (1.14)	2.93*** (1.08)
I feel overwhelmed because my workload seems endless	2.47 (1.12)	2.90 (1.10)	2.18*** (1.03)
N	**1,996**	**807**	**1,226**

T-test for difference between L&D nurses and doulas: † $p < 0.10$, *$p < 0.05$, **$p < 0.01$, ***$p < 0.001$.
[a]Item is reverse coded in subscale.

Independent variables that are relevant for burnout include measures of work–family conflict, work overload, and emotional intelligence. To measure work–family conflict, the survey asked respondents to rate their agreement with the following: "I have trouble balancing the time demands of my maternity work with my family responsibilities and other obligations." To measure work overload, the survey asked L&D nurses if they work "fewer," "as many," or "more" hours than they would prefer in an average month, and it asked doulas if they have "fewer," "as many," or "more" clients than they would prefer in an average month. We coded responses that indicated that they had more clients or worked more hours than they would prefer as having work overload. We created a subscale for emotional regulation using the EI scale from the measurement tool that Schutte and colleagues developed (Schutte et al., 1998). The internal consistency reliability of the emotional regulation subscale was strong for the whole sample ($\alpha = 0.84$) and within roles (nurses $\alpha = 0.82$, doulas $\alpha = 0.85$) (Table A1 presents descriptive statistics for the individual EI measures).

Additional independent variables include attitudinal measures about birth and obstetric practices. The MSS asked respondents the primary source of their views about childbirth, and we include dichotomous measures for whether a positive or negative experience with their own birth was an important source of their attitudes (1 = yes). The survey measured attitudes toward obstetric practices with 5-point Likert scales from 1 (strongly disagree) to 5 (strongly agree). We constructed standardized scales with ranges of 0–10, ranked from extremely negative to extremely positive, for attitudes toward epidural analgesia, induction, and cesarean delivery (see Table A2). The scale for attitudes toward epidural analgesia had moderate to strong internal reliability. The scales for attitudes toward induction and cesarean delivery had weaker internal reliability but we retained these scales because a Cronbach's alpha near 0.7 is common for attitudinal scales and we expected attitudes about standard obstetric practices to influence MSWs' experience of emotional burnout in a birth culture where these interventions are common (Kline, 2000; Liva et al., 2012). Witnessing unethical mistreatment may also be related to secondary trauma and emotional burnout, and the survey asked MSWs how often they witnessed several forms of unethical mistreatment using a 4-point scale from 1 (never) to 4 (often). These measures included the frequency with which nurses and doulas witnessed care providers make racially derogatory remarks, use extra procedures due to race or ethnicity, use sexually degrading language, engage in procedures without consent, or engage in procedures explicitly against a woman's wishes. We also included measures of the practice environment in which MSWs support labor. We asked all survey respondents, "About what percentage of the births that you attend result in cesarean section?" This was a continuous variable ranging from 0% to 95%. Finally, we asked L&D nurses if the hospital they worked at had a wellness program that was available to them.

Methods

We treat emotional burnout as a continuous measure and we used Ordinary Least Squares (OLS) multiple regression analysis with robust standard errors to analyze this variable. OLS regression is a generalized linear modeling technique that models the linear effects of predictor variables on an interval-level response variable, like the emotional burnout subscale. While our models exhibited very strong conformity with OLS assumptions, robust standard errors adjust for a collection of minor concerns about failure to meet OLS assumptions. (Plots of the unadjusted residuals demonstrated that the models conformed very well to OLS assumptions of uncorrelated and normally distributed error terms and simple standard errors were essentially the same.) The models examine the linear relationship between independent variables (predictors) and emotional burnout.

We conducted separate analyses for nurses and doulas. For each group, the first model examines the relationship between emotional burnout and demographic characteristics; the second adds measures of work/family conflict, overload, and emotional regulation; the third model includes attitudinal measures specific to maternity care; and the final model includes ethical violations and features of the practice environment, including the availability of hospital wellness programs for nurses. Although the total sample included 1,569 doulas and 1,012 nurses, we excluded 85 nurses who did not work primarily at one hospital, and 120 nurses and 343 doulas with missing values on one or more variables. (The variable with the most missing values was the dependent variable, so multiple imputation of missing values was inappropriate.) The analyses include 807 nurses and 1,226 doulas. Using a power analysis for multiple regression, we determined the minimum sample sizes to estimate a medium effect size with an alpha of 0.05 using 24 predictor variables (nurse model) or 23 predictor variables (doula model), to be 306 and 301, respectively. The sample sizes for the models are significantly larger than these minimum sizes, and have >99% power to reject the null hypothesis if a relationship is present.

RESULTS

Table 2 presents the descriptive statistics and metrics for all variables in the models. *T*-tests reveal that L&D nurses and doulas are significantly different on most measures. Nurses have higher average household incomes, are much more likely to feel overworked, and have more positive views of induction, epidural analgesia, and cesarean delivery (although both groups tend to have negative views of cesarean delivery). Nurses also report attending a significantly higher percentage of cesarean deliveries than doulas. Doulas' views about birth are shaped by their own birth experiences much more frequently than nurses'

Table 2. Descriptive Statistics for Nurses and Doulas in the Maternity Support Survey.

Variable	Metric	All % or Mean (SD)	Nurses % or Mean (SD)	Doulas % or Mean (SD)
Dependent variable				
Emotional burnout	10 = low, to 50 = high	19.53 (4.89)	21.24 (5.21)	18.39*** (4.32)
Independent variables				
Age	In years	43.71 (11.93)	47.80 (10.84)	41.23*** (11.97)
White	1 = Yes	94.1%	94.7%	93.6%
HH income	1 = <$20k to 7 = $150k +	4.68 (1.60)	5.42 (1.18)	4.20*** (1.65)
Education	1 = HS or less to 5 = Doctorate	2.87 (0.82)	3.02 (0.73)	2.77*** (0.85)
Married	1 = Yes	70.8%	71.3%	70.8%
Region				
Northeast	1 = Yes	16.5%	17.7%	15.8%†
Midwest	1 = Yes	21.0%	23.2%	19.9%†
South	1 = Yes	21.0%	24.9%	18.9%**
West (reference)	1 = Yes	25.9%	22.6%	27.7%**
Canada	1 = Yes	11.8%	7.9%	14.1%***
Work/family conflict	1 = Strongly disagree, to 5 = Strongly agree	2.79 (1.10)	2.74 (1.07)	2.81† (1.11)
Overwork (more than desired)	(1 = Yes)	12.0%	25.7%	3.2%***
EI (emotional regulation)	10 = Low, to 50 = High	41.75 (4.11)	40.84 (3.97)	42.38*** (4.11)
Views shaped by positive birth	1 = Yes	39.8%	35.2%	42.3%**
Views shaped by negative birth	1 = Yes	8.5%	5.5%	10.4%***
Positive about epidurals	Scale 0–10	3.65 (2.29)	5.42 (2.00)	2.48*** (1.45)
Positive about induction	Scale 0–10	2.49 (1.81)	3.64 (1.73)	1.72*** (1.31)
Positive about cesareans	Scale 0–10	1.94 (1.28)	2.54 (1.35)	1.55*** (1.02)
Unethical Mistreatment				

Racist remarks	1 = Never, to 4 = Often	1.44 (0.72)	1.52 (0.76)	1.39*** (0.69)
Extra procedures due to race	1 = Never, to 4 = Often	1.50 (0.84)	1.32 (0.69)	1.63*** (0.92)
Sexist remarks	1 = Never, to 4 = Often	1.38 (0.66)	1.28 (0.57)	1.46*** (0.72)
Procedures without informed consent	1 = Never, to 4 = Often	2.82 (0.95)	2.85 (0.98)	2.81 (0.92)
Procedures against explicit wishes	1 = Never, to 4 = Often	1.75 (0.80)	1.60 (0.74)	1.86*** (0.82)
Births by C-section	% of births	16.32 (13.24)	23.30 (12.82)	11.90*** (11.51)
Hospital wellness program	1 = Yes	—	87.2%	—
N		**1,996**	**807**	**1,226**

† $p < 0.10$, *$p < 0.05$, **$p < 0.01$, ***$p < 0.001$.

views. Because L&D nurses and doulas offer different types of support and have substantially different education and training for their maternity support roles, we analyze them separately. (Results of models that aggregate both groups of MSWs are available from the first author and have substantially similar results.)

Table 3 presents the results of OLS regression models for emotional burnout among L&D nurses. Model 1 is a base model with only demographic variables, which explain 3.3% of the variation in burnout among nurses. In this model, age, education, and marital status are significantly and negatively associated with emotional burnout, which is consistent with prior research. The relationship between age and burnout may be a selection effect, in which workers who are less resilient to burnout may leave the profession early (Brewer & Shapard, 2004). Marital status has been shown to be a protective factor for burnout, as well as other mental health outcomes (Carr & Springer, 2010; Killian, 2008).

Model 2 adds measures of work/family conflict, perceived overwork, and emotional intelligence, and this model explains 39% of the variance in burnout among nurses. Accordingly, work–family conflict and overwork are positively associated with burnout (p <0.001), supporting H_1 (more work–family conflict is associated with more emotional burnout) and H_2 (working more hours than one wants to is associated with higher levels of burnout). Supporting H_3, emotional intelligence is a protective factor, so that nurses with higher levels of emotional regulation had lower levels of burnout. Marital status remained significant in Model 2, but age is no longer significant once other measures are included.

Model 3 adds attitudinal measures, and explains 41% of the variance in nurse burnout. In this model, more positive views of labor induction are associated with lower levels of burnout (contradicting H_5) while more positive views of cesarean delivery are associated with higher levels of burnout among nurses (supporting H_5). Birth views that were shaped by personal birth experiences were not associated with burnout among nurses, failing to support H_{4A} and H_{4B}.

The full model (Model 4) includes frequency of witnessing unethical mistreatment, percent of births by cesarean, and the availability of a hospital-based wellness program, and explains 43% of the variance in burnout. This model reveals that witnessing sexist remarks and violations of informed consent is associated with higher levels of burnout among nurses, offering support to H_6. In particular, the unethical mistreatment effects indicate that L&D nurses who witness more frequent violations of informed consent experience more emotional burnout. Accordingly, a lack of informed consent may not only harm laboring women, but also the support workers caring for them. However, witnessing forms of unethical mistreatment based on race (racist remarks and the use of extra procedures due to a woman's race or ethnicity) had no significant effects.

Table 3. OLS Regression Models Predicting Emotional Burnout Among L&D Nurses.

	Model 1	Model 2	Model 3	Model 4
Age	−0.04* (0.02)	0.00 (0.01)	0.00 (0.01)	0.00 (0.01)
White	0.85 (0.81)	0.52 (0.63)	0.42 (0.64)	0.20 (0.64)
HH income	0.07 (0.16)	0.04 (0.13)	0.08 (0.13)	0.00 (0.13)
Education	−0.53* (0.24)	−0.26 (0.19)	−0.24 (0.19)	−0.39* (0.20)
Married	−1.60** (0.46)	−1.27** (0.37)	−1.27** (0.38)	−1.00** (0.36)
Northeast	−0.44 (0.56)	−0.35 (0.42)	−0.40 (0.42)	−0.51 (0.42)
Midwest	−0.71 (0.52)	−0.77† (0.42)	−0.82† (0.43)	−0.76† (0.42)
South	0.18 (0.53)	0.03 (0.41)	−0.12 (0.42)	−0.34 (0.40)
Canada	−0.47 (0.75)	−0.02 (0.65)	0.27 (0.64)	0.52 (0.64)
Work/family conflict		1.63*** (0.15)	1.62*** (0.15)	1.55*** (0.15)
Overwork		1.64*** (0.34)	1.53*** (0.34)	1.51*** (0.33)
EI (emotional regulation)		−0.52*** (0.04)	−0.51*** (0.04)	−0.51*** (0.04)
Views shaped by positive birth			−0.40 (0.31)	−0.29 (0.30)
Views shaped by negative birth			0.76 (0.56)	0.47 (0.53)
Positive view of epidurals			0.12 (0.09)	0.14 (0.09)
Positive view of induction			−0.28** (0.11)	−0.11 (0.11)
Positive view of cesareans			0.27* (0.13)	0.25† (0.13)
Racist remarks				0.08 (0.22)
Extra procedures due to race				−0.09 (0.23)
Sexist remarks				0.50† (0.29)
Procedures without informed consent				0.38* (0.18)
Procedures against explicit wishes				0.46† (0.24)
% C-sections				0.03* (0.01)
Hospital wellness program				−0.94* (0.42)
Constant	24.76*** (1.54)	38.99*** (1.93)	38.34*** (2.05)	36.03*** (2.13)
N	807	807	807	807
Adjusted R^2	0.03	0.39	0.40	0.43

† $p < 0.10$, *$p < 0.05$, **$p < 0.01$, ***$p < 0.001$.

Supporting H_7, Model 4 also reveals that nurses who attend a high percentage of cesarean deliveries have higher average levels of burnout ($p < 0.001$), so that every 1% rise in cesarean deliveries was associated with an average increase of 0.3 points on the burnout scale. There was also a significant and negative association with hospital wellness programs, indicating that nurses who worked at a hospital that has a wellness program had lower levels of burnout (supporting H_8).

Table 4 presents the results of parallel models for emotional burnout among doulas, and illustrates both similarities with and differences from L&D nurses.

Table 4. OLS Regression Models Predicting Emotional Burnout Among Doulas.

	Model 5	Model 6	Model 7	Model 8
Age	−0.03** (0.01)	−0.01 (0.01)	−0.01 (0.01)	−0.01† (0.01)
White	−0.60 (0.59)	−0.73 (0.51)	−0.69 (0.51)	−0.63 (0.50)
HH income	0.00 (0.08)	−0.07 (0.07)	−0.08 (0.07)	−0.10 (0.07)
Education	0.37* (0.15)	0.08 (0.13)	0.08 (0.13)	0.03 (0.13)
Married	−0.62† (0.34)	−0.84** (0.28)	−0.82** (0.28)	−0.48† (0.28)
Northeast	0.39 (0.36)	0.40 (0.32)	0.37 (0.32)	0.00 (0.31)
Midwest	0.20 (0.34)	0.21 (0.30)	0.24 (0.29)	0.15 (0.28)
South	0.20 (0.37)	0.39 (0.31)	0.38 (0.31)	0.10 (0.30)
Canada	0.66 (0.45)	0.16 (0.38)	0.24 (0.37)	0.21 (0.36)
Work/family conflict		1.42*** (0.10)	1.43*** (0.10)	1.32*** (0.10)
Overwork		1.79† (0.91)	1.73† (0.91)	1.63† (0.86)
EI (emotional regulation)		−0.36*** (0.03)	−0.35*** (0.03)	−0.35*** (0.03)
Views shaped by positive birth			−0.41† (0.21)	−0.21 (0.21)
Views shaped by negative birth			0.94** (0.35)	0.97** (0.34)
Positive view of epidurals			0.13† (0.07)	0.16* (0.07)
Positive view of induction			−0.10 (0.09)	−0.01 (0.09)
Positive view of cesareans			0.16 (0.11)	0.18† (0.10)
Racist remarks				0.36† (0.20)
Extra procedures due to race				−0.01 (0.15)
Sexist remarks				0.50** (0.15)
Procedures without informed consent				0.46** (0.14)
Procedures against explicit wishes				0.32* (0.16)
% C-sections				0.03** (0.01)
Constant	19.45*** (0.85)	31.00*** (1.55)	30.20*** (1.62)	27.28*** (1.62)
N	1,226	1,226	1,226	1,226
Adjusted R^2	0.02	0.31	0.32	0.37

† $p < 0.10$, *$p < 0.05$, **$p < 0.01$, ***$p < 0.001$.

Model 5 explains 2% of the variance in doula burnout and reveals that age and marriage are both negatively associated with doula burnout, so that younger and unmarried doulas suffer from less burnout than older and married doulas. In contrast, education is associated with greater burnout for doulas. However, the effects of age and education disappear in Model 6, which adds measures of work–family conflict, work overload, and emotional intelligence, and explains 31% of the variance in doula burnout. This model is consistent with Model 2 for nurses in Table 3, with marital status and EI being associated with lower levels of burnout, while work/family conflict and work overload are associated with higher burnout. The magnitude of the effect of EI is weaker for doulas than for nurses, even though doulas had higher average EI scores and their training focuses on developing EI.

Results of Model 7 in Table 4 differs from Model 3 for nurses. While attitudes toward birth based on personal experience had no effect on burnout among nurses, they had the expected effects on doulas (H_{4A} and H_{4B}) and views based on negative birth experiences had particularly strong effects for doulas. In contrast, attitudes toward obstetric procedures had little effect for doulas, possibly because doulas held quite consistently negative views of these practices. However, relatively more positive views of epidural analgesia were associated with slightly higher average levels of burnout, contradicting H_5. In the full model, which explains 37% of the variance, greater frequency of witnessing unethical mistreatment in the form of racist and/or sexist remarks and lack of informed consent are associated with higher levels of burnout among doulas, as is attending a higher percentage of cesarean deliveries (supporting H_6 and H_7).

DISCUSSION

Emotional burnout and compassion fatigue are serious problems in caring occupations because they may encourage workers to distance themselves from their work and their patients. This study examines emotional burnout among two types of MSWs who support mothers during L&D. MSWs are particularly likely to suffer from emotional burnout because emotional experience, regulation of emotion, and emotional labor are important aspects of maternity support work (Kirkham, 1999). While L&D nurses and doulas lack authority in the medical model of birth, they have significant contact with laboring women and are likely to connect with the people they serve (Corbett & Callister, 2000; Davis-Floyd, 2001, 2004; Jordan, 1993; Mann & Cowburn, 2005; Wear, 2006). MSWs' training and the work that they do with mothers and infants encourages continuous emotional engagement. The combination of lack of authority with high emotional engagement makes MSWs vulnerable to negative emotional experiences (Kemper, 1991).

To summarize, nurses reported higher average levels of burnout than doulas. Work/family conflict and work overload were sources of burnout for both groups of MSWs, while emotional regulation was a form of emotional intelligence that protected both groups from burnout. More frequently witnessing incidences of mistreatment clearly contributed to higher levels of burnout for both groups of MSWs, suggesting that mistreatment not only harms laboring women but also the workers who support them. MSWs also experienced more burnout when they attended a higher percentage of deliveries via cesarean section. This suggests that working in hospitals where cesarean deliveries are more common increases emotional stress among MSWs.

There were also some differences between nurses and doulas in the effects of experiential knowledge and attitudes toward common obstetric practices. Doulas whose own birth experiences shaped their attitudes experienced less burnout if they had positive birth experiences and more burnout if they had negative birth experiences. However, experience as a basis for views about birth had no effect on nurses' levels of burnout. The findings also reveal a relationship between attitudes toward medical procedures and emotional burnout, although this relationship is more complicated that the original hypothesis suggested it would be. For nurses, more negative views of labor induction are associated with higher levels of burnout, as we hypothesized (H_5). However, more positive attitudes toward cesarean deliveries are associated with higher levels of burnout, in contradiction to H_5. A similar effect occurs for doulas, although this effect only approaches statistical significance ($p < 0.1$). For doulas, more positive views of epidural analgesia are associated with higher levels of burnout, in contradiction to H_5. In thinking about how to make sense of findings that contradicted our hypothesis, we must consider that the causal relationship may also be reversed: MSWs may develop more positive views of obstetric procedures, especially those that reduce demands for one-on-one care, as a coping strategy to reduce burnout. Thus, the more that MSWs become emotionally burned out, the more they may accept the organizational benefits of medical technologies (or become resigned to them). In other words, MSWs who are more burned out may experience a sense of depersonalization with clients and patients, leading to less negative views of cesarean sections.

We also found that L&D nurses who worked at a hospital that had a wellness program reported lower levels of burnout, suggesting that hospital programs that aim to reduce workers' emotional stress can effectively reduce burnout. Thus, care workers in organizations that offer programs to help them to manage stress have lower average rates of burnout, providing evidence for the benefits of these programs. These findings have important healthcare policy implications because emotional burnout is relatively common in caring occupations and it can contribute to high turnover and lower quality of care. MSWs with individual or organizational coping mechanisms and supports in place are more protected from burnout.

Limitations and Future Research

The MSS is the first cross-national survey to examine the under-studied roles and views of MSWs in the United States and Canada. The survey obtained a large number of responses, but a limitation of the data is that the recruitment methods resulted in a nonrandom sample and made it impossible to calculate a response rate because the population-size denominator is unknown. Most MSS respondents were members of professional organizations that assisted with the study, but many MSWs are not members of these specific organizations. As a result, the data may not be generalizable to all L&D nurses and doulas in the United States and Canada.

CONCLUSION

Emotional burnout and compassion fatigue are ongoing challenges in healthcare. Support workers face serious demands that produce negative outcomes for themselves and their patients. Without proper attention to the emotional demands placed on those who provide support, the healthcare field will be unable to provide sufficient care to those who need it. The results from the MSS highlight factors that influence emotional burnout among MSWs, including work–family conflict, overwork, emotional intelligence, and the frequency of unethical mistreatment of laboring women. Our data illustrate that MSWs' attitudes about controversial medical procedures like cesarean sections and induction are tied to their experiences of emotional burnout. Both nurses and doulas with more positive views of cesarean delivery were more burned out, but negative views of other procedures like induction are associated with greater emotional burnout among L&D nurses. It is possible that increased use of medical technologies in obstetric practices have led to "emotional deskilling" (Bone, 2008).

The findings also establish a link between witnessing mistreatment of laboring women and burnout, revealing that traumatic incidents can have negative emotional consequences for both patients and the workers who care for them. Campaigns such as ImprovingBirth.org's #breakthesilence aim to inform more people about mistreatment in maternity care, revealing that ethical violations and mistreatment are quite common (Roth et al., 2014, 2016). With greater awareness of this problem, patients and care workers hope to reduce the incidence of trauma and accordingly, emotional burnout, which can result from repeated exposure to mistreatment.

REFERENCES

Anonymous. (2015). Our family secrets. *Annals of Internal Medicine*, *163*, 321.

Beck, C. T., & Gable, R. K. (2012). A mixed methods study of secondary traumatic stress in labor and delivery nurses. *Journal of Obstetric, Gynecologic, & Neonatal Nursing*, *41*(6), 747–760.

Beckstead, J. (2002). Confirmatory factor analysis of the Maslach burnout inventory among Florida nurses. *International Journal of Nursing Studies*, *39*, 785–792.

Bone, D. (2008). Epidurals not emotions: The care deficit in US maternity care. In B. Hunter & R. Deery (Eds.), *Emotions in midwifery and reproduction* (pp. 56–72). Hampshire, UK: Palgrave Macmillan.

Brewer, E. W., & Shapard, L. (2004). Employee burnout: A meta-analysis of the relationship between age or years of experience. *Human Resource Development Review*, *3*(2), 102–123.

Canadian Institute for Health Information. (2012). Health indicators. Ottawa, Ontario: CIHI.

Cancian, F., & Oliker, S. (2000). *Caring and gender*. Walnut Creek, CA: Alta Mira Press.

Carr, D., & Springer, K. W. (2010). Advances in families and health research in the 21st century. *Journal of Marriage and Family*, *72*, 743–761.

Corbett, C., & Callister, L. C. (2000). Nursing support during labor. *Clinical Nursing Research*, *9*(1), 70–83.

Davies, B. L., & Hodnett, E. (2002). Labor support: Nurses' self-efficacy and views about factors influencing implementation. *JOGNN*, *31*(1), 48–56.

Davis-Floyd, R. (2001). The technocratic, humanistic, and holistic paradigms of childbirth. *International Journal of Gynecology and Obstetrics*, *75*, S5–S23.

Davis-Floyd, R. E. (2003). *Birth as an American rite of passage* (2nd ed.). Berkeley, CA: University of California Press.

Davis-Floyd, R. (2004 [1992]). *Birth as an American rite of passage*. Berkeley, CA: University of California Press.

Deitrick, L. M., & Draves, P. R. (2008). Attitudes towards doula support during pregnancy by clients, doulas and labor-and-delivery nurses: A case study from Tampa, Florida. *Human Organization*, *67*(4), 397–406.

DONA International. (2014). "What is a doula?" DONA International. Retrieved from http://www.dona.org/mothers/index.php. Accessed on August 4, 2014.

Ekström, A., Guttke, K., Lenz, M., & Wahn, E. H. (2011). Long term effects of professional breastfeeding support – An intervention. *International Journal of Nursing and Midwifery*, *3*(8), 109–117.

Eley, D., Eley, R., Bertello, M., & Rogers-Clark, C. (2012). Why did I become a nurse? Personality traits and reasons for entering nursing. *Journal of Advanced Nursing*, *68*, 1546–1555.

Erickson, R. J., & Grove, W. J. C. (2007). Why emotion matters: Age, agitation, and burnout among registered nurses. *Online Journal of Issues in Nursing*, *13*, 1.

Figley, C. R. (1983). Catastrophes: An overview of family reaction. In C. Figley & H. McCubbin (Eds.), *Stress and the family* (11th ed.). New York, NY: Brunner/Mazel.

Figley, C. R. (1995). Compassion fatigue as secondary traumatic stress disorder: An overview. In C. R. Figley (Ed.), *Compassion fatigue*. New York, NY: Brunner/Mazel.

Figley, C. R. (2002). Compassion fatigue: Psychotherapists' chronic lack of self-care. *JCLP/In Session: Psychotherapy in Practice*, *58*(11), 1433–1441.

Flamm, B. L., Berwick, D. M., & Kabcenell, A. (1998). Reducing cesarean section rates safely: Lessons from a 'breakthrough series' collaborative. *Birth*, *25*(2), 117–124.

Goldberg, L. (2002). Rethinking the birthing body: Cartesian dualism and perinatal nursing. *Journal of Advanced Nursing*, *37*(5), 446–451.

Graham, I., Logan, J., Davies, B., & Nimrod, C. (2004). Changing the use of electronic fetal monitoring and labor support: A case study of barriers and facilitators. *Birth*, *31*(4), 293–301.

Henley, M. M. (2015). Alternative and authoritative knowledge: The role of certification for defining expertise among doulas. *Social Currents*, *2*(3), 260–279.

Henley, M. M. (2016). *Science and service: Doulas and the legitimacy of alternative knowledge systems*. Department of Sociology, University of Arizona. Unpublished Manuscript.

Hochschild, A. (1983). Exploring the managed heart and feeling management: From private to commercial uses. In *The managed heart: Commercialization of human feeling* (pp. 3–23 and 89–136). Berkeley, CA: University of California Press.

Hochschild, A. R. (1979). Emotion work, feeling rules, and social structure. *American Journal of Sociology*, *85*, 551–575.

Hodnett, E. D., S. Gates, G. Hoymeyr, & C. Sakala (2013). *Continuous support for women during childbirth. Cochrane Database of Systematic Reviews*. Retrieved from http://www.cochrane.org/CD003766/PREG_continuous-support-for-women-during-childbirth. Accessed on January 4, 2015.

Huynh, T., Alderson, M., & Thompson, M. (2008). Emotional labor underlying caring: An evolutionary concept analysis. *Journal of Advanced Nursing*, *64*(2), 195–208.

Jordan, B. (1993). *Birth in four cultures: A crosscultural investigation of childbirth in Yucatan, Holland, Sweden, and the United States*. Prospect Heights, IL: Waveland Press.

Kemper, T. (1991). Predicting emotions from social relations. *Social Psychology Quarterly*, *54*, 330–342.

Kirkham, M. (1999). The culture of midwifery in the National Health Service in England. *Journal of Advanced Nursing*, *30*(3), 732–739.

Kennell, J., Klaus, M., McGrath, S., Robertson, S., & Hinkley, C. (1991). Continuous emotional support during labor in a US hospital: A randomized controlled trial. *JAMA*, *265*(17), 2197–2201.

Killian, K. D. (2008). Helping till it hurts? A multimethod study of compassion fatigue, burnout, and self-care in clinicians working with trauma survivors. *Traumatology*, *14*(2), 32–44.

Klaus, M. H., Kennell, J. H., & Klaus., P. H. ([1993] 2012). *The doula book: How a trained labor companion can help you have a shorter, easier, and healthier birth* (3rd ed.). Boston, MA: Da Capo Lifelong Books.

Kline, P. (2000). *The handbook of psychological testing*. New York, NY: Routledge.

Kozhimannil, K. B., Hardeman, R. R., Alarid-Escudero, F., Vogelsang, C. A., Blauer-Peterson, C., & Howell, E. A. (2016). Modeling the cost-effectiveness of doula care associated with reductions in preterm birth and cesarean delivery. *Birth*. Retrieved from http://onlinelibrary.wiley.com/doi/10.1111/birt.12218/. Accessed on January 26, 2016.

Kravits, K., McAllister-Black, R., Grant, M., & Kirk, C. (2010). Self-care strategies for nurses: A psycho-educational intervention for stress reduction and the prevention of burnout. *Applied Nursing Research*, *23*(3), 130–138.

Laine, C., Taichman, D. B., & laCombe, M. A. (2015). On being a doctor: Shining a light on the dark side. *Annals of Internal Medicine*, *163*(4), 320. doi:10.7326/M15-1144.

Langer, A., Campero, L., Garcia, C., & Reynoso, S. (1998). Effects of psychosocial support during labour and childbirth on breastfeeding, medical interventions, and mothers' wellbeing in a Mexican public hospital: A randomized clinical trial. *British Journal of Obstetrics and Gynecology*, *105*, 1056–1063.

Lantz, P., Low, M., Kane, L., Varkey, S., & Watson, R. L. (2005). Doulas as childbirth paraprofessionals: Results from a national survey. *Women's Health Issues*, *15*(3), 109–116.

Larsen, D., Stamm, B. H., & Davis, K. (2002). Telehealth for prevention and intervention of the negative effects of caregiving. *Traumatic StressPoints*, *16*(4), 1–2. Retrieved from https://www.istss.org/education-research/traumatic-stresspoints/2002-fall/telehealth-for-prevention-and-intervention-of-the.aspx. Accessed on June 21, 2004.

Lawler, J. (2006). *Behind the screens: Nursing, somology and the problem of the body*. Australia: Sydney University Press.

Lee, R. T., & Ashforth, B. E. (1990). On the meaning of Maslach's three dimensions of burnout. *Journal of Applied Psychology*, *75*(6), 743–747.

Liu, S., Liston, R. M., Joseph, K. S., Heaman, M., Sauve, R., & Kramer., M. S. (2007). Maternal mortality and severe morbidity associated with low-risk planned cesarean delivery versus planned vaginal delivery at term. *CMAJ*, *175*, 455–460.

Liva, S. J., Hall, W. A., Klein, M. C., & Wong, S. T. (2012). Factors associated with differences in Canadian perinatal nurses' attitudes toward birth practices. *JOGNN*, *41*(6), 761–773.

Mann, S., & Cowburn, J. (2005). Emotional labour and stress within mental health nursing. *Journal of Psychiatric and Mental Health Nursing*, *12*(2), 154–162.

Mander, R. (2001). *Supportive care and midwifery*. Osney Mead, Oxford: Blackwell Science Ltd.

Manning-Orenstein, G. (1998). A birth intervention: The therapeutic effects of doula support versus Lamaze preparation on first-time mothers' working models of caregiving. *Alternative Therapies in Health and Medicine*, *4*(4), 73–81.

Martin, J. A., Hamilton, B. E., Ventura, S. J., Osterman, M. J. K., & Mathews, T. J. (2013). *Births: Final data for 2011, in National Vital Statistics Reports*. Hyattsville, MD: National Center for Health Statistics.

Maslach, C. (2003). *Burnout: The cost of caring*. Los Altos, CA: Malor Books.

Maslach, C., & Jackson, S. E. (1981). The measurement of experienced burnout. *Journal of Occupational Behaviour*, *2*, 99–113.

McGrath, S. K., & Kennell, J. H. (2008). A randomized controlled trial of continuous labor support for middle-class couples: Effect on cesarean delivery rates. *Birth*, *35*(2), 92–97.

McNiven, P., Hodnett, E. D., & O'Brien-Pallas, L. L. (1992). Supporting women in labor: A work sampling study of the activities of intrapartum nurses. *Birth*, *19*(1), 3–9.

Medland, J., Howard-Ruben, J., & Whitaker, E. (2004). Fostering psychosocial wellness in oncology nurses: Addressing burnout and social support in the workplace. *Oncology Nursing Forum*, *31*(1), 47–54.

Melvin, C. S. (2012). Professional compassion fatigue: What is the true cost of nurses caring for the dying. *International Journal of Palliative Nursing*, *18*(12), 606–611.

Mikolajczak, M., Menil, C., & Luminet, O. (2007). Explaining the protective effect of trait emotional intelligence regarding occupational stress: Exploration of emotional labour processes. *Journal of Research in Personality*, *41*(5), 1107–1117.

Miller, K. I., Stiff, J. B., & Ellis, B. H. (1988). Communication and empathy as precursors to burnout among human service workers. *Communication Monographs*, *55*(3), 250–265.

Monari, F., Di Mario, S., Facchinetti, F., & Basevi, V. (2008). Obstetricians' and midwives' attitudes toward cesarean section. *Birth*, *35*(2), 129–135.

Morris, T. (2013). *Cut it out: The C-section epidemic in America*. New York, NY: New York University Press.

Morton, C. H., & Clift, E. G. (2014). *Birth ambassadors: Doulas and the re-emergence of woman-supported birth in America*. Amarillo, TX: Praeclarus Press.

Olde, E., van der Hart, O., Kleber, R., & van Son, M. (2006). Posttraumatic stress following childbirth: A review. *Clinical Psychology Review*, *26*, 1–16.

Payant, L., Davies, B., Graham, I. D., Peterson, W. E., & Clinch, J. (2008). Nurses' intentions to provide continuous labor support to women. *Journal of Obstetric, Gynecologic, & Neonatal Nursing*, *37*, 405–414.

Peeters, M. C. W., Montgomery, A., Bakker, A. B., & Schaufeli, W. B. (2005). Balancing work and home: How job and home demands are related to burnout. *International Journal of Stress Management*, *12*(1), 43–61.

Perry, B., Toffner, G., Merrick, T., & Dalton, J. (2011). An exploration of the experience of compassion fatigue in clinical oncology nurses. *Canadian Oncology Nursing Journal*, *2*, 91–97.

Pines, A. M., & Aronson, E. (1988). *Career burnout: Causes and cures*. New York, NY: Free Press.

Reime, B., M. C. Klein, Kelly, A., Duxbury, N., Saxell, L., Liston, R., & Wong, V. (2004). Do maternity care provider groups have different attitudes towards birth? *BJOG: An International Journal of Obstetrics and Gynaecology*, *111*(12), 1388–1393.

Roth, L. M., N. Heidbreder, M. M. Henley, M. Marek, M. Sessions, J. Torres, & C. H. Morton. (2014). *Maternity support survey: A report on the cross-national survey of doulas, childbirth educators, and labor and delivery nurses in the United States and Canada*.

Roth, L. M., M. M. Henley, M. Seacrist, J. M. C. Torres, & C. H. Morton. (2016). *Bearing witness: U.S. and Canadian maternity support workers' observations of ethical violations in childbirth*. Unpublished manuscript.

Sandelowski, M. (1984). *Pain, pleasure and American childbirth: From the twilight sleep to the read method, 1914–1960*. Westport, CT: Greenwood Press.

Schiller, R. (2015). The scandal of the doctors who upload selfies taken next to women's vaginas during childbirth. *Vice*. Retrieved from http://www.vice.com/en_uk/read/doctors-taking-selfies-of-women-post-labour-shows. Accessed on July 13, 2015.

Schutte, N. S., Malouff, J. M., Hall, L. E., Haggerty, D. J., Cooper, J. T., Golden, C. J., & Dornheim., L. (1998). Development and validation of a measure of emotional intelligence. *Personality and Individual Differences*, *25*, 167–177.

Shirom, A., Nirel, N., & Vinokur, A. D. (2010). Work hours and caseload as predictors of physician burnout: The mediating effects by perceived workload and by autonomy. *Applied Psychology*, *59*(4), 539–565.

Simkin, P. (1991). Just another day in a woman's life? Women's long-term perceptions of their first birth experience. Part I. *Birth*, *18*(4), 203–210.

Simonds, W., Rothman, B. K., & Norman, B. M. (2007). *Laboring on: Birth in transition in the United States*. New York, NY: Routledge.

Smith, A. C., & Kleinman, S. (1989). Managing emotions in medical school: Students' contacts with the living and the dead. *Social Psychology Quarterly*, *52*, 56–69.

Smith, P. (1992). *The emotional labour of nursing*. London: Macmillan.

Stamm, B. H. (2010). *The concise proQOL manual*, 2nd ed. Pocatello, ID: ProQOL.org.

Townsend, S. M., & Campbell, R. (2009). Organizational correlates of secondary traumatic stress and burnout among sexual assault nurse examiners. *Journal of Forensic Nursing*, *5*, 97–106.

Wear, D. (2006). Making fun of patients: medical students' perceptions and use of derogatory and cynical humor in clinical settings. *Academic Medicine*, *81*(5), 454–462.

Zadeh, S., Gamba, N., Hudson, C., & Wiener, L. (2012). Taking care of care providers: A wellness program for pediatric nurses. *Journal of Pediatric Oncology Nursing*, *29*(5), 294–299.

Zaers, S., Waschke, M., & Ehlert., U. (2008). Depressive symptoms and symptoms of post-traumatic stress disorder in women after childbirth. *Journal of Psychosomatic Obstetrics and Gynaecology*, *29*, 61–71.

APPENDIX

Table A1. Descriptive Statistics for Emotional Intelligence and Emotional Regulation Subscale.

	All Mean (SD)	Nurses Mean (SD)	Doulas Mean (SD)
When I am faced with obstacles, I remember times I faced similar obstacles and overcame them	4.12 (0.61)	4.10 (0.59)	4.13 (0.63)
Other people find it easy to confide in me	4.35 (0.63)	4.18 (0.65)	4.46*** (0.59)
I know why my emotions change	4.07 (0.66)	3.96 (0.65)	4.14*** (0.65)
When I experience a positive emotion, I know how to make it last	3.90 (0.73)	3.81 (0.71)	3.98*** (0.73)
I seek out activities that make me happy	4.24 (0.63)	4.15 (0.64)	4.31*** (0.62)
I present myself in a way that makes a good impression on others	4.27 (0.58)	4.17 (0.56)	4.34*** (0.59)
I have control over my emotions	3.91 (0.69)	3.86 (0.69)	3.94* (0.69)
I motivate myself by imagining a good outcome to tasks I take on	4.01 (0.74)	3.92 (0.77)	4.07*** (0.72)
I compliment others when they have done something well	4.50 (0.53)	4.42 (0.54)	4.56*** (0.52)
I help other people feel better when they are down	4.39 (0.56)	4.28 (0.55)	4.46*** (0.56)
A	**0.84**	**0.82**	**0.85**
N	**1,996**	**807**	**1,226**

***$p < 0.001$.

Table A2. Attitude Scales.

Scale	Subscale Items (1 = Strongly Disagree, to 5 = Strongly Agree)	α
Epidural analgesia	Epidurals should be routinely offered to all women in labor	0.80
	Epidurals conserve maternal energy for the second stage of labor	
	Epidurals interfere with the normal progress of labor (reverse coded)	
	Epidurals increase the risk of cesarean delivery (reverse coded)	
Induction	Induction is safe as part of a standardized protocol	0.67
	Induction increases the need for epidural analgesia (reverse coded)	
	Inductions increase the cesarean rate (reverse coded)	
Cesarean Delivery	Cesareans prevent urinary incontinence	0.71
	Cesareans are safer for babies than vaginal births	
	Vaginal birth often compromises a woman's sexual functioning after birth	
	Cesareans are as safe for women as vaginal births	
	Women should be able to choose CS, even in absence of medical indication	
	For a woman with a previous CS, scheduled repeat CS is the best for her health	
	For a woman with a previous CS, scheduled repeat CS reduces litigation risk	
	A woman who is a good candidate for VBAC should be able to attempt it if she desires	

"LOST IN TRANSLATION": HOW CLINICIANS MAKE SENSE OF STRUCTURAL BARRIERS TO DIABETES CARE AMONG US LATINOS WITH LIMITED ENGLISH PROFICIENCY

Claudia Chaufan, Mi-Kyung "Miki" Hong and Alicia Fernandez

ABSTRACT

We explored how clinicians assisting low-income US Latino patients with diabetes and limited English proficiency (LEP) made sense of language-discordant care in the context of the social determination of health.

We interviewed 14 physicians in an urban teaching hospital, recorded and transcribed the interviews, and read transcripts to identify themes and interpret meanings. We used a mixed qualitative approach and drew from the Marxian tradition that illuminates how the dynamic of the clinical encounter tends to reproduce the social order by excluding its critical appraisal.

Participants believed that language barriers undermine the quality of the clinical encounter and diabetes outcomes, were eager to serve disadvantaged patients, and were well schooled in the social determination of health and its

Health and Health Care Concerns among Women and Racial and Ethnic Minorities
Research in the Sociology of Health Care, Volume 35, 127–143

ISSN: 0275-4959/doi:10.1108/S0275-495920170000035007

role in diabetes inequalities. However, they appeared unable to conceptualize macro-level changes that may achieve greater health equity.

The structure of medical discourse appears to limit the ability of individual clinicians to conceptualize and engage in social change on behalf patients. Recent debates in primary care indicate that this limitation is currently being challenged. Health services for persons with diabetes and limited English proficiency in the United States and elsewhere require significant improvements in interpreter services. At a broader level, clinicians should consider stepping beyond the limited, traditional role of medical/behavioral advisor to engage in political action toward greater social equity, which would result in better health.

Research in the various dimensions of language discordance is largely quantitative thus the need for qualitative studies to inform practice and policy.

Keywords: Social determination of health; language-discordant care among US Latinos; politics of diabetes inequalities

> Medicine is a social science and politics is nothing else but medicine on a large scale. Medicine as a social science, as the science of human beings, has the obligation to point out problems and to attempt their theoretical solution; the politician, the practical anthropologist, must find the means for their actual solution
>
> Rudolf Virchow (1848), Mackenbach (2009).

INTRODUCTION

Multiple structural factors cause, and reproduce, health inequities among US Latinos and other US minorities, including inadequate access to health services, institutional discrimination, and poverty (Centers for Disease Control & Prevention, 2011; Chaufan, Davis, & Constantino, 2011; Raphael et al., 2011). One such factor is language-discordant care, that is, care in which clinicians and patients are not proficient in the same language. In the context of a dominant, Anglo-Saxon culture, patients with limited English proficiency (LEP) tend to have worse access to preventive services (Harlan, Bernstein, & Kessler, 1991; Pearson, Zhao & Ford, 2011), experience increased risk of medical errors and misdiagnoses (Flores, Abreu, Olivar, & Kastner, 1998), and are more likely to be discharged from the hospital with lesser understanding discharge instructions (Diamond & Reuland, 2009). All these tend to undermine the quality of care that patients receive and affect clinical outcomes (Hornerberger et al., 1996; Wilson, Chen, Grumbach, Wang, & Fernandez, 2005).

Care across the language divide may be especially impaired in the case of US Latinos, the fastest growing US minority, given that a significant number of them – 21 out of 52 million – report speaking English less than "very well" (Ryan, 2011) and, as other US minorities with LEP, tend to be quite poor (Zong & Batalova, 2015). Poverty compounds the harmful health effects of language barriers. Because diabetes, highly prevalent among Latinos, is a complex disease that imposes significant demands on patients, including lifestyle changes and complex treatment plans (Fernandez et al., 2004, Peek, Cargill, & Huang, 2007; Timmins, 2002), US Latinos with LEP are especially vulnerable to the effects of language discordance on diabetes care and outcomes.

Research in the various dimensions of language discordance is largely quantitative (Diamond et al., 2014; Hsu et al., 2006; Schenker, Wang, Selig, Ng, & Fernandez, 2007; Stern et al., 2012). Quantitative studies can tell *that* such outcomes exist and *whether* they are good or poor, yet cannot illuminate *how* they come about, thus the need for qualitative studies to inform practice and policy. As an example, our own qualitative research has revealed features of language-discordant care that we had not anticipated given our quantitative research: we found that while low-income, LEP Latino patients with diabetes preferred to receive care from language concordant clinicians – all else equal – because it enabled them to "be themselves" and to better communicate their concerns, they did not believe that language discordance *per se* made a difference to the quality of care they received, which they attributed to the competence of their clinician.

Nor did they believe that language discordance *per se* influenced diabetes outcomes, which they overwhelmingly attributed to their own ability to comply with clinicians' directives. Patients taking responsibility for *poor* outcomes was paradoxically, and inadvertently, encouraged by clinicians' praise of patients successfully implementing lifestyle changes, seen as largely, and primarily, responsible for *favorable* outcomes. Maybe not coincidentally, patients in this study also tended to downplay structural barriers to treatment, such as family or work obligations, or financial barriers (Chaufan, Fielding, Chesla, & Fernandez, 2015), whose negative effects on diabetes outcomes are well established (Chaufan et al., 2011; Dinca Panaitescu et al., 2011; Ross, Bradley, & Busch, 2006).

Having evaluated in that prior study the perspectives of patients and having found how patients made – or rather, failed to make – sense of language-discordant care as one element within a broader complex of structural barriers, in this study our goal was to understand the perspective of clinicians – especially to shed light on how clinicians make sense of language-discordant care within the broader context of the social determination of health (Breilh, 2015). We also elaborated on the implications of our findings for the goals of reducing diabetes and other health inequities. The study is part of a broader research program on the politics of diabetes inequalities.

METHODS

Sample Description

We interviewed a convenience sample of 14 primary care clinicians, about one third of them bilingual and two thirds of them requiring interpreter services, at a major, urban, teaching and public hospital in northern California that largely serves the needs of low-income populations. The hospital counts with award-winning interpreter services. Inclusion criteria for participants were presence in the hospital diabetes registry as being the primary care clinician of Latino patients with diabetes and LEP.

Research Approach and Design, Data Collection, and Data Analysis

Theoretically, we drew from the Marxian tradition that illuminates how the dynamic of the clinical encounter tends to reproduce the social order by excluding its critical appraisal (Waitzkin, 1989). Methodologically, we applied a qualitative, mixed approach (Barbour, 1998; Patton, 1999), drawing from interpretive phenomenology (Chesla, 1995), grounded theory (Charmaz, 1990), and thematic analysis (Aronson, 1995). Qualitative approaches attempt to make sense of the human experience by examining *how* things come into being rather than *whether* or *that* they do (Anderson, 1998). Therefore sample size and generalizability matter less than the ability of a study to shed light on the processes underlying quantitative findings (Berg, 2004).

Potential participants were identified through the hospital's diabetes registry and later contacted by the first author via email. There were no language proficiency exclusions, so Spanish fluent and non-Spanish fluent physicians were contacted indistinctly. Those who agreed to participate were subsequently invited to schedule a meeting with the first author, who interviewed clinicians in their offices. Interviews lasted between 30 and 50 minutes, and were digitally recorded, transcribed, and analyzed. After providing written informed consent, participants completed a brief interviewer-administered questionnaire eliciting demographic, professional, and language proficiency-related information. This portion of the meeting lasted 5 minutes on average. The remainder of the session was devoted to a semistructured interview designed to elicit participants' narratives of direct experience of language-discordant care and reflections on this experience, addressing three overarching questions: (a) how does language concordance/discordance influence the quality of the clinical encounter and diabetes outcomes; (b) how do language barriers interact with other barriers encountered by low-income populations; and (c) what practice and structural changes could improve diabetes outcomes and reduce diabetes inequalities more generally.

Because the sample size was small, we conducted our analysis using only a word processor (Microsoft Office Word, 2007). The first author read the original transcripts in their entirety and identified emergent interpretive/analytic themes. Then the second author reviewed the transcripts and identified selected passages that illuminated these themes, while at the same time remaining open to new themes and identifying significant words or smaller units that may or not fit these themes (a more grounded approach). Next, the first and second authors met to discuss emerging themes and texts that illuminated or contradicted those themes, and developed interpretations of the meaning of the identified words, small units, or selected passages for participants, resolving discrepancies by consensus. The third author, an expert in language-discordant care among Latinos, oversaw the investigation and made recommendations concerning the implications of the findings for research, practice, and policy. The first author drafted the initial manuscript that was later expanded by the second author, leading to subsequent drafts, in turn read by all authors who provided feedback in an iterative fashion until completion of a manuscript for submission. The Committee for Human Research at the University of California San Francisco approved the study and York University in Toronto provided the space and resources to complete the analysis.

FINDINGS

Out of 14 participants, there were equal numbers of men and women. Most of them were faculty (64%, *N*: 9), and the remainder residents (36%, *N*: 5). The majority of them (71%, *N*: 10) had graduated within the last 15 years, whereas a minority (29%, *N*: 4) had been in clinical practice for over 15 years. The majority (64%, *N*: 9) identified as "white," whereas a significant minority (29%, *N*: 4) as Asian, and the remainder (7%, *N*: 1) as African–American. None of the clinicians identified as Hispanic or as belonging to "other" races/ethnicities. The self-reported Spanish fluency of most participants (64%, *N*: 9) ranged from fair to none, whereas a minority (36%, *N*: 5) self-reported their Spanish fluency as very good to excellent (Table 1).

Barriers to Care and the Limits of Medical Discourse

Our interpretation of clinicians' interviews yielded three significant findings:

> First, clinicians identified language discordance as influencing both the quality of care they were able to deliver and diabetes outcomes, independently from other factors. If we contrast this perspective with that of patients in our earlier study (Chaufan et al., 2015), both clinicians and patients

Table 1. Characteristics of Physician Participants.

Physician Characteristics	% (*N*)
Rank	
Faculty	64 (9)
Resident	36 (5)
Years since graduation	
≤ 15 years	71 (10)
> 15 years	29 (4)
Gender	
Female	50 (7)
Male	50 (7)
Race/Ethnicity	
African–American	7 (1)
Asian	29 (4)
White	64 (9)
Hispanic	0 (0)
Other/Unknown	0 (0)
Spanish Fluency	
Very good to excellent	36 (5)
Fair to none	64 (9)

resembled in that they agreed that their ability to "be themselves" was significantly impaired by language discordance, yet at the same time differed in how they evaluated its clinical relevance: clinicians generally believed language-discordant care influences outcomes, whereas patients did not.

Second, clinicians showed a strong commitment to provide the best care to their patients. As our earlier study shows, this commitment was effectively communicated to patients even across the language divide – patients in our research site reported that they felt that their physicians "cared" (Chaufan et al., 2015). Moreover, clinicians regularly reflected upon the quality of care they provide and appeared trained to identify the social determination of health, such as how diabetes status or outcomes may be affected by poverty.

Third, and most notably, despite clinicians' awareness of the social determination of health, they appeared unable to imagine scenarios that *even in the presence of language barriers may lead to better diabetes outcomes and lesser inequalities*. Much like patients blamed themselves for poor diabetes outcomes, clinicians, when invited to produce an unconstrained "wish list" of changes that could improve their patients' outcomes, identified micro-level changes (i.e., causes of poor outcomes in relation to themselves, their patients, or the doctor–patient relationship worth changing) or at most changes at the level of operations within medical establishments. They did not express a desire, or call, for changes at the level of health systems or policy (e.g., a universal healthcare system with no barriers to access based on varying eligibility criteria such as income level or residency status), much less at the level of broader social conditions (e.g., elimination or at least a significant reduction of poverty that may lead to better health regardless of language issues) – at least not explicitly. Only one participant, and only when prompted in that direction, proposed that "may be a South American, with limited English proficiency but of higher socioeconomic status, would have less trouble seeking and finding quality care – they would have access to greater resources". Following C. Wright Mills (Wright Mills, 1959), we propose that participants lacked a "sociological imagination" that would enable them to relate "biography and history," identify the social determination of health as a "fundamental cause" (Link & Phelan, 1995), and imagine scenarios alternative to current circumstances.

In the following sections, we expand on these interpretive/analytic themes after which we move on to elaborate on their implications for diabetes inequalities and health inequities more broadly.

"There is something lost in translation": Deep difference in language-discordant care.

Virtually all participants agreed that barriers to quality care and good outcomes pervaded the clinical encounter with low-income, LEP patients, largely barriers due to the diminished quality of the communication in the patient-clinician dyad. In the words of two participants:

> [This patient's] English is pretty good, but I think there are some nuances that get lost, especially concerning the specifics of her diabetes care which is when do you use your sliding scale and when shouldn't you, and if your sugar is less level, how much should you give yourself? So I think there probably was something that was lost in translation. (Participant #2)

> In English I can use nuances, I can think about what is the best way to say this. In Spanish, I don't necessarily have five different ways of saying something. I have one, maybe I have two. (Participant #1)

In language-discordant encounters, clinicians felt that it was harder for them to "get" the patient, to convey to the patient that they care about them, to address nonmedical issues, and to communicate nuances. All these factors often led clinicians to stick to medical topics and avoid more complex, including personal, topics, even on occasions when they felt that information about the latter may help improve outcomes more than the medical ones.

Clinicians also feared that language-discordant encounters were less conducive to patients developing trust, a justified concern, as mistrust is not uncommon among a population often subjected to discriminatory treatment (Institute of Medicine, 2002). They also sensed that patients were more cautious when working through an interpreter, as they may doubt whether their concerns were being properly relayed to their clinician, a worry that was confirmed in our earlier, patient study (Chaufan et al., 2015). Finally, they felt that patients became more passive when not communicating in their own language and were less disposed to being proactive with their own diabetes care. As another participant compellingly put it:

> My patients with whom I speak Spanish, they come in and they just yack and yack and yack, and they tell me, the Cubanos come in there with their whole... and I'm like, "Time out baby". Whereas, when I've got an interpreter, I am driving the ship, I decide when the patient talks and how much they talk and often it's not a lot. I think the patient's centeredness, obviously, then suffers and the relationship suffers because I love to hear people's stories about whatever's going on, and I'm not benefiting from that either. I think it affects it profoundly. Diabetes is the window into all health and health communication. (Participant #8)

Clinicians also observed that low-income LEP patients tend to have a "respectful and deferential" attitude that leads them to expect instructions from clinicians rather than to take personal initiative. In the words of another participant:

> Patients are so respectful and deferential. It's not good, they should be like I want this or I want that, but unfortunately it doesn't happen a ton with ... again this is a generalization, but [I see it in] LEP Latino patients. (Participant #13)

Finally, a few participants lamented their own limited language skills and expressed a desire to speak at least one additional language so as to be able to better serve underserved populations. In sum, limitations inherent in themselves, their patients, or the doctor–patient relationship given the nature of the language-discordant clinical encounter were multiple, and participants generally believed that these *could not but impair* both the quality of the care delivered and clinical outcomes.

"No level playing field with respect to time": The level of health care establishments.

Clinicians were also keen to share their experience of barriers at the level of their own hospital establishment, barriers that impaired their ability to provide good care to their patients. These included the fact that interpreters are not always available, especially after clinical hours and often when they are most needed, that many interpreters are poorly trained, that the equipment often malfunctions and takes away precious time, and that even when interpreter services are in place and of good quality, the time of the consultation is effectively "cut in half." In the words of two participants:

> Being able to speak the language doubles your appointment length. By using a translator, basically your time with the patient is cut in half, the ability to ask the number of questions you can ask, the number of things you can explain, because it takes twice the amount of time because everything is being translated to use the interpreter. (Participant #4)

> What I'd like to know, actually I'd really like to know, does it take 1.5 times the amount of time? Does it take two times the amount of time or 2.5 or three. I don't really know what the factor, the ... What is the exponential factor of time needed to actually communicate with

> the same level of quality, just from a technical linguistic standpoint? Leaving aside trust and leaving aside the other emotional aspects of it. If you wanted to ask these 10 questions related to diabetes self-care, how long would it take you to do that mediated through an interpreter, as opposed to not? (Participant #8)

Clinicians also identified language barriers in factors other than interpreter services. For instance, one clinician mentioned that medication labeling and instructions are often not available in the language spoken by patients, which significantly undermines the quality of the care that this participant felt able to deliver, as confirmed by the literature (Hsu et al., 2006). Clinicians were also aware of the complexity of securing access to care within the fragmented US healthcare system, identified as "insurance issues," (participant #6) which made it hard for patients to receive adequate and timely care that clinicians would otherwise be perfectly competent to provide.

"A higher socio-economic status would help": The social determination of health.

Importantly, clinicians were well aware of barriers at the societal level contributing to inequalities in diabetes outcomes. They discussed the multiple constraints faced by patients living in poverty to pursue the lifestyle changes and adhere to the complex treatment required by diabetes, and in one case wondered how class (articulated as "socioeconomic" status) might make a difference to diabetes care and outcomes, even in the presence of language barriers. As one participant, after being prompted by the investigator, pondered:

> Question: If you had an upper income or upper class patient who speaks Spanish only and not English?
>
> Answer: Sure. I can think of cases like that. They generally have ... those patients, let's say it's someone who, for example, someone who had just moved here from a South American country and was wealthy, but had no American insurance. They're just odd-speaking, that person would have a better understanding of their healthcare because they are probably more educated ... or their health problem, because they are more educated with a better understanding of where to go to get the things that they needed, especially ancillary services, may have a better understanding of things like dietary changes. (Participant #9)

In certain cases issues of class were construed as "culture," with one participant suggesting that sharing the culture of patients helped this participant understand their plight. As they put it, in the context of a discussion on social barriers to diabetes care:

> I'm from XX and I have a lot of African–American patients from XX...I can enter a sort of zone where I so get those patient's and I even start talking like someone from XX and they do too. They mimic that back to me. I can sort of intuit what's going on in their heads (sic) so much better because I understand where they are coming from. It's not a matter of me being from XX or not, it's me understanding the sort of cultural background. Those problems happen regardless of language; it's culture, right? [...] You change your manner of speaking. It's much more intimate than I usually use. [...] I mean this might sound like blah, but I can feel it when we are there, when we really are sort of seeing eye-to-eye. [...] I don't

> get that with Spanish speaking patients and I don't know if it's because I have a much more difficult time channeling that cultural background […] or if it's the language. (Participant #5)

This participant was clearly tapping into how language construes class broadly understood, a well-studied topic in the sociological literature (Bourdieu, 1991).

Other acknowledged socioeconomic constraints mentioned by participants included lack of adequate transportation to reach healthcare services, inability to take time from a precarious job to keep a medical appointment, and significant financial hardship in securing a proper diet. Participants also pointed out that their LEP Latino patients seemed overall poorer than their English-speaking counterparts, and that the cultural divide with them felt harder to bridge.

"I need to learn 10 new languages": Social change and the limits of medical discourse.

Finally, when prompted for what changes they could imagine – no material limits imposed – that could improve their patients' diabetes outcomes and overall health, participants had a range of wishes (this was a probe used by investigators): they relayed their desire to have better language skills – as one participant put it, "learn 10 new languages" – in addition to counting on greater number of resources in the language of their patients – from health staff, to educational brochures, to workshops that could train willing family members as interpreters. They also reiterated their desire to have longer scheduled appointments and to visit some patients in their homes, both features – longer appointments and home visits – identified in the literature as strengthening clinical practice (Dugdale, Epstein, & Pantilat, 1999; Kao, Conant, Soriano, & McCormick)

However, and as mentioned earlier, virtually no participant ventured beyond the middle level of the medical establishment or, at most, of patients' health insurance status. Only one participant wondered how different the patient situation might be if their socioeconomic status were higher – and only after being prompted.

DISCUSSION

In this study of how clinicians experience language-discordant care in the context of broader structural barriers to care, we found an overlap between the experience of clinicians and patients (in our former study) in that both valued language concordance because it allowed them to communicate their feelings better, and both tended to identify barriers to diabetes outcomes as embedded either in the dynamics of the language-discordant clinical encounter or in features intrinsic to participants – in the case of patients, their ability or lack thereof to follow the recommendations of their clinician, and in the case of clinicians, their limited foreign language proficiency. Clinician participants were also able to identify and articulate the need for change at the mezzo-level of institutions – the medical establishment and the coverage of services.

It was clear to authors that participants were eager to deliver good care, cared about the quality of the clinical encounter, and seemed clinically very competent (the first and last authors are physicians with experience in diabetes care). We also found that clinicians often went above the call of duty, for instance, by staying after hours to improve the quality of the care they provide. Further, clinicians seemed mindful of structural barriers, aware of the cumbersome nature of US healthcare system – which they construed as "insurance problems" – and sympathetic to how the significant poverty of their patients often impairs their ability to meet the demands of the treatment of diabetes. That said, we identified gaps, issues that are "lost in translation," *beyond* the loss of ability to "be oneself" experienced by participants in a language-discordant clinical encounter.

First, clinicians in our study believed that a "good patient" is one who is engaged, takes responsibility for their own care, and isn't "too respectful and deferential". In contrast, patients in our study believed that a "good patient" is he or she who follows clinicians' instructions. Indeed, they thought of a "good clinician" as one who is solidly medically trained and tells them "what to do," including "what changes to make" in their health behaviors. They were reluctant to decide on their own, and didn't unless they believed that the instructions were inappropriate or misguided from a medical point of view. The mismatch may lead to misunderstandings that ultimately impair the development of a trusting relationship, if clinicians fail to grasp what counts as "a good doctor" or "a good patient" *for the patient*. Cultural and class differences, when clinicians are typically members of the dominant culture and class, as in our study, are bound to exist in language-discordant clinical encounters. Mindfulness about these issues would go a long way in enabling patients to trust, an issue considered very important by clinicians in our sample, as in the medical literature more generally (Pearson & Raeke, 2000).

At the level of the health system, clinicians may be more concerned than patients about the availability of professionally trained interpreters, although perspectives vary both within patients and clinicians. Generally, it appears that, if patients feel comfortable, they prefer to "muddle through" a conversation across the language divide in order to avoid the presence of a third party, with whom they often have reservations given the importance they attribute to medical training. In other words, patients may share certain private information with clinicians precisely because they have respect and deference to clinicians' medical training, which interpreters in principle lack (Chaufan et al., 2015).

When prompted to state what changes they could imagine – no material limits imposed – that could improve their patients' diabetes outcomes and overall health, participants seemed unable to articulate changes beyond the level of medical establishments: not a single one noted that "insurance problems" are directly related to the fact that the US healthcare system is organized on the basis of commercial insurance, which dumps "special populations" (e.g., elderly, disabled, poor, veterans, aboriginals) on the state, even as the state outsources its obligation *back onto commercial insurers* (e.g., Medicare "Advantage" plans, commercial, HMO plans for Medicaid patients) (Chaufan, 2015). Eligibility for these plans is extremely constrained (e.g., proving "poverty" or another kind of need is increasingly cumbersome) and even in the best case scenario much of the financial burden is placed on the shoulder of patients (often construed as "customers"). The situation is unique among wealthy nations and imposes increasing barriers to care (Davis, Stremikis, Schoen, & Squires, 2014), undermining health equity.

Moreover, not a single participant *spontaneously* proposed that maybe if something were done at the systemic level to decrease poverty and inequality, the health condition of many LEP patients with diabetes and comorbidities might improve. Only one participant speculated – and only after prompted by the interviewer – that if their patients were better off, that is, had "higher socioeconomic status," they would likely experience fewer barriers to quality diabetes care whatever their English proficiency.

Our study has limitations, many of them shared with qualitative studies as extensively discussed elsewhere, including in our own work (Barbour, 2001; Chaufan et al., 2011, 2015; Patton, 1999). From our point of view, one important limitation was that our data collection time was limited – we spent at most 50 minutes with each participant, we could not explore their views over time, we could not observe actual interactions between participants in both studies, nor were we able to solicit or receive feedback from participants themselves, all strategies that would have strengthened our analysis and conclusions (Patton, 1999).

That being said, we now move on to elaborate on why we conclude that, despite the fact that participants in our study were well schooled in the social determination of health, they appeared unable to imagine "utopias," locate language barriers within patients' broader social disadvantage, and articulate alternatives from *without* the clinical encounter or establishment that could significantly improve clinical outcomes independently of them, that is, to generalize the case of that "wealthy patient from South America," imagined as doing significantly better regardless of English proficiency.

Following Howard Waitzkin (1989), we argue that the language of medicine itself has a built-in incapacity to allow "social issues" to operate other than as *contexts*, rather than *causes*, which may have limited the ability of participants to articulate ideas that may have lurked in their minds. As a result of this, and much like patient participants in our earlier study, clinician participants in the study failed to see, in the words of C. Wright Mills, the connection between "private troubles" and "public issues" (Wright Mills, 1959), which in turn made it harder for them to conceptualize language barriers as one element in the broader context of the social determination of their patients' health. Such conceptualization may have allowed participants to realize that better care and outcomes among LEP Latino patients with diabetes may require more than greater competencies on the part of participants (e.g., better language skills on their part or a more proactive attitude on the part of patients), or better interpreter services (already top-level in our research site) and necessitate changes at a macro level, such as a major re-examination of power in society toward greater social equality and less poverty at best, or a major overhaul of a dysfunctional healthcare system toward more equitable access at the very least.

Waitzkin also argues – and we agree – that it is generally accepted that the role of clinicians is limited to offering medical, or at most, behavioral, advice, so when structural inequalities are "diagnosed," such as precarious employment preventing patients to show up at a medical visit or follow a proper diet, they are not acknowledged as a legitimate site of medical intervention. This is because the very nature of medical discourse renders social change "unthinkable" – it simply does not fall under the jurisdiction of clinicians, even when such change is transparently what would lead to better health (Waitzkin, 1989). But as indicated by recent debates in the "trenches" of primary care, limiting the role of clinicians to that of a medical/behavioral advisor, especially in the face of increasing social inequality, may no longer be necessary or desirable: as noted by Deputy Commissioner of the New York City Department of Health, Dr. Aletha Maybank, "fighting for social and health justice is not what I went to medical school for, but it has now become the driving force behind my work." (Maybank, 2017).

PRACTICE AND POLICY IMPLICATIONS AND RECOMMENDATIONS

At the more immediate level, we conclude that, first, linguistic training matters. There is a need for more clinicians with solid language skills to communicate with an increasingly linguistically diverse population in the United States, if for no other reason than both patients and clinicians feel more comfortable, and, as evidence shows, language concordance in itself is conducive to better health outcomes (Fernandez et al., 2011). Second, if clinicians are not fluent in the language of their patients, professional, high-quality interpreter services become critical (Karliner, Jacobs, Chen, & Mutha, 2007). However, it is also critical that other services be accessible to enhance the quality of the care of LEP patients. The lack of informational material and bilingual staff cannot fail to impair the comfort, if not the outcomes, of patients, especially as they face the challenge of overly complex healthcare services. Third, an increasing complex and fragmented system of insurance – that remains at best a patchwork of plans, private and public, or public yet outsourced to commercial vendors, even after major health reform – adds insult to injury to the healthcare experience of low-income LEP patients. Health equity cannot be achieved without substantial structural change at that level.

At the level of longer-lasting social change, training of health professionals in the political and social determination of health matters. Its implications on diabetes status, outcomes, and inequalities, as well as on health inequities more broadly, is hardly any longer a matter of debate (Chaufan et al., 2011; Raphael, 2006, 2015) but rather of public policy and political will, and a topic of increasing popularity in clinical training and practice (Klein et al., 2010; Naz, Rosenberg, Andersson, Labonté, & Andermann, 2016). However, the question remains, what type of training would truly transform medical practice? Indeed, participants in the study seemed sensitive to, and well trained in, the social determination of health in general, and as it pertains to diabetes in particular. However, we identified a gap between their knowledge and their ability to relate those "public issues" with the "private troubles" of their patients, which interfered with their ability to engage in social change that could truly improve the conditions of their patients.

Therefore, even when prompted to simply imagine changes at any level that could better their patients' health and overall well-being, they seemed unable to articulate changes beyond the level of medical establishments – they did not even tread into the territory of the notoriously inequitable US medical system (Davis et al., 2014). In so doing, clinicians inadvertently naturalized the very structures that prevent their patients from achieving the best health that the hard and conscientious work of clinicians can contribute to.

We conclude that emphasis on structural barriers to diabetes care during and beyond medical education may prepare clinicians to affect change in the lives of individual patients. However, we also propose that real engagement with social change will require that clinicians, especially those treating disorders requiring substantial patient engagement such as diabetes, reconceptualize medicine as a social science that, not only as more recent debates indicate, but also as proposed by Rudolph Virchow over 150 years ago, should "point out problems and attempt their theoretical solutions" beyond the boundaries of the profession. In so doing, clinicians may be able to partner with the "politician and practical anthropologist," as citizens, in transforming power relations toward greater equity and better health.

ACKNOWLEDGMENTS

The authors thank the patients, medical personnel, and staff who kindly volunteered their time and expertise to our project. The first author also thanks her students whose questions and concerns are a continuing source of inspiration. Funding was provided by 3R01DK090272-02S1 and K24DK102057 from the National Institute of Diabetes and Digestive and Kidney Diseases (NIDDK).

REFERENCES

Anderson, R. (1998). How do we know? Reflections on qualitative research in diabetes. *Diabetes Care*, *21*(9), 1387–1388.

Aronson, J. (1995). A pragmatic view of thematic analysis. *The Qualitative Report*, *2*(1). Retrieved from http://nsuworks.nova.edu/cgi/viewcontent.cgi?article=2069&context=tqr. Accessed on March 2012.

Barbour, R. S. (1998). Mixing qualitative methods: Quality assurance or qualitative quagmire? *Qualitative Health Research*, *8*(3), 352–361.

Barbour, R. S. (2001). Checklists for improving rigour in qualitative research: A case of the tail wagging the dog? *BMJ*, *322*(7294), 1115–1117.

Berg, B. L. (2004). *Qualitative research methods for the social sciences*. New York, NY: Pearson.

Bourdieu, P. (1991). *Language and symbolic power*. Cambridge: Polity Press.

Breilh, J. (2015). La determinación social de la salud como herramienta de transformación hacia una nueva salud pública (salud colectiva). *Revistas Facultad Nacional Salud Pública*, *31*(suppl. 1), 14–27.

Centers for Disease Control and Prevention. (2011). *CDC Health Disparities and Inequalities Report*. Retrieved from http://www.cdc.gov/mmwr/pdf/other/su6001.pdf. Accessed on December 14, 2013.

Charmaz, K. (1990). 'Discovering' chronic illness: Using grounded theory. *Social Science & Medicine*, *30*(11), 1161–1172.

Chaufan, C. (2015). Why do Americans still need single-payer health care after major health reform? *International Journal of Health Services*, *45*(1), 149–160.

Chaufan, C., Davis, M., & Constantino, S. (2011). The twin epidemics of poverty and diabetes: Understanding diabetes disparities in a low-income Latino and immigrant neighborhood. *Journal of community Health*, *36*, 1032–1043.

Chaufan, C., Fielding, H., Chesla, C. A., & Fernandez, A. (2015). "It's not the doctor – it's me": How self blame obscures language and other structural barriers to diabetes care among low-income Latinos with limited English proficiency. *Research in the Sociology of Health Care*, *33*, 187–208.

Chesla, C. A. (1995). Hermeneutic phenomenology: An approach to understanding families. *Journal of Family Nursing*, *1*(1), 63–78.

Davis, K., Stremikis, K., Schoen, D., & Squires, K. (2014). *Mirror, mirror on the wall: How the U.S. health care system compares internationally – 2014 An update*. New York, NY: The Commonwealth Fund. Retrieved from http://www.commonwealthfund.org/~/media/files/publications/fundreport/2014/jun/1755_davis_mirror_mirror_2014.pdf. Accessed on June 19, 2014.

Diamond, L., & Reuland, D. (2009). Describing physician language fluency: Deconstructing medical Spanish. *JAMA*, *301*(4), 426–428.

Diamond, L., Sukyung, C., Ferguson, W., Gonzalez, J., Jacobs, E. A., & Gany, F. (2014). Relationship between Self-assessed and tested non-English language proficiency among primary care providers. *Medical Care*, *52*(5), 435–438.

Dinca Panaitescu, S., Dinca Panaitescu, M., Bryant, T., Daiski, I., Pilkington, B., & Raphael, D. (2011). Diabetes prevalence and income: Results of the Canadian community health survey. *Health Policy*, *99*(2), 116–123.

Dugdale, D. C., Epstein, R., & Pantilat, S. Z. (1999). Time and the patient–physician relationship. *Journal of General Internal Medicine*, *14*(suppl. 1), S34–S40.

Fernandez, A., Schillinger, D., Grumbach, K., Rosenthal, A., Stewart, A., Wang, F., & Pérez-Stable, E. (2004). Physician language ability and cultural competence. *Journal of General Internal Medicine*, *19*(2), 167–174.

Fernandez, A., Schillinger, D., Warton, E. M., Adler, N., Moffet, H. H., Schenker, Y., ... Karter, A. J. (2011). Language barriers, physician-patient language concordance, and glycemic control among insured Latinos with diabetes: The Diabetes Study of Northern California (DISTANCE). *Journal of General Internal Medicine*, *26*(2), 170–176.

Flores, G., Abreu, M., Olivar, M., & Kastner, B. (1998). Access barriers to health care for Latino children. *Archives of Pediatrics & Adolescent Medicine*, *152*(11), 1119–1125.

Harlan, L., Bernstein, A., & Kessler, L. (1991). Cervical cancer screening: Who is not screened and why? *American Journal of Public Health*, *81*(7), 885–890.

Hornerberger, J. C., Gibson, C. D. J., Wood, W., Dequeldre, C., Corso, I., Palla, B., & Bloch, D. A. (1996). Eliminating language barriers for non-English-speaking patients. *Medical Care*, *34*(8), 845–856.

Hsu, W. C., Cheung, S., Ong, E., Wong, K., Lin, S., Leon, K., ... King, G. L. (2006). Identification of linguistic barriers to diabetes knowledge and glycemic control in Chinese Americans with diabetes. *Diabetes Care*, *29*(2), 415.

Institute of Medicine. (2002). *Unequal treatment: What healthcare providers need to know about racial and ethnic disparities in health care*. Retrieved from https://www.nap.edu/read/10260/chapter/10261. Accessed October 13, 2013.

Kao, H., Conant, R., Soriano, T., & McCormick, W. The past, present, and future of house calls. *Clinics in Geriatric Medicine*, *25*(1), 19–34.

Karliner, L. S., Jacobs, E. A., Chen, A. H., & Mutha, S. (2007). Do professional interpreters improve clinical care for patients with limited English proficiency? A systematic review of the literature. *Health Services Research*, *42*(2), 727–754.

Klein, M. D., Kahn, R. S., Baker, R. C., Fink, E. E., Parrish, D. S., & White, D. C. (2010). Training in social determinants of health in primary care: Does it change resident behavior? *Academic Pediatrics*, *11*(5), 387–393.

Link, B., & Phelan, J. (1995). Social conditions as fundamental causes of disease. *Journal of Health and Social Behavior*, *35*, 80–94.

Mackenbach, J. P. (2009). Politics is nothing but medicine at a larger scale: Reflections on public health's biggest idea. *Journal of Epidemiology and Community Health*, *63*(3), 181–184.

Maybank, A. (2017). Moving beyond the hospital walls: Health activism in 2017. *Huffington Post, January 5*. Retrieved from http://www.huffingtonpost.com/aletha-maybank-md-mph/moving-beyond-the-hospita_b_13960130.html.

Naz, A., Rosenberg, E., Andersson, N., Labonté, R., & Andermann, A. (2016). Health workers who ask about social determinants of health are more likely to report helping patients: Mixed-methods study. *Canadian Family Physician*, *62*(11), e684–e693.

Patton, M. (1999). Enhancing the quality and credibility of qualitative analysis. *Health Services Research*, *34*(5 Pt 2), 1189–1208.

Pearson, S. D., & Raeke, L. H. (2000). Patients' trust in physicians: Many theories, few measures, and little data. *Journal of General Internal Medicine*, *15*(7), 509–513.

Pearson, W. S., Zhao, G., & Ford, E. S. (2011). An analysis of language as a barrier to receiving influenza vaccinations among an elderly Hispanic population in the United States. *Advances in Preventive Medicine*, *2011*, 6, 2011. doi:10.4061/2011/298787

Peek, M. E., Cargill, A., & Huang, E. S. (2007). Diabetes health disparities: A systematic review of health care interventions. *Medical Care Research and Review*, *64*(5 suppl.), 101S–156S.

Raphael, D. (2006). social determinants of health: Present status, and answer questions, and future directions. *International Journal of Health Services*, *26*(4), 651–677.

Raphael, D. (2015). The political economy of health: A research agenda for addressing health inequalities in Canada. *Canadian Public Policy*, *41*(suppl. 2), S17–S25.

Raphael, D., Daiski, I., Pilkington, B., Bryant, T., Dinca-Panaitescu, M., & Dinca-Panaitescu, S. (2011). A toxic combination of poor social policies and programmes, unfair economic arrangements and bad politics: The experiences of poor Canadians with Type 2 diabetes. *Critical Public Health*, *22*(2), 127–145.

Ross, J. S., Bradley, E. H., & Busch, S. H. (2006). Use of health care services by lower-income and higher-income uninsured adults. *JAMA*, *295*(17), 2027–2036.

Ryan, C. (2011). Language use in the United States: 2011. American community surveys report. Retrieved from http://www.census.gov/prod/2013pubs/acs-2022.pdf

Schenker, Y., Wang, F., Selig, S., Ng, R., & Fernandez, A. (2007). The impact of language barriers on documentation of informed consent at a hospital with on-site interpreter services. *Journal of General Internal Medicine*, *22*(2), 294–299.

Stern, R. J., Fernandez, A., Jacobs, E. A., Neilands, T. B., Weech-Maldonado, R., Quan, J., … Seligman, H. K. (2012). Advances in measuring culturally competent care: A confirmatory factor analysis of CAHPS-CC in a safety-net population. *Medical Care*, *50*, S49–S55.

Timmins, C. L. (2002). The impact of language barriers on the health care of Latinos in the United States: A review of the literature and guidelines for practice. *The Journal of Midwifery & Womens Health*, *47*(2), 80–96.

Waitzkin, H. (1989). A critical theory of medical discourse: Ideology, social control, and the processing of social context in medical encounters. *Journal of Health and Social Behavior*, *30*(2), 220–239.

Wilson, E., Chen, A. H., Grumbach, K., Wang, F., & Fernandez, A. (2005). Effects of limited English proficiency and physician language on health care comprehension. *Journal of General Internal Medicine*, *20*(9), 800–806.

Wright Mills, C. (1959). *The sociological imagination*. London: Oxford University Press.

Zong, J., & Batalova, J. (2015). *The Limited English proficient population in the United States*. Migration Policy Institute. July 8. Retrieved from http://www.migrationpolicy.org/article/limited-english-proficient-populationunited-states. Accessed December 26, 2016.

RACIAL RESIDENTIAL SEGREGATION AND THE DISTRIBUTION OF AUXILIARY HEALTH CARE PRACTITIONERS ACROSS URBAN SPACE

Kathryn Freeman Anderson

ABSTRACT

Scholarship has demonstrated important consequences of segregation on health and health care outcomes, yet the mechanisms behind this association remain poorly understood. Several recent studies have shown inequities in the distribution of a wide variety of health-related organizations across urban neighborhoods, which may account for some portion of this negative health association. Though, within this literature, relatively little attention has been given to the distribution of health care facilities in particular.

Here, I consider how segregation is related to the distribution of several auxiliary health care practitioners in a series of spatial regression models of zip codes across the United States using data from the 2010 US Census and County Business Patterns (CBP).

I find that both Black and Latino segregation is negatively related to the density of a number of auxiliary health care practitioners, including mental health providers, dentists, physical/occupational/speech therapists, chiropractors, optometrists, podiatrists, and miscellaneous health care practitioners.

Health and Health Care Concerns among Women and Racial and Ethnic Minorities
Research in the Sociology of Health Care, Volume 35, 145–167

ISSN: 0275-4959/doi:10.1108/S0275-495920170000035008

However, this association is reduced (in certain instances to non-significance) with the inclusion of socioeconomic indicators, chiefly the percent of college educated individuals and the unemployment rate of the zip code. This is association is reduced for both Black and Latino segregation, with a larger reduction in the size of the effects for Latino segregation.

This research suggests that segregation plays an important role in the distribution of health care facilities, but that policy and public health interventions should focus on the intersection between racial residential segregation and socioeconomic considerations.

Keywords: Residential segregation; health care; urban sociology; race/ethnicity

INTRODUCTION

Research demonstrates that racial/ethnic minority communities experience a wide variety of poor physical health and mortality outcomes. For instance, both Black and Latino segregation has been linked to higher mortality rates, infant health outcomes, poor self-rated health, and nutrition and obesity (Anderson & Fullerton, 2014; Collins & Williams, 1999; Ellen, Cutler, & Dickens, 2000; Polednak, 1997; Subramanian, Acevedo-Garcia, & Osypuk, 2005; Williams & Collins, 2001). However, within this work, the mechanisms which could produce such an association have seldom been theoretically explored or empirically tested (White, Haas, & Williams, 2012; Williams & Collins, 2001). In this study, I examine one possible mechanism – the distribution of health care services – and examine how racial residential segregation may be related to the density of such establishments across urban neighborhoods. Specifically, I examine a wide variety of auxiliary health care practitioners, which may be considered to be "optional" services and are often not covered by traditional health care insurance programs. Such establishments include mental health practitioners, dentist's offices, physical/occupational/speech therapists, chiropractors, optometrists, podiatrists, and miscellaneous health services (which include a large of number of alternative and homeopathic health practitioners). These types of organizations can play a vital role in overall health and well-being, as well as be related to functional ability and the management of health symptoms and chronic conditions. Thus, an inequitable distribution of such resources may help us to understand important differences in health outcomes across such communities.

Though previous work has considered the distribution of other health-related and health care services, this is the first to consider these types of establishments (Anderson, 2017; Beaulac, Kristjansson, & Cummins, 2009;

Hayanga, Waljee, Kaiser, Chang, & Morris, 2009). Moreover, this study advances the extant literature on segregation and the distribution of health-related service providers by moving beyond the Black–White paradigm to consider how these patterns may play out for other racial/ethnic minority groups in the United States. Specifically, I address two major research questions. First, what is the relationship between racial/ethnic residential segregation and the density of auxiliary health care providers? Essentially, do racial/ethnic minority segregated communities have fewer of such establishments compared to their White or more integrated counterparts? And, second, what other area-level social and demographic factors can help account for this association? I will address these questions in a study of auxiliary health care practitioners across the United States using a series of spatial regression models. First, I review the extant literature on the topic and discuss the theoretical frameworks which could help us to understand why such an association may exist.

LITERATURE REVIEW AND THEORETICAL FRAMEWORK

Segregation and Health-Related Organizations

Recent work, largely in the area of public health, has seen an explosion of interest in the distribution of certain health-related resources across urban space and how this may differ by a variety of urban social conditions. This is particularly notable in the so-called food deserts literature, which examines the distribution of food resources across urban neighborhoods, such as grocery stores and restaurants (Beaulac et al., 2009; Walker, Keane, & Burke, 2010). Though this literature of course finds some particular nuances and caveats to the issues, on the whole, this literature demonstrates that poor and minority communities are less likely to have a variety of such resources, and that where present, are lower in quality when compared their predominately White and affluent counterparts (Algert, Agrawal, & Lewis, 2006; Alwitt & Donley, 1997; Bower, Thorpe Jr, Rohde, & Gaskin, 2014; Horowitz, Colson, Hebert, & Lancaster, 2004; Moore & Diez Roux, 2006; Morland, Wing, Roux, & Poole, 2002; Powell, Slater, Mirtcheva, Bao, & Chaloupka, 2007; Schuetz, Kolko, & Meltzer, 2012; Smiley et al., 2010). In a related set of studies, some work also shows a similar disparity in the distribution of physical recreation sites, with poor and minority communities again being less likely to have an adequate number of such resources (Estabrooks, Lee, & Gyurcsik, 2003; Moore, Roux, Evenson, McGinn, & Brines, 2008; Popkin, Duffey, & Gordon-Larsen, 2005; Wilson, Kirtland, Ainsworth, & Addy, 2004).

Additionally, moving beyond those resources which have a more proximate relationship to health outcomes, sociological research demonstrates important inequalities in the distribution of a number of other community establishments which may be related to health more distally. For example, such establishments include retail, non-profit social services, employment opportunities, civic associations, religious organizations, and mental health and substance abuse centers (Allard, 2009; Allard, Rosen, & Tolman, 2003; Allard, Tolman, & Rosen, 2003; Anderson, 2017; Galaskiewicz, Mayorova, & Duckles, 2013; Kissane, 2010; Marwell & Gullickson, 2013; Sampson, 2012; Small & McDermott, 2006; Small & Stark, 2005; Small, 2009). Though most of these studies have not addressed the community health component directly, they inform the present study and show important disparities across segregated communities and other facets of urban social disadvantage.

Furthermore, other work demonstrates that the lack of such facilities has consequences for the residents of those areas. For instance, research has linked food and recreational deserts to a number of issues related to diet quality, recreational activity, and health outcomes. Specifically, such studies have demonstrated that the distribution of food stores and supermarkets is related to personal food choices, such as fruit and vegetable consumption, and how these choices may be related to overall diet quality (Blitstein, Snider, & Evans, 2012; Jetter & Cassady, 2006; Laraia, Siega-Riz, Kaufman, & Jones, 2004; Morland et al., 2002). Similarly, other studies have shown that these constrained diet choices are related to greater BMI and rates of obese in those communities with limited food options (Bader et al., 2013; Gibson, 2011; Inagami, Cohen, Finch, & Asch, 2006; Morland, Diez Roux, & Wing, 2006; Ohri-Vachaspati et al., 2013; Zick et al., 2009). With regard to physical recreation, several studies have shown that the lack of physical recreation sites in a community is related to lower rates of physical activity and greater BMI (Black, Macinko, Dixon, & Fryer, 2010; Gordon-Larsen, Nelson, Page, & Popkin, 2006). Though these findings are somewhat preliminary and more work should be done on the consequences of the inequitable distribution of resources, these studies provide some evidence that understanding the distribution of such resources is important for scholarship on area or neighborhood based health inequalities.

Limitations of the Empirical Literature

Despite this recent attention to the distribution of health-related organizations across neighborhoods, there has been relative inattention to the case of health care facilities in particular (for a few exceptions see Anderson (2017) and Hayanga, Kaiser et al. (2009)). Some extant work has examined segregation within the health care system itself, both in terms of access to and utilization of facilities, as well as racial segregation and discrimination in the delivery of health care to certain communities (Smedley & Stith, 2003; Smith, Feng, Fennell, Zinn, & Mor, 2007; White et al., 2012). In a related study, Black and

Latino residents of areas with a high percentage of racial minorities were less likely to perceive barriers to obtaining the necessary health care (Haas et al., 2004). However, in general, this literature has not examined the spatial dynamics of how segregation is related to the locational decision making of health care facilities and how residents of segregated communities access and utilize health care resources. Only a limited number of studies have directly examined racial residential segregation and the distribution of health care related facilities (Anderson, 2017; Hayanga, Kaiser et al., 2009; Hayanga, Waljee et al., 2009). For example, in two studies on the topic, Hayanga and colleagues found disparities in the distribution of a number of surgical facilities and practitioners at the county level for Black segregation (Hayanga, Kaiser et al., 2009; Hayanga, Waljee et al., 2009). Relatedly, Anderson (2017) found that both Black and Latino segregation at the zip code level are related to a decrease in the number of generalist physicians, hospitals, and outpatient facilities, though much of this association was accounted for by several socioeconomic factors. It is clear that more work on this topic is needed, especially to examine a greater variety of health care facilities. In this study, I examine seven different types of auxiliary health care practitioners, including non-physician mental health professionals, dentists, chiropractors, physical/occupational/speech therapists, optometrists, podiatrists, and miscellaneous health providers. As these types of resources may be considered "elective" and are often not covered by traditional insurance plans, we may be more likely to observe a disparity in the distribution of such establishments by racial residential segregation.

Furthermore, in much of this literature, there is relatively less attention placed on the conceptualization/measurement of key social variables, especially racial residential segregation. Most of these studies measure segregation through ethnic density scores, which essentially reflect the proportion of a certain group over a defined area (zip code, county, etc.) However, segregation has multiple dimensions and implies not just the concentration of a group, but also the extent to which that group may be clustered across geographical space (Massey & Denton, 1988, 1989). Relatedly, ethnic density scores, especially when used in a nation-wide analysis, fail to capture important metropolitan or regional variations in the relative numbers of such groups. For example, in the US-Mexico border region, the percentage of Latinos in any given area is higher, and the use of ethnic density scores would then simply become an analysis of the border region versus the rest of the United States rather than capturing patterns of segregation within a metropolitan area or region, which is what segregation is typically understood to mean.

Additionally, much of the thinking, theorizing, and empirical analysis of these issues is highly focused on the Black case and on how Black–White segregation may produce such an association. It is unclear from much of this literature how or why we might observe this association for other minority groups in the United States and what the implications of such an association might be for those residents. As Latinos are now the largest racial/ethnic minority group in the United States, and a group which is becoming increasingly more segregated over time, this is an important oversight (Fischer, Stockmayer, Stiles, & Hout, 2004; Iceland, 2004). As such, this study considers the segregation of the three largest racial/ethnic minority groups: Blacks, Latinos, and Asians. A discussion of the theoretical implications of segregation for these groups follows here.

Theories of Segregation and Urban Outcomes

While the theoretical literature on segregation and the distribution of organizations specifically is quite scant, we can turn to broader theories of segregation from urban sociology in an attempt to shed light on these associations. In general, the theoretical perspectives on segregation and its consequences fall into two main theoretical camps. The first of these camps is the place stratification perspective which emphasizes the role of racism and discrimination in perpetuating segregation and any negative effects it might have for the community (Charles, 2003; Logan, 1978; Massey & Denton, 1993). In essence, the argument is that segregation acts as a comprehensive system of stratification which is driven by discriminatory processes (Massey & Denton, 1993). As such, these areas have lower quality housing, goods and services, and community support, which is not driven principally or exclusively by the socioeconomic conditions of such neighborhoods (Krivo, Peterson, Rizzo, & Reynolds, 1998; Massey & Denton, 1993; Massey, Gross, & Shibuya, 1994). As it relates to organizations more specifically, from this perspective, we would expect such areas to have fewer organizational resources due to the same racially discriminatory processes which produce segregation (Massey & Denton, 1993; Small & McDermott, 2006). For example, service providers may avoid such areas because of the racialized expectations about predominantly minority areas, or related phenomena, such as the concentration of crime and social problems which follows the condition of segregation, concentrated poverty, and social isolation.

Most of the theorizing from the place stratification perspective is focused on the case of Black segregation, and it is often unclear as to whether or not these ideas can be readily applied to other racial/ethnic minority groups (Charles, 2003). However, key to this thinking is the marginalization of a group in social and physical space. Scholarship on other groups, Latinos in particular, demonstrates the increasing racialization of the group, as well as their social marginalization (Alba, Logan, & Stults, 2000; Brown, 2007; Massey, 2009; Ortiz & Telles, 2012). Moreover, research demonstrates that Latinos and Asians have become increasingly more segregated over time in the United States with the growth of these populations, though their rates of segregation remain considerably less than that of Black Americans (Alba, Denton, Leung, & Logan, 1995; Fischer et al., 2004; Iceland, 2004). It remains to be fully explored whether or not the place stratification perspective can be readily applied to the case of other groups, which is one of the aims of the analysis here. From this perspective, we can derive the following hypothesis about the relationship between residential segregation and the distribution of auxiliary health care practitioners:

> **H1:** As the segregation of racial/ethnic minorities across urban areas increases, the density of auxiliary health care practitioners will decrease, regardless of the socioeconomic conditions in such areas.

However, the other main theoretical camp on segregation is the spatial assimilation perspective, which conversely emphasizes the role of socioeconomic factors in residential segregation (Charles, 2003). From this perspective, such thinkers argue that it is not the minority status per se of such communities which is driving segregation, but rather the fact that racial/ethnic minorities tend to be of lower socioeconomic status which is driving their spatial clustering (Logan, Alba, & Zhang, 2002). Thus, these processes are not driven by racial discrimination and social exclusion, but by the financial inability of such groups to be able to live in closer proximity to predominantly White areas. As such groups achieve socioeconomic parity with Whites, we then should observe lower rates of racial residential segregation. Some work, particularly on the case of Latinos and Asians, supports this notion (Iceland & Scopilliti, 2008; Massey & Fischer, 1999; Waters & Jimenez, 2005). As it relates to the distribution of organizations specifically, though, we might expect that such communities lack adequate health care facilities because there is not a market for such services given the clustering of poverty and low socioeconomic status in such areas. From this perspective then, we would derive the following hypothesis:

> **H2:** As the segregation of racial/ethnic minorities across urban areas increases, its effect on the density of auxiliary health care practitioners will be null, after accounting for the socioeconomic standing of such communities.

A related perspective, the immigrant enclave perspective, emphasizes the role of immigration in these processes as well. Similar to the spatial assimilation camp, the immigrant enclave perspective argues that it is the immigrant status of such minority communities, particularly Latino and Asian communities, which keeps them isolated (Logan et al., 2002). However, with assimilation and socioeconomic attainment, such social isolation will dissipate. Further, as it relates to organizations, such communities may actually be more likely to have a greater density of organizations, as the immigrant enclave itself provides space and opportunity for within-community entrepreneurship (Aldrich & Waldinger, 1990; Logan et al., 2002; Portes & Bach, 1985). Essentially, the immigrant community itself provides a forum and a ready clientele for entrepreneurial endeavors, especially given the unique role and motivations of the immigrant community. From this perspective, we then get the following alternative hypothesis:

> **H3:** As the segregation of racial/ethnic minorities across urban areas increases, the density of auxiliary health care practitioners will also increase, especially when accounting for immigration.

In the analysis that follows, I test these hypotheses in a nation-wide examination of zip codes across the United States in order to test the association between racial residential segregation and the distribution of a variety of auxiliary health care practitioners. I also test this association for the three largest racial/ethnic minority groups in order to examine how this process may differ across groups, especially as they relate to the theoretical perspectives discussed above. First, I detail the methodological considerations here.

DATA AND METHODS

Data

In order to examine the distribution of auxiliary health care practitioners across urban space, I combine three main data sources, all of which come from the US Census and are measured at the zip code unit of analysis. These include the 2010 CBP, the 2010 full decennial Census, and the 2008–2012 American Community Survey (ACS). The CBP provides counts of business establishments from Internal Revenue Service (IRS) tax records and are organized by North American Industry Classification System (NAICS) codes, and these counts are used as the dependent variables across all analyses. The smallest geographical unit for which these counts are available is at the zip code level. I combine this source using the zip code identification code with these two other Census sources. I use the 2010 decennial Census for all basic demographic and population data, and the 2008–2012 ACS for socioeconomic indicators. The ACS is only available at a small geographical unit of analysis, like the zip code, when combined into 5 years in order to get a large enough sample size to be representative. As such, I use the 2008–2012 version of this survey in order to have 2010 as the midpoint year to pair with the other data sources.

I combine these three sources and use the zip code as the unit of analysis. However, not all zip codes are included. As this is an analysis of urban social dynamics, I exclude any zip code which does not belong to a metropolitan area according to the Office of Management and Budget (OMB) definitions. However, as the OMB definitions are by county and thus include many areas on the fringes of metropolitan areas, I also further exclude any zip code which does not have at least 200 residents so as to eliminate non-residential areas, and any zip code which does not have a population density of at least 0.15 persons per square kilometer. I also exclude Hawaii and Alaska as being non-contiguous portions of the United States as this has implications for spatial analysis. Using these three exclusion criteria, the final sample size of included zip codes is 8,644 (down from 33,120 in the full sample).

Dependent Variables

The dependent variables all come from the CBP data source and reflect the number of establishments in a zip code per 10,000 people. I went through the NAICS codebook to include any code for a health services-related organization which is not primarily a physician (MD or DO) practice, not generalist in nature, outpatient, non-residential, primarily based around health practitioners, and which provides health-related services directly to a patient. Using these exclusion/inclusion criteria, this leaves seven different types of auxiliary health care practitioners. These include: *mental health practitioners* (621330), *dentists* (621210), *physical, occupational and speech therapists, and audiologists* (621340), *chiropractors* (621310), *optometrists* (621320), *podiatrists* (621391), and *miscellaneous health practitioners* (621399). The miscellaneous category includes a wide variety of non-physician health practitioners, such as naturopaths, homeopaths, midwives, nurse's offices, respiratory therapists, dieticians, acupuncturists, and hypnotherapists to name a few examples.

Independent Variables

The main independent variables in this analysis are a set of variables measuring segregation at the zip code level of analysis. These are derived from measures of percent Black, percent Latino, and percent Asian, all of which come from the 2010 US Census and which reflect the three largest racial/ethnic minority groups in the United States. In order to capture both the concentration and clustering across space of such groups (as opposed to just density), I calculated a clustering measure for each of these groups which takes into account both the percent of that group in a zip code (concentration), as well as the extent to which that zip code is physically adjacent to other zip codes which also have high numbers of that group (clustering) (Anderson, 2017). The measure is specifically calculated using the following formula:

$$C_i = x_i \sum_{j=1,\, j \neq i}^{n} w_{ij} x_j$$

where x_i is the variable for feature i, x_j is the variable for feature j, and w_{ij} is the spatial weight between features i and j. Essentially, it is the product of the percent of the group in a zip code and average percent of the same group in adjacent zip codes (using a k-2 nearest neighbor spatial weight matrix). For a substantive interpretation of this variable, high values on this measure would indicate that a zip code has a high percentage of a group who reside within the zip code, and that same zip code is surrounded by zip codes which also have a high percentage of that group. Furthermore, I then group-mean centered the variable by the means for the metropolitan area, in order to contextualize the variable to the metropolitan area. Of note, this is not a macro-level measure of segregation, such as the popular indices of segregation or dissimilarity, which give an indication of the extent of segregation in a metropolitan area or region (Massey & Denton, 1988, 1989). Rather, this measure provides an indication of how to code for which areas within a particular context are segregated. In this study, I include three measures for the three largest racial/ethnic minority groups: *percent Black clustering*, *percent Latino (of any race) clustering*, and *percent Asian clustering*.

I also account for a number of other variables which could account for the effect of the clustering measure of the percent of racial/ethnic minorities in an area. First, I include a variable for the *percent foreign born* of any racial/ethnic group (or immigration). Next, I include a number of socioeconomic variables, including *percent in poverty* (below federal poverty line), *percent with a college degree or higher*, and *percent unemployed.* Finally, I include several demographic control variables, including *percent age 65 and above*, and *percent of vacant housing units*. I checked for multicollinearity using the variance inflation factor and it was not found to be a problem for the included independent variables. All independent variables are treated as continuous, and are group-mean centered around the means for the metropolitan area in order to account for the clustering by metropolitan areas, which is a technique used by Sampson and colleagues (Sampson, Morenoff, & Earls, 1999). Descriptive statistics for all variables used can be found in Table 1.

METHODS

For the analysis, I estimate a series of spatial error models (SEM) which is a type of spatial regression model which accounts for spatial autocorrelation in the errors. One of the assumptions of regression is that the observations are independent of one another. However, as these units are geographical and spatially contiguous, these units likely influence each other in some way. In order to address this violation, the spatial error model includes a term (lambda), which measures the intensity of spatial dependence across the residuals (Anselin, Florax, & Rey, 2004). In particular, I estimate a series of SEM using a k-2 nearest neighbor spatial weight matrix, which was the spatial weight matrix which best maximized global Moran's I (a measure of spatial

Table 1. Descriptive Statistics for Variables Used in Statistical Models of Organizational Densities.

Variable Name	Mean	SD	Range	Description
Dependent Variables				
Mental Health Professionals	0.85	3.64	0 to 162.27	Mental health professionals per 10,000 people
Dentist's Offices	5.34	15.63	0 to 896.74	Dentist's offices per 10,000 people
Physical Therapists	1.23	2.25	0 to 96.15	Physical/occupational/speech therapists per 10,000 people
Chiropractors	1.44	3.78	0 to 221.67	Chiropractors per 10,000 people
Optometrists	0.78	2.10	0 to 91.46	Optometrists per 10,000 people
Podiatrists	0.38	1.40	0 to 81.52	Podiatrists per 10,000 people
Miscellaneous Health	0.58	2.18	0 to 135.87	Miscellaneous health practitioners per 10,000 people
Independent Variables				
% Black Clustering	442.08	1129.79	0 to 9082.58	Clustering measure of percent Black
% Latino Clustering	477.17	1159.11	0 to 9554.16	Clustering measure of percent Latino
% Asian Clustering	67.61	225.67	0 to 3599.23	Clustering measure of percent Asian
% Foreign Born	13.41	12.15	0 to 77.50	Percent born outside of the United States
% in Poverty	14.35	12.09	0 to 100	Percent below federal poverty line
% College Educated	32.84	18.98	0 to 100	Percent with a college degree or higher
% Unemployed	6.02	3.01	0 to 50.50	Percent unemployed
% Age 65 and Up	12.94	6.68	0 to 93.50	Percent age 65 and up
% Vacant Housing	9.44	8.08	0 to 100	Percent of vacant homes

Note: $N = 8{,}644$.

autocorrelation). This was determined to be the most appropriate model according to a series of Lagrange Multiplier tests. I also use Kelejian-Prucha robust standard errors to account for significant heteroskedasticity present in the models (Kelejian & Prucha, 2010).

Furthermore, I estimate three main sets of models. First, I estimate a series of models with just the segregation variables included in order to capture the gross effects of segregation on the distribution of auxiliary health care practitioners (see Table 2). Next, I add the other independent variables in order to analyze the extent to which these variables change (if at all) the relationship between the segregation variables and the outcomes (see Table 3). Finally, I ran a series of models for each of the dependent variables which introduce the key independent variables one-by-one in order to examine specifically where the change in the effect may be coming from. These findings are discussed in the results section below.

Table 2. Coefficients and (Standard Errors) from Spatial Error Models of Organizational Densities.

Variable Name	Mental Health Professionals[a]	Dentist's Offices	Physical Therapists	Chiropractors	Optometrists	Podiatrists	Misc. Health Services
Independent Variables							
% Black Clustering	−0.129***	−0.824***	−0.200***	−0.223***	−0.102***	−0.045***	−0.091***
	(0.023)	(0.085)	(0.015)	(0.020)	(0.010)	(0.007)	(0.009)
% Latino Clustering	−0.207***	−0.946***	−0.265***	−0.254***	−0.137***	−0.067***	−0.133***
	(0.037)	(0.105)	(0.022)	(0.032)	(0.029)	(0.009)	(0.013)
% Asian Clustering	0.372	4.513	0.037	1.293	0.623	0.024	0.450*
	(0.678)	(2.719)	(0.185)	(1.415)	(0.325)	(0.046)	(0.198)
Constant	0.728***	5.264***	1.214***	1.425***	0.768***	0.374***	0.572***
	(0.146)	(0.179)	(0.026)	(0.044)	(0.024)	(0.016)	(0.025)
Lambda	0.167	0.072**	0.092***	0.083*	0.079*	0.040	0.059***
	(0.173)	(0.023)	(0.020)	(0.035)	(0.038)	(0.027)	(0.015)
Rho	0.084						
	(0.163)						
Pseudo R^2	0.190	0.010	0.019	0.013	0.010	0.003	0.007

Notes: $N = 8{,}644$. $^{*}p < .05$, $^{**}p < .01$, $^{***}p < .001$ (two-tailed). The coefficients for percent Black clustering, percent Latino clustering, and percent Asian clustering are multiplied by 1,000 for the ease of presentation.

[a]This model is a spatial autocorrelation (or SAC) model which accounts for both spatial error (lambda) and spatial lag (rho) effects as this was found to be the most appropriate model for this dependent variable.

Table 3. Coefficients and (Standard Errors) from Spatial Error Models of Organizational Densities.

Variable Name	Mental Health Professionals[a]	Dentist's Offices	Physical Therapists	Chiropractors	Optometrists	Podiatrists	Misc. Health Services
Independent Variables							
% Black Clustering	−0.041	−0.341***	−0.078***	−0.174***	−0.043**	−0.012	−0.053***
	(0.024)	(0.092)	(0.023)	(0.034)	(0.016)	(0.008)	(0.014)
% Latino Clustering	0.013	−0.353	−0.100*	−0.044	−0.032	−0.065*	−0.073
	(0.053)	(0.376)	(0.044)	(0.133)	(0.040)	(0.026)	(0.046)
% Asian Clustering	0.104	2.788	−0.194	1.391	0.516	−0.170*	0.150
	(0.578)	(3.485)	(0.236)	(1.819)	(0.412)	(0.082)	(0.247)
% Foreign Born	0.002	0.089	0.013	−0.006	0.005	0.011*	0.014
	(0.009)	(0.067)	(0.007)	(0.025)	(0.007)	(0.005)	(0.008)
% in Poverty	0.016*	0.075*	0.011*	0.005	0.006	0.008**	0.006
	(0.008)	(0.031)	(0.005)	(0.011)	(0.004)	(0.003)	(0.003)
% College Educated	0.022***	0.116***	0.023***	0.019***	0.013***	0.005***	0.019***
	(0.006)	(0.018)	(0.003)	(0.004)	(0.003)	(0.001)	(0.002)
% Unemployed	−0.041	−0.266*	−0.025	−0.045	−0.046	−0.024*	0.001
	(0.025)	(0.130)	(0.018)	(0.042)	(0.025)	(0.011)	(0.019)
% Age 65 and Above	0.021	0.216***	0.067*	0.014	0.013	0.029*	0.010
	(0.019)	(0.062)	(0.030)	(0.015)	(0.015)	(0.013)	(0.007)
% Vacant Housing	0.036	0.112	0.000	0.052	0.026	−0.001	0.022*
	(0.029)	(0.080)	(0.013)	(0.037)	(0.015)	(0.006)	(0.011)

Table 3. (*Continued*)

Variable Name	Mental Health Professionals[a]	Dentist's Offices	Physical Therapists	Chiropractors	Optometrists	Podiatrists	Misc. Health Services
Constant	0.424***	5.284***	1.217***	1.427***	0.769***	0.374***	0.574***
	(0.112)	(0.174)	(0.025)	(0.043)	(0.024)	(0.015)	(0.024)
Lambda	−0.323	0.055*	0.066**	0.071*	0.073	0.033	0.044**
	(0.181)	(0.023)	(0.021)	(0.034)	(0.037)	(0.025)	(0.014)
Rho	0.443***						
	(0.123)						
Pseudo R^2	0.264	0.040	0.076	0.032	0.034	0.025	0.031

Notes: $N = 8{,}644$. $*p < .05$, $**p < .01$, $***p < .001$ (two-tailed). The coefficients for percent Black clustering, percent Latino clustering, and percent Asian clustering are multiplied by 1,000 for the ease of presentation.

[a]This model is a spatial autocorrelation (or SAC) model which accounts for both spatial error (lambda) and spatial lag (rho) effects as this was found to be the most appropriate model for this dependent variable.

RESULTS

Turning to the results in Table 2, I first examine the gross effects of segregation on the distribution of auxiliary health care practitioners. What is readily clear from this table is that both Black and Latino segregation are significantly negatively associated with each of the dependent variables. In some cases, the size of the effect is quite large, especially in the case of dentist's offices, physical/occupational/speech therapists, and chiropractors. Substantively, this indicates that as the concentration and clustering of Blacks and Latinos increases across urban zip codes, the distribution of all seven types of auxiliary health care practitioners' decreases. In essence, the more racially segregated a community, the less likely they are to have these types of establishments. This finding does not apply to Asian segregation, though. The coefficient is not significant, with the exception of miscellaneous health care practitioners, and in this case, the coefficient is actually positive. This indicates that Asian segregation is generally unrelated to the distribution of auxiliary health care practitioners across space, except in one instance in which such communities are more likely to have such facilities.

This picture changes somewhat, though, when examining the full results in Table 3. Most notably, the coefficients for Black clustering for mental health professionals and for podiatrists are no longer significant, and almost all of the coefficients for the Latino clustering measure drop to non-significance, with the exception of physical/occupational/speech therapists and podiatrists. Substantively, the size of these effects (even when still significant) are also considerably smaller across the board for both Black and Latino clustering for each of the dependent variables. This suggests that these other independent variables can account for at least some portion of the significant association between racial/ethnic minority segregation and the distribution of auxiliary health care practitioners.

Moreover, when examining the results for the other variables, some patterns are evident. First, socioeconomic indicators are evidently related to these associations. Indeed, the percent of college educated individuals in a zip code has a significant and substantively large association across all of the dependent variables. Specifically, the effects are all positive, indicating that a higher percentage of a college educated population, the greater the density of these types of auxiliary health care establishments. This result is not unexpected, as highly educated individuals are more likely to have the means to afford such services and more information on the need for such services. However, the flip side of educational attainment as a socioeconomic indicator is measure of socioeconomic deprivation. Here, I include both the unemployment rate and the percent of people living in poverty. The variable for unemployment is only significant for two dependent variables (dentist's offices, and podiatrists). In these two cases, the variable is negative, meaning that the higher the unemployment rate, the lower the density of dentist's offices and podiatrists in urban neighborhoods. In the case of poverty, though, these results diverge from the theoretical expectations. The variable is significant for four out of the seven dependent variables (mental health professionals, dentist's offices, physical/occupational/speech therapists, and podiatrists), yet in all of these cases, the coefficient is actually positive. This means that the greater the percentage of the population living in poverty in a zip code, the greater the density of these four types of auxiliary health services. In terms of the other theoretically pertinent variables, the variable for percent foreign born is only significant in one instance, for the dependent variable for podiatrists. In this case, it is significant and positive, indicating that a higher percentage of foreign born population (or immigration), the greater density of podiatrists in a zip code.

In order to better understand the relationships between these variables, and how each of the explanatory independent variables may alter or mitigate the association between racial residential segregation and health, I also ran a series of six models for each of the dependent variables and added the other independent variables one-by-one (results not shown here, available upon request). In the case of Black segregation, the coefficients in the full model were reduced to non-significance for mental health professionals and podiatrists. In the case of mental health professionals, when introducing the variables one-by-one, the coefficient is greatly reduced and non-significant once including the variables for percent college educated and the unemployment rate. In the case of podiatrists, the reduction in the effect is greatest with the inclusion of the unemployment rate. In terms of the other dependent variables, where the coefficient for Black segregation was not reduced to non-significance, there were also notable reductions in the size of the coefficient in the case of optometrists with the inclusion of the unemployment rate, and in the case of miscellaneous health providers with the inclusion of percent college educated.

For Latino segregation, understanding what is driving the reduction in the effects is perhaps more important as the coefficient is reduced to non-significance for five out of the seven dependent variables in the full models. In this case, the percent of college educated individuals in a zip code seems to be the most substantial variable included in the models. This variable reduces the coefficient for Latino segregation to non-significance for mental health practitioners, dentist's offices, optometrists, and miscellaneous health practitioners. Furthermore, the variable for percent foreign born also seems to have an important association here. In the case of mental health practitioners and chiropractors, the inclusion of this variable is significant and positive, and reduces the size of the coefficient for Latino segregation to non-significance. In sum, for Latino segregation, the reduction in the size of the effects seems to be largely driven by percent of college educated in a zip code and the extent of immigration.

DISCUSSION AND CONCLUSIONS

The central aim of this study is to examine the relationship between racial residential segregation and the distribution of a wide variety of auxiliary health care practitioners across urban neighborhoods in the United States. Some limited work has been conducted which demonstrates a negative association between racial/ethnic segregation and certain generalist health care providers and facilities, yet little is known about the assortment of non-physician health care practitioners who provide a variety of important health services to individuals. Indeed, here we may expect a greater disparity across communities as these types of providers are often considered to be optional health-related services, and are frequently not covered by traditional health insurance.

Here, I find that racial/ethnic residential segregation is related to a lack of a wide variety of such providers across urban space for both Black and Latino segregation, though Asian segregation seems to be unrelated to this distribution. However, after including a number of other area-level independent variables, these associations are notably reduced indicating that these other area-level factors are accounting for some of the association between segregation and the density of auxiliary health care practitioners. In the case of Black segregation, the coefficients remain significant for most of the seven outcomes, with the exception of mental health practitioners and podiatrists, but the size of the effect is smaller in all cases, even when still significant. The reduction in the size of the effect here seems to be largely driven by the percent of the population which is college educated and the unemployment rate. This result largely affirms Hypothesis 1, or the place stratification perspective, that segregation will be related to fewer health-related organizations, regardless of the socioeconomic conditions of such areas. Though, this also suggests some partial support for Hypothesis 2, or the spatial assimilation perspective, in that socioeconomic indicators, particularly education, accounts for some of this relationship. For Latino segregation, this association is reduced to non-significance for almost all of the dependent variables, with the exception of physical/occupational/speech therapists and podiatrists. In this case, the variables for percent college educated and in a few cases percent foreign born reduce the size of the effect. This seems to provide more support for Hypothesis 2, or the spatial assimilation perspective, in the case of Latinos as the effect drops out for most of the dependent variables (though it remains for two of out the seven types). Further, the positive results for immigration in certain cases provide some additional partial support for Hypothesis 3, or the immigrant enclaving perspective. Thus, it is clear that racial/ethnic residential segregation is related to the patterns of the locations of auxiliary health care practitioners, but that economic and social factors can help account for this finding in certain cases.

These results are in keeping with much of the current literature on racial residential segregation and the density of a wide variety of health-related organizations and service providers. Such work has found important disparities in the distribution of a number of health-related organizations by racial/ethnic segregation and density, in addition to some work on health care specifically (Anderson, 2017; Beaulac et al., 2009; Gordon-Larsen et al., 2006; Hayanga, Kaiser et al., 2009; Morland et al., 2002). Further, much of this work is highly focused on the case of Black Americans and finds a stronger association with Black segregation than for other groups (though often other groups are not considered). In general, the findings presented here are in keeping with such trends.

However, I also examine the case of Latino and Asian segregation, and include a number of other area-level independent variables which may account for this association. I find rather strong effects of Latino segregation in the gross effects across all seven types of auxiliary health care practitioners. And, further, I find that this association for both Black and Latino segregation is mitigated by the inclusion of key variables for certain outcomes. For Black segregation, this reduction is largely driven by education and unemployment, and for Latino segregation, by education and to a lesser extent immigration. Moreover, unlike previous studies, I find no substantial negative effects of poverty, which is where much of the previous literature is focused when it comes to analyzing the sociodemographic factors which could be related. Where significant, the coefficient for percent in poverty is significant and positive, indicating that a higher level of poverty is related to a greater density of establishments, which runs counter to much of the theoretical thinking and empirical findings on the association of socioeconomic indicators and the density of such establishments. Further, the inclusion of poverty does not notably reduce the size of the association of the segregation variables with the density of establishments, indicating that poverty is not a factor which can help explain away the association. Though this may seem quite counterintuitive, it is in line with several studies on the distribution which use these same data and find that segregation is more strongly related with the density of establishments than poverty (Anderson, 2017; Small & McDermott, 2006).

In sum, this study presents several important advances in our understanding of the association between racial/ethnic segregation and the density of health-related community organizations and service providers. First, it considers a number of different kinds of health care practitioners, all of which have not been previously tested in the extant literature. Further, I examine auxiliary health care practitioners, which are often overlooked, but which play an important role in health maintenance and recovery. An inequitable distribution may be especially important for certain types of health providers with whom patients may need to visit frequently or consistently for certain ailments, such as mental health practitioners, physical/occupational/speech therapists, chiropractors, and a number of alternative medicine providers which fall under the miscellaneous category. The lack of such facilities from within the immediate community may in these cases be an important barrier to their use, even when necessary. Second, I also give careful consideration to important measurement issues that are frequently overlooked in the literature on the distribution of health-related organizations. Principally, I examine segregation through the use of a geographically informed clustering coefficient which measures two dimensions of segregation: clustering and concentration. This measure is also contextualized to the particular dynamics of the metropolitan area at large. This provides a more dynamic measurement of segregation and the manner in which it may impact the distribution of organizations. Finally, I consider the segregation of several racial/ethnic minority groups in the United States, namely Blacks, Latinos, and Asians, of which Latinos and Asians are often ignored in this literature. Though I find no substantial effects for Asian segregation, I do observe several important patterns for the segregation of Latinos, which is now the largest minority group in the country and a group which is becoming increasingly segregated over time. Thus, their inclusion is important for understanding this association.

Although this study presents these advances in the literature, the analysis also meets with certain limitations. First of all, the unit of analysis is limited to the zip code level, which may not be the most intuitive way to consider how people interact with their local context. Individuals and their movements are not bound by their zip codes, especially if the individual lives on the edges of the zip code. However, this was the smallest unit of analysis available in the CBPs data on counts of establishments. Relatedly, and perhaps more importantly, this analysis does not actually account for the use patterns and behavior of individuals living within these segregated areas. The analysis makes the assumption that people are more likely to utilize resources which are in close proximity to them, and that the lack of local service provision may provide a barrier to their use. However, this analysis only examines the distribution of people and establishments and does not directly measure or analyze who and under what circumstances people are patronizing such establishments. For some individuals with greater resources, this distance may not be a barrier to access. Moreover, the analysis does not relate the distribution of such facilities to any kind of individual or community-level health outcomes. The analysis suggests that the lack of auxiliary health care practitioners in a community could help account for the divergent health patterns that we observe across communities, but this is not directly tested here. Future research should consider in more detail the actual movement of people throughout metropolitan space, their utilization of health-related organizations, and in turn how this may affect their physical and mental health outcomes.

In sum, the results presented here demonstrate that racial/ethnic residential segregation is related to the lack of a variety of auxiliary health care practitioners, including mental health professionals, dentist's offices, physical/occupational/speech therapists, chiropractors, optometrists, podiatrists, and miscellaneous health practitioners for both Black and Latino segregation. However, this relationship is partially attenuated for certain types of practitioners with the inclusion of sociodemographic indicators, with a stronger reduction in the effects for Latino segregation. These findings show a disparity in urban neighborhood access to health care practitioners, which may be vital to certain health outcomes and behaviors. Such results indicate that in order to address racial/ethnic inequities in service provision and health, residential segregation should be an important consideration.

REFERENCES

Alba, R. D., Denton, N. A., Leung, S. J., & Logan, J. R. (1995). Neighborhood change under conditions of mass immigration - The New-York-City Region, 1970–1990. *International Migration Review*, *29*(3), 625–656. doi:10.2307/2547497

Alba, R. D., Logan, J. R., & Stults, B. J. (2000). The changing neighborhood contexts of the immigrant metropolis. *Social Forces*, *79*(2), 587–621. doi:10.2307/2675510

Aldrich, H. E., & Waldinger, R. (1990). Ethnicity and entrepreneurship. *Annual Review of Sociology*, *16*, 111–135.

Algert, S. J., Agrawal, A., & Lewis, D. S. (2006). Disparities in access to fresh produce in low-income neighborhoods in Los Angeles. *American Journal of Preventive Medicine*, *30*(5), 365–370. doi:10.1016/j.amepre.2006.01.009

Allard, S. W. (2009). *Out of reach: place, poverty, and the new American welfare state*. New Haven, CT: Yale University Press.

Allard, S. W., Rosen, D., & Tolman, R. M. (2003). Access to mental health and substance abuse services among women receiving welfare in Detroit. *Urban Affairs Review*, *38*(6), 787–807. doi:10.1177/1078087403038006002

Allard, S. W., Tolman, R. M., & Rosen, D. (2003). Proximity to service providers and service utilization among welfare recipients: The interaction of place and race. *Journal of Policy Analysis and Management*, *22*(4), 599–613. doi:10.1002/pam.10157

Alwitt, L. F., & Donley, T. D. (1997). Retail stores in poor urban neighborhoods. *Journal of consumer affairs*, *31*(1), 139–164.

Anderson, K. F. (2017). Racial residential segregation and the distribution of health-related organizations in urban neighborhoods. *Social Problems*, *64*(2), 256–276. doi: 10.1093/socpro/spw058

Anderson, K. F., & Fullerton, A. S. (2014). Residential segregation, health, and health care: Answering the Latino question. *Race and Social Problems*, *6*(3), 262–279. doi:10.1007/s12552-014-9125-2

Anselin, L., Florax, R. J. G. M., & Rey, S. J. (2004). *Advances in spatial econometrics: Methodology, tools and applications*. Berlin: Springer-Verlag.

Bader, M. D. M., Schwartz-Soicher, O., Jack, D., Weiss, C. C., Richards, C. A., Quinn, J. W. … Rundle, A. G. (2013). More neighborhood retail associated with lower obesity among New York City public high school students. *Health & Place*, *23*(0), 104–110. doi:http://dx.doi.org/10.1016/j.healthplace.2013.05.005

Beaulac, J., Kristjansson, E., & Cummins, S. (2009). A systematic review of food deserts, 1966-2007. *Preventing Chronic Disease*, *6*(3), 10.

Black, J. L., Macinko, J., Dixon, L. B., & Fryer, G. E., Jr. (2010). Neighborhoods and obesity in New York City. *Health & Place*, *16*(3), 489–499. doi:10.1016/j.healthplace.2009.12.007

Blitstein, J. L., Snider, J., & Evans, W. D. (2012). Perceptions of the food shopping environment are associated with greater consumption of fruits and vegetables. *Public Health Nutrition*, *15*(06), 1124–1129. doi:10.1017/S1368980012000523

Bower, K. M., Thorpe Jr, R. J., Rohde, C., & Gaskin, D. J. (2014). The intersection of neighborhood racial segregation, poverty, and urbanicity and its impact on food store availability in the United States. *Preventive Medicine*, *58*(1), 33–39. doi:10.1016/j.ypmed.2013.10.010

Brown, S. K. (2007). Delayed spatial assimilation: Multigenerational incorporation of the Mexican-origin population in Los Angeles. *City & Community*, *6*(3), 193–209. doi:10.1111/j.1540-6040.2007.00213.x

Charles, C. Z. (2003). The dynamics of racial residential segregation. *Annual Review of Sociology*, *29*, 167–207. doi:10.1146/annurev.soc.29.010202.100002

Collins, C. A., & Williams, D. R. (1999). Segregation and mortality: The deadly effects of racism? *Sociological Forum*, *14*(3), 495–523. doi:10.1023/a:1021403820451

Ellen, I. G., Cutler, D. M., & Dickens, W. (2000). Is segregation bad for your health?: The case of low birth weight. Brookings-Wharton Papers on Urban Affairs, 203–238.

Estabrooks, P. A., Lee, R. E., & Gyurcsik, N. C. (2003). Resources for physical activity participation: Does availability and accessibility differ by neighborhood socioeconomic status? *Annals of Behavioral Medicine*, *25*(2), 100–104. doi:10.1207/s15324796abm2502_05

Fischer, C. S., Stockmayer, G., Stiles, J., & Hout, M. (2004). Distinguishing the geographic levels and social dimensions of US metropolitan segregation, 1960-2000. *Demography*, *41*(1), 37–59. doi:10.1353/dem.2004.0002

Galaskiewicz, J., Mayorova, O. V., & Duckles, B. M. (2013). Studying the roles of non-profits, government, and business in providing activities and services to youth in the Phoenix metropolitan area. *Annals of the American Academy of Political and Social Science*, *647*, 50–82. doi:10.2307/23479095

Gibson, D. M. (2011). The neighborhood food environment and adult weight status: Estimates from longitudinal data. *American Journal of Public Health*, *101*(1), 71–78. doi:10.2105/AJPH.2009.187567

Gordon-Larsen, P., Nelson, M. C., Page, P., & Popkin, B. M. (2006). Inequality in the built environment underlies key health disparities in physical activity and obesity. *Pediatrics*, *117*(2), 417–424. doi:10.1542/peds.2005-0058

Haas, J. S., Phillips, K. A., Sonneborn, D., McCulloch, C. E., Baker, L. C., Kaplan, C. P., ... Liang, S.-Y. (2004). Variation in access to health care for different racial/ethnic groups by the racial/ethnic composition of an individual's county of residence. *Medical Care*, *42*(7), 707–714.

Hayanga, A. J., Kaiser, H. E., Sinha, R., Berenholtz, S. M., Makary, M., & Chang, D. (2009). Residential segregation and access to surgical care by minority populations in US counties. *Journal of the American College of Surgeons*, *208*(6), 1017–1022. doi:10.1016/j.jamcollsurg.2009.01.047

Hayanga, A. J., Waljee, A. K., Kaiser, H. E., Chang, D. C., & Morris, A. M. (2009). Racial clustering and access to colorectal surgeons, gastroenterologists, and radiation oncologists by African Americans and Asian Americans in the United States: A county-level data analysis. *Archives of Surgery*, *144*(6), 532–535. doi:10.1001/archsurg.2009.68

Horowitz, C. R., Colson, K. A., Hebert, P. L., & Lancaster, K. (2004). Barriers to buying healthy foods for people with diabetes: Evidence of environmental disparities. *American Journal of Public Health*, *94*(9), 1549–1554.

Iceland, J. (2004). Beyond Black and White – Metropolitan residential segregation in multi-ethnic America. *Social Science Research*, *33*(2), 248–271. doi:10.1016/s0049-089x(03)00056-5

Iceland, J., & Scopilliti, M. (2008). Immigrant residential segregation in US metropolitan areas, 1990-2000. *Demography*, *45*(1), 79–94. doi:10.1353/dem.2008.0009

Inagami, S., Cohen, D. A., Finch, B. K., & Asch, S. M. (2006). You are where you shop: Grocery store locations, weight, and neighborhoods. *American Journal of Preventive Medicine*, *31*(1), 10–17. doi:http://dx.doi.org/10.1016/j.amepre.2006.03.019

Jetter, K. M., & Cassady, D. L. (2006). The availability and cost of healthier food alternatives. *American Journal of Preventive Medicine*, *30*(1), 38–44. doi:http://dx.doi.org/10.1016/j.amepre.2005.08.039

Kelejian, H. H., & Prucha, I. R. (2010). Specification and estimation of spatial autoregressive models with autoregressive and heteroskedastic disturbances. *Journal of Econometrics*, *157*(1), 53–67. doi:10.1016/j.jeconom.2009.10.025

Kissane, R. J. (2010). "We call it the badlands": How social-spatial geographies influence social service use. *Social Service Review*, *84*(1), 3–28. doi:10.1086/652988

Krivo, L. J., Peterson, R. D., Rizzo, H., & Reynolds, J. R. (1998). Race, segregation, and the concentration of disadvantage: 1980-1990. *Social Problems*, *45*(1), 61–80. doi:10.1525/sp.1998.45.1.03x0157a

Laraia, B. A., Siega-Riz, A. M., Kaufman, J. S., & Jones, S. J. (2004). Proximity of supermarkets is positively associated with diet quality index for pregnancy. *Preventive Medicine*, *39*(5), 869–875. doi:http://dx.doi.org/10.1016/j.ypmed.2004.03.018

Logan, J. R. (1978). Growth, politics, and the stratification of places. *American Journal of Sociology*, *84*(2), 404–416.

Logan, J. R., Alba, R. D., & Zhang, W. Q. (2002). Immigrant enclaves and ethnic communities in New York and Los Angeles. *American Sociological Review*, *67*(2), 299–322. doi:10.2307/3088897

Marwell, N. P., & Gullickson, A. (2013). Inequality in the spatial allocation of social services: Government contracts to non-profit organizations in New York City. *Social Service Review*, *87*(2), 319–353. doi:10.1086/670910

Massey, D. S. (2009). Racial formation in theory and practice: The case of Mexicans in the United States. *Race and social problems*, *1*(1), 12–26.

Massey, D. S., & Denton, N. A. (1988). The dimensions of residential segregation. *Social Forces*, *67*(2), 281–315. doi:10.2307/2579183

Massey, D. S., & Denton, N. A. (1989). Hypersegregation in United-States metropolitan areas - Black and Hispanic segregation along five dimensions. *Demography*, *26*(3), 373–391. doi:10.2307/2061599

Massey, D. S., & Denton, N. A. (1993). *American apartheid: Segregation and the making of the underclass*. Cambridge, MA: Harvard University Press.

Massey, D. S., & Fischer, M. J. (1999). Does rising income bring integration? New results for blacks, Hispanics, and Asians in 1990. *Social Science Research*, *28*(3), 316–326. doi:10.1006/ssre.1999.0660

Massey, D. S., Gross, A. B., & Shibuya, K. (1994). Migration, segregation, and the geographic concentration of poverty. *American Sociological Review*, *59*(3), 425–445. doi:10.2307/2095942

Moore, L. V., & Diez Roux, A. V. (2006). Associations of neighborhood characteristics with the location and type of food stores. *American Journal of Public Health*, *96*(2), 325–331. doi:10.2105/AJPH.2004.058040

Moore, L. V., Roux, A. V. D., Evenson, K. R., McGinn, A. P., & Brines, S. J. (2008). Availability of recreational resources in minority and low socioeconomic status areas. *American Journal of Preventive Medicine*, *34*(1), 16–22. doi:10.1016/j.amepre.2007.09.021

Morland, K., Wing, S., Roux, A. D., & Poole, C. (2002). Neighborhood characteristics associated with the location of food stores and food service places. *American Journal of Preventive Medicine*, *22*(1), 23–29. doi:10.1016/s0749-3797(01)00403-2

Morland, K., Diez Roux, A. V., & Wing, S. (2006). Supermarkets, other food stores, and obesity: The atherosclerosis risk in communities study. *American Journal of Preventive Medicine*, *30*(4), 333–339. doi:http://dx.doi.org/10.1016/j.amepre.2005.11.003

Ohri-Vachaspati, P., Lloyd, K., DeLia, D., Tulloch, D., & Yedidia, M. J. (2013). A closer examination of the relationship between children's weight status and the food and physical activity environment. *Preventive Medicine*, *57*(3), 162–167. doi:http://dx.doi.org/10.1016/j.ypmed.2013.05.009

Ortiz, V., & Telles, E. (2012). Racial identity and racial treatment of Mexican Americans. *Race and social problems*, *4*(1), 41–56.

Polednak, A. P. (1997). *Segregation, poverty, and mortality in urban African Americans*. New York, NY: Oxford University Press.

Popkin, B. M., Duffey, K., & Gordon-Larsen, P. (2005). Environmental influences on food choice, physical activity and energy balance. *Physiology & Behavior*, *86*(5), 603–613. doi:10.1016/j.physbeh.2005.08.051

Portes, A., & Bach, R. L. (1985). *Latin journey: Cuban and Mexican immigrants in the United States*. Berkeley, CA: University of California Press.

Powell, L. M., Slater, S., Mirtcheva, D., Bao, Y., & Chaloupka, F. J. (2007). Food store availability and neighborhood characteristics in the United States. *Preventive Medicine*, *44*(3), 189–195. doi:10.1016/j.ypmed.2006.08.008

Sampson, R. J. (2012). *Great American city: Chicago and the enduring neighborhood effect*. Chicago, IL: The University of Chicago Press.

Sampson, R. J., Morenoff, J. D., & Earls, F. (1999). Beyond social capital: Spatial dynamics of collective efficacy for children. *American Sociological Review*, *64*(5), 633–660. doi:10.2307/2657367

Schuetz, J., Kolko, J., & Meltzer, R. (2012). Are poor neighborhoods "retail deserts?" *Regional Science and Urban Economics*, *42*(1–2), 269–285. doi:10.1016/j.regsciurbeco.2011.09.005

Small, M. L. (2009). *Unanticipated gains: Origins of network inequality in everyday life*. New York, NY: Oxford University Press.

Small, M. L., & McDermott, M. (2006). The presence of organizational resources in poor urban neighborhoods: An analysis of average and contextual effects. *Social Forces*, *84*(3), 1697–1724. doi:10.1353/sof.2006.0067

Small, M. L., & Stark, L. (2005). Are poor neighborhoods resource deprived? A case study of child-care centers in New York. *Social Science Quarterly*, *86*(5), 1013–1036. doi:10.1111/j.0038-4941.2005.00334.x

Smedley, B. D., & Stith, A. Y. (2003). *Unequal treatment: Confronting racial and ethnic disparities in health care*. Washington, DC: National Academies Press.

Smiley, M. J., Diez Roux, A. V., Brines, S. J., Brown, D. G., Evenson, K. R., & Rodriguez, D. A. (2010). A spatial analysis of health-related resources in three diverse metropolitan areas. *Health & Place*, *16*(5), 885–892. doi:10.1016/j.healthplace.2010.04.014

Smith, D. B., Feng, Z., Fennell, M. L., Zinn, J. S., & Mor, V. (2007). Separate and unequal: Racial segregation and disparities in quality across U.S. nursing homes (2007). *Health Affairs*, *26*(6), 1794–1794.

Subramanian, S. V., Acevedo-Garcia, D., & Osypuk, T. L. (2005). Racial residential segregation and geographic heterogeneity in black/white disparity in poor self-rated health in the US: A multilevel statistical analysis. *Social Science & Medicine*, *60*(8), 1667–1679. doi:10.1016/j.socscimed.2004.08.040

Walker, R. E., Keane, C. R., & Burke, J. G. (2010). Disparities and access to healthy food in the United States: A review of food deserts literature. *Health & Place*, *16*(5), 876–884. doi:10.1016/j.healthplace.2010.04.013

Waters, M. C., & Jimenez, T. R. (2005). Assessing immigrant assimilation: New empirical and theoretical challenge. *Annual Review of Sociology*, *31*, 105–125.

White, K., Haas, J. S., & Williams, D. R. (2012). Elucidating the role of place in health care disparities: The example of racial/ethnic residential segregation. *Health Services Research*, *47*(3pt2), 1278–1299. doi:10.1111/j.1475-6773.2012.01410.x

Williams, D. R., & Collins, C. (2001). Racial residential segregation: A fundamental cause of racial disparities in health. *Public Health Reports*, *116*(5), 404–416. doi:10.1016/s0033-3549(04)50068-7

Wilson, D. K., Kirtland, K. A., Ainsworth, B. E., & Addy, C. L. (2004). Socioeconomic status and perceptions of access and safety for physical activity. *Annals of Behavioral Medicine*, *28*(1), 20–28. doi:10.1207/s15324796abm2801_4

Zick, C. D., Smith, K. R., Fan, J. X., Brown, B. B., Yamada, I., & Kowaleski-Jones, L. (2009). Running to the store? The relationship between neighborhood environments and the risk of obesity. *Social Science & Medicine*, *69*(10), 1493–1500. doi:http://dx.doi.org/10.1016/j.socscimed.2009.08.032

PART IV
RACIAL AND ETHNIC MINORITIES AND HEALTH AND HEALTH CARE

NATIVITY, RACE–ETHNICITY, AND DUAL DIAGNOSIS AMONG US ADULTS

Magdalena Szaflarski, Shawn Bauldry, Lisa A. Cubbins and Karthikeyan Meganathan

ABSTRACT

This study investigated disparities in dual diagnosis (comorbid substance use and depressive/anxiety disorders) among US adults by nativity and racial–ethnic origin and socioeconomic, cultural, and psychosocial factors that may account for the observed disparities.

The study drew on data from two waves of the National Epidemiological Survey on Alcohol and Related Conditions. Racial–ethnic categories included African, Asian/Pacific Islander, European, Mexican, Puerto Rican, and other Hispanic/Latino. Substance use and depressive/anxiety disorders were assessed per DSM-IV. A four-category measure of comorbidity was constructed: no substance use or psychiatric disorder; substance use disorder only; depressive/anxiety disorder only; and dual diagnosis. The data were analyzed using multinomial logistic regression.

The prevalence of dual diagnosis was low but varied by nativity, with the highest rates among Europeans and Puerto Ricans born in US states, and the lowest among Mexicans and Asians/Pacific Islanders. The nativity and racial–ethnic effects on likelihood of having dual diagnosis remained significant after all adjustments.

Health and Health Care Concerns among Women and Racial and Ethnic Minorities
Research in the Sociology of Health Care, Volume 35, 171–191

ISSN: 0275-4959/doi:10.1108/S0275-495920170000035009

The limitations included measures of immigrant status, race–ethnicity, and stress and potential misdiagnosis of mental disorder among ethnic minorities.

This new knowledge will help to guide public health and health care interventions addressing immigrant mental and behavioral health gaps.

This study addressed the research gap in regard to the prevalence and correlates of dual diagnosis among immigrants and racial–ethnic minorities. The study used the most current and comprehensive data addressing psychiatric conditions among US adults and examined factors rarely captured in epidemiologic surveys (e.g., acculturation).

Keywords: Immigrants; race–ethnicity; mental health; substance abuse; comorbidity

INTRODUCTION

The foreign-born population in the United States is growing rapidly and is becoming more diverse (Camarota, 2012). Past research (Escobar & Vega, 2006; Escobar, Hoyos Nervi, & Gara, 2000) indicates that when most immigrants enter the United States, their risk of alcohol and drug abuse is lower and their quality of mental health is higher than the native population, even among those of the same race–ethnicity. However, the longer immigrants are in the United States, the greater are their risks for substance abuse and psychiatric disorders.

There has been a growing interest in the co-occurrence of substance use disorders (SUDs) and nonsubstance use psychiatric disorders (Vega, Sribney, & Achara-Abrahams, 2003). This comorbidity, referred to as *dual diagnosis*, is most common for mood disorders, especially depression. For example, in the United States, the lifetime prevalence of illicit drug abuse is estimated at 19.4% in mood disorders and 24% in major depressive disorder (Kessler et al., 2003; Volkow, 2004). Further, the presence of drug abuse has been shown to increase the risk for depression five-fold (Regier et al., 1990). Dual diagnosis is of great concern because it is often associated with a higher psychopathological severity, poor physical and social functioning, more emergency admissions, increased rates of psychiatric hospitalization, and self-destructive behavior including suicides (Hirschfield, Hasin, Keller, Endicott, & Wunder, 1990; Murphy, 1990; Regier et al., 1990; Torrens, Martin-Santos, & Samet, 2006). In addition, comorbid drug users have an increased rate of risk behaviors and sexually transmitted infections (e.g., HIV), more psychosocial impairments such as unemployment and homelessness, and high rates of violent and criminal behavior (Torrens et al., 2006). Clinical management of individuals with dual diagnosis is challenging because of the presence of multiple conditions which tend to be refractory.

Very little information is available on how foreign- and US-born groups differ in their risks for co-occurring SUDs and depressive and anxiety disorders. Immigrant mental health literature is also generally limited because many studies are cross-sectional or fail to consider potential effects of acculturation, social ties, or discrimination on immigrant mental health. To better understand the impact of immigration on the co-occurrence of SUD's and depressive and anxiety disorders, we investigated whether and how comorbidity between SUD's and depressive and anxiety disorders varies by nativity, race–ethnicity, and a range of potential explanatory factors. In addressing these questions, our analyses were conducted for six different groups of racial–ethnic descent: African, Asian/Pacific Islander, European, Mexican, Puerto Rican, and other Hispanic/Latino, using data from Wave 1 and Wave 2 of the *National Epidemiologic Survey on Alcohol and Related Conditions* (NESARC).

BACKGROUND

The conceptual framework for the study drew on existing theoretical perspectives and research on alcohol and illicit drug use, substance abuse and psychiatric disorders, dual diagnosis, and immigrant and minority health.

Nativity, Immigrant Characteristics, and Substance Abuse

There is longstanding evidence of differences in substance use and abuse between native- and foreign-born individuals in the United States (Malzberg, 1964; Odegaard, 1932), usually showing higher levels of use among the US-born. Patterns of alcohol and drug use, however, vary considerably across ethnicity and country of origin. Research on the new immigrants of the past 40 years indicates that drinking among Mexican–American men is more frequent and of a higher quantity than among immigrant Mexican men in the United States (Gilbert, 1991), consistent with studies showing that drinking among US Latinos as a general population becomes heavier with each additional generation (Rebhun, 1998). Further, US-born Hispanics 12 to 74 years old have higher marijuana and cocaine use compared to foreign-born (Amaro, Whitaker, Coffman, & Heeren, 1990). Notably, there is some evidence that drinking among immigrant Mexican women is even less common than among women who remain in Mexico, though as with men, these women's alcohol use increases across subsequent generations (Gilbert, 1991). National data suggest that foreign-born Latinos are less likely than are US-born Latinos to experience SUDs in the last year (Alegria, Mulvaney-Day, et al., 2007).

Similar to Hispanic immigrants, Asian immigrants tend to have lower rates of SUDs than the general population (Breslau & Chang, 2006), but some alcohol use patterns vary by country of origin, gender, and generation since immigration (Marshall, Schell, Elliott, Berthold, & Chun, 2005; Rebhun, 1998). Some exceptions are found among immigrant Japanese women who tend to have higher rates of moderate and heavy drinking than women in Japan, and immigrant Japanese men have *higher* rates of drinking than American-born Japanese men (Rebhun, 1998).

Few studies have considered the impact of nativity status on alcohol and other drug abuse among individuals of African descent. Research using the National Survey of American Life (NSAL) (2001–2003) data indicate that among those of African descent nativity status is significantly related to the likelihood of any SUD in the past year, with the risk being lower for foreign-born men and women (Williams et al., 2007).

Nativity, Immigrant Characteristics, and Psychiatric Disorders

Similar to alcohol and other drug use, the prevalence of substance use, depressive, and anxiety disorders tends to vary between the native- and foreign-born groups. Foreign-born typically have a lower risk than US-born of having most types of psychiatric and substance use disorders, except there is no nativity effect for Puerto Ricans and Cuban-Americans with respect to mood (e.g., depression) and anxiety disorders (Alegria, Canino, Stinson, & Grant, 2006; Grant et al., 2004). Studies focusing specifically on immigrants from Latin American countries have also shown that foreign-born Latinos are less likely to have psychiatric disorders than their US-born non-Hispanic counterparts (Alegria, Mulvaney-Day, et al., 2007). However, among Asian Americans, US-born are at greater risk for mood and anxiety disorders than are foreign-born Asian Americans (Breslau & Chang, 2006), with those entering the United States at older ages having the lowest risk. However, foreign birth does not offer permanent immunity, and the rates of disorders appear to increase with length of time in the United States for the foreign-born of both Latino (Vega, Kolody, Aguilar-Gaxiola, & Catalano, 1999) and Asian descents (Breslau & Chang, 2006; Breslau et al., 2007).

Few studies have examined psychiatric disorders among African immigrants. One study reported lower rates of depression for foreign-born Caribbean and African women compared to their US-born African American counterparts (Miranda, Siddique, Belin, & Kohn-Wood, 2005). Another study showed that foreign-born men of African descent are less likely than their US-born counterparts to have had any mood disorder in the last year, though no difference was found for women (Williams et al., 2007). Similarly, immigrant status had no relationship with having any anxiety disorder in the last year for either men or women of African descent.

Nativity, Immigrant Characteristics, and Dual Diagnoses

Only a few studies have addressed the relationship between foreign-born status and the co-occurrence of substance abuse and mood and anxiety disorders. Among these, Vega and colleagues analyzed data from a California sample of Mexican-descent adults (Vega et al., 2003). They found that being foreign-born reduced the risk of lifetime comorbid SUDs and mood and anxiety disorders. In another study, Turner and Gil (Turner & Gil, 2002) analyzed data on psychiatric and substance use disorders among young adults in South Florida. They found that nativity was not related to lifetime comorbidity of substance use or psychiatric disorders among Cubans with any disorders. However, foreign-born Other Hispanics who had experienced a SUD or psychiatric disorder at some point in their life were less likely to experience an additional disorder than were comparable US-born Other Hispanics. Finally, a more recent study has found US-born Latino women and men to be much more likely than their foreign-born counterparts to report dual diagnoses (Vega, Canino, Cao, & Alegria, 2009).

Correlates of Substance Abuse and Mental Health Problems

Immigrant mental health is known to be shaped by socioeconomic, cultural, and psychosocial factors, which can be intertwined. With respect to socioeconomic factors, immigrants typically seek economic opportunities in the United States and a chance to attain higher standards of living. Many immigrants are at economic disadvantage before entry to the United States. That disadvantage often continues in the host country due to limited employment opportunities, low-pay work, discrimination, and segregation. In past research, socioeconomic factors provided some explanation for the association of nativity, race–ethnicity, and alcohol use/abuse or depressive disorders (Szaflarski et al., 2016; Szaflarski, Cubbins, & Ying, 2011).

In terms of cultural factors, immigrant health is known to be shaped by the process of acculturation, or experiences that immigrants have after the arrival in the host country that can protect against or exacerbate mental health problems. Acculturation may involve learning the language and adapting lifestyles of the host country, but different forms of acculturation – assimilation, integration, separation, or marginalization – can lead to different outcomes (Berry, 1992, 2001). Several studies indicate that acculturation increases the risk of substance abuse for both foreign- and US-born Hispanics. For example, among Hispanics the likelihood of marijuana and cocaine use increases with the use of English, such that the risk of drug use is lowest among those who primarily speak Spanish and highest among those who speak only English (Amaro et al., 1990). However, other data show that greater proficiency in the English language *lowers* the risks of psychiatric disorders among men of Asian descent (Takeuchi, Alegria, Jackson, & Williams, 2007). Other research shows that acculturative stress may increase the risk of dual diagnosis among Puerto Ricans (Conway, Swendsen, Dierker, Canino, & Merikangas, 2007). Racial–ethnic identity is another indicator of acculturation and refers to a person's subjective sense of belonging to a certain group or culture (Phinney, 1990). Some research shows little association between racial–ethnic identity and depression once gender and socioeconomic status are controlled (Cuellar & Roberts, 1997). In contrast, having a stronger racial–ethnic identity has been found to buffer the negative impact of discrimination on psychological distress (Sellers, Caldwell, Schmeelk-Cone, & Zimmerman, 2003).

Acculturative experience intertwined with major life changes can result in stress which can manifest itself in poor mental health, feelings of alienation, and psychosomatic symptoms (Berry, 1992). Stress is often assessed as stressful life events, perceived stress, and chronic stress (Taylor & Turner, 2002). Chronic stress associated with both drug abuse and depression has been suggested to account for some of their comorbidity while acute stress has been linked to episodes of depression and relapse in drug abuse (Volkow, 2004).

Discrimination and prejudice are additional stressors that have been linked to increased substance use (Yen, Ragland, Greiner, & Fisher, 1999a, 1999b) and adverse mental health risk (Gee, Ryan, Laflamme, & Holt, 2006; Williams & Williams-Morris, 2000; Williams, Neighbors, & Jackson, 2003). Other research suggests that while discrimination may heighten psychological distress, it has less of an impact on depression than recent and chronic stressors such as lifetime adversity or traumatic events (Taylor & Turner, 2002). Traumatic events (Wheaton, 1999; Williams et al., 2003), such as death in a family or job loss, are known to contribute to substance use and abuse (Cooper, Russell, Skinner, Frone, & Mudar, 1992), though their effects may vary by race–ethnicity (Kessler & Neighbors, 1986).

Social ties in the host country can also shape immigrant mental health. Research has found that having a perception of high social support has beneficial effects on mental health by reducing psychological distress and buffering the impact of stressful events (Ritsner & Ponizovsky, 2003; Turner & Marino, 1994) and can reduce the nativity effect on psychiatric disorders (Alegria, Mulvaney-Day, et al., 2007). However, immigrants may have less support than US natives and varying levels based on ethnicity (Rodriguez & DeWolfe, 1990).

As documented here, past studies provide some evidence that foreign-born status reduces the risks of dual diagnosis. The studies, however, often draw on relatively small regional samples and/or on a single racial–ethnic group, and most analyses are of lifetime occurrences rather than co-occurrence within a recent and more limited time frame. There is also still much to learn about the correlates of dual diagnoses by nativity and racial–ethnic background. The current study addresses some of these gaps.

METHODS

Data

The data for the study were drawn from Wave 1 and Wave 2 of the *National Epidemiologic Survey on Alcohol and Related Conditions* (NESARC), a representative sample of the US civilian, noninstitutionalized population of individuals 18 years or older (Grant et al., 2009; Grant, Kaplan, Shepard, & Moore, 2003; Ruan et al., 2008). The NESARC sampling procedures included over-sampling of non-Hispanic Black and Hispanic households and within households over-sampling of 18 to 24 year olds. The sample sizes for Wave 1 (2001–2002) and Wave 2 (2004–2005) were 43,093 and 34,653, respectively. The analysis sample consists of respondents with nonmissing data for all covariates ($N = 30{,}322$). Preliminary analyses showed no differences in results whether or not multiple imputation was used to address missing values.

Measurement

Dependent Variable

Substance (alcohol and illicit drug) abuse or dependence and nonsubstance use psychiatric disorders – depressive disorders (major depressive disorder and dysthymia) and anxiety disorders (panic with/without agoraphobia, social phobia, specific phobia, and general anxiety disorder) – were assessed using DSM-IV criteria (American Psychiatric Association, 2000). NESARC's diagnostic classifications were based on the Alcohol Use Disorder and Associated Disability Interview Schedule – DSM-IV Version (AUDADIS-IV) (Grant & Dawson, 2006; Ruan et al., 2008). Based on the diagnostic questions, the NESARC constructed dichotomous variables for Wave 2-based diagnoses of substance abuse/dependence, depressive, and anxiety disorders during the last 12 months. We used these indicators to construct a four-category measure of comorbidity: (0) no substance abuse/dependence or psychiatric (depressive or anxiety) disorder, (1) substance abuse/dependence disorder only, (2) psychiatric disorder only, and (3) dual diagnosis (substance abuse/dependence co-occurring with a depressive/anxiety disorder).

Independent Variables

Nativity was defined as US-born (referent) versus foreign-born. *Racial–ethnic origin* was based on self-reported country of origin or racial–ethnic descent (59 categories). We created six racial–ethnic groups: African, European, Asian/Pacific Islander, Mexican, Puerto Rican, and other Hispanic/Latino.

Several socioeconomic factors were assessed. *Education* was a categorical measure with categories defined by the highest grade completed (less than high school, high school or GED [referent category], some college, and college graduate). *Employment status* was divided into three categories: not working, working part-time, and working full-time (referent category). NESARC assessed *household income* by using 21 categories. The categories were recoded to their midpoint values (divided by $10,000); the top category was determined by a Pareto approximation (Hout, 2004). *Insurance coverage* was a binary variable indicating coverage and no coverage (referent category).

Cultural factors included indicators of acculturation and discrimination. *Years in the US* was the difference between year of entry and year of birth for foreign-born and a value of 0 for US-born respondents (with age included in all models). Measures of *language preference* and *racial–ethnic social preference* were constructed based on the Brief Acculturation Rating Scale II (ARSMA-II) (Coronado, Thompson, McLerran, Schwartz, & Koepsell, 2005; Cuellar & Roberts, 1997; Deyo, Diehl, Hazoda, & Stern, 1985; Solis, Marks, Garcia, & Shelton, 1990) and the East Asian Acculturation Measure (Barry, 2001). Seven questions on language preference asked respondents about which language they generally read and speak; spoke as a child; usually speak at home; usually think in; usually speak with friends; and watch/listen to in TV/radio programming. Response categories used a 5-point scale and were: only non-English language; more non-English language than English; both equally; more English than non-English language; and only English. Factor analysis was used to generate a single factor on language preference (Cronbach's $\alpha = 0.97$). Higher values indicate greater acculturation.

The NESARC questions on *racial–ethnic social preference* asked respondents about the race–ethnicity of their close friends; people at the social gatherings and parties they prefer to attend; the people they visit with; and their children's friends if they could choose. The pattern of possible responses was coded as: all from my racial–ethnic group; more from my racial–ethnic group than other racial–ethnic groups; about half and half; more from other racial–ethnic groups than from my racial–ethnic group; and all from other racial–ethnic groups. Factor analysis produced a score measure of racial–ethnic social preference (Cronbach's $\alpha = 0.833$). Higher values indicate greater acculturation.

For *racial–ethnic orientation* we used questions in the NESARC that were adapted from other scales of racial–ethnic identity (Barry, 2002; Phinney, 1990; Rahim-Williams et al., 2007). Respondents were asked how strongly they agreed or disagreed that they have a strong sense of self as a member of their racial–ethnic group; identify with other people from their racial–ethnic group; racial–ethnic heritage is important in their life; and are proud of their racial–ethnic heritage. The scale's Cronbach's α was 0.829. Higher values on the measure indicate less identification with one's own racial–ethnic group, reflecting greater acculturation and assimilation. Data on acculturation were collected for all respondents regardless of nativity.

Perceived racial–ethnic discrimination was assessed by asking respondents about how often they experienced discrimination related to their race or ethnicity in a variety of situations during the last 12 months. These include experiencing discrimination in their ability to obtain health care or health insurance; in how they are treated when they got health care; in public, (on the street, in stores, or in restaurants); in any other situation (jobs, school or training program, in courts or with police, or obtaining housing); being called a racist name because of their race–ethnicity; and being made fun of, picked on, pushed, shoved, hit, or threatened with harm because of their race–ethnicity. Factor analysis was used to generate two factors indicating perceived discrimination related to health care (Cronbach's $\alpha = 0.75$) and other aspects of life (e.g., in jobs, schooling, housing, in businesses, or by police; Cronbach's $\alpha = 0.75$).

Psychosocial factors included measures of social networks, social support, and social stress. *Social Network Index* (Cohen, Doyle, Skoner, Rabin, & Gwaltney, 1997) indicates the total number of different types of people respondents see or talk to on the phone or via internet at least once every 2 weeks. The responses were used to create continuous indicators for the number of close ties (e.g., children, parents) and instrumental ties (e.g., teachers, co-workers) respondents have in their social network. Higher values indicate a larger network.

Social support was assessed by using the Interpersonal Support Evaluation List (ISEL12); (Cohen & Hoberman, 1983; Cohen, Mermelstein, Kamarck, & Hoberson, 1985) which had six questions on how true it is respondents could find someone to help them or join them in a variety of situations, including: help with daily chores if sick, seek advice about handling problems with family, go to a movie, deal with personal problems, have lunch, and get ride if stranded 10 miles from home. Factor analysis was used to create a scale of level of social support (Cronbach's $\alpha = 0.79$). Higher values indicate higher levels of social support.

Stressful life events was the total number of the following 12 events that respondents reported experiencing in the 12 months prior to the interview: any family member or close friend died; any family or close friend had serious illness or injury; moved/anyone new came to live with you; fired or laid off from a job; unemployed and looking for a job for more than a month; trouble with their boss or a co-worker; changed job, job responsibilities, or work hours; marital separation or divorce or breakup of a steady relationship; had problems with neighbor, friend, or relative; financial crisis, declaration of bankruptcy, or being unable to pay their bills; respondent or family member had serious trouble with the police or law; and respondent or family member being crime victim.

To assess *perceived social stress* respondents were asked how often, in the past year, they have felt that they were not able to control the important things in their life; felt confident about their ability to handle personal problems; felt things were going their way; and felt difficulties piling up so high that they could not overcome them. The response categories for each question were: never, sometimes, fairly often, and very often. Factor analysis was used to construct two perceived stress measures: stress related to personal life and a lack of control in life (Cronbach's α of 0.64 and 0.70, respectively).

Control Variables
Sociodemographic and health-related control variables included age, gender, marital status, number of children in household, region of residence, community type, smoking, and religiosity.

ANALYSIS

The data were analyzed using weighted multinomial logistic regression models with adjustments for complex survey design. A series of models were estimated that introduced successive sets of covariates. Model 1 included just the indicators for racial–ethnic origins and nativity along with the sociodemographic covariates. Model 2 included the socioeconomic covariates. Model 3 included the cultural covariates. Model 4 included the social support and social stress covariates. Finally, Model 5 included all of the covariates in a single model. In all models, dual diagnosis was treated as the referent category.

We assessed the extent to which socioeconomic, cultural, social support and social stress factors accounted for the observed racial–ethnic origin- and nativity-based disparities in comorbid conditions by calculating predicted probabilities based on Models 1 and 5 along with confidence intervals and comparing the predicted probabilities. This approach is preferred to comparing coefficients across models (Long, 1997).

All statistical analyses were conducted using SAS software (version 9.3; SAS Institute, Cary, NC). Specifically, the survey-related procedures SURVEY MEANS, SURVEYFREQ, SURVEYREG, and SURVEYLOGISTIC. For all regression models, odds ratios (OR) are reported along with two-tailed significance tests.

FINDINGS

The prevalence of dual diagnosis was relatively low, but it was three times as high among the US-born (3.1%) compared to foreign-born respondents (1.1%;

Table 1. Prevalence of Dual Diagnoses by Nativity and Racial–Ethnic Origin.

		Comorbidity Status (%)			
	N	Neither	Subst. only	Psych. Only	Both
Nativity					
Nonimmigrant	25526	74.5%	8.6%	13.8%	3.1%
Immigrant	4796	83.9%	4.2%	10.7%	1.1%
Racial–Ethnic Origin					
Africa	6178	76.3%	7.9%	13.4%	2.4%
Asia/Pacific Islands	1016	83.1%	4.2%	10.8%	2.0%
Europe	17204	74.9%	8.5%	13.6%	3.1%
Mexico	3327	77.7%	8.5%	12.1%	1.7%
Puerto Rico	719	73.5%	6.2%	17.3%	3.0%
Other Hispanic/Latino	1878	78.5%	6.2%	13.2%	2.1%
Total	30322	75.8%	8.1%	13.4%	2.8%

Notes: Percentages weighted by NESARC sample weights. Design-based F-statistic for nativity = 48.76, p-value < 0.001. Design-based F-statistic for racial-ethnic origin = 4.29, p-value < 0.0001.

see Table 1). With respect to racial–ethnic origin, the lowest prevalence was found among Mexicans (1.7%) while the highest was found among Europeans (3.1%) and Puerto Ricans (3.0%). We now turn to an examination of these bivariate differences in a multivariate framework.

Dual diagnosis versus neither SUD nor psychiatric disorder. The first five columns of Table 2 report the odds ratios for the series of models introducing successive sets of covariates for the contrast between dual diagnosis (the referent) versus having neither a SUD nor psychiatric disorder. From Model 1 we see that even after controlling for the sociodemographic and health-related covariates, people of African (OR = 1.36) and Mexican origin (OR = 1.44) as well as immigrants (OR = 2.38) are more likely to have neither a SUD nor a psychiatric disorder than a dual diagnosis relative to people of European origin and nonimmigrants, respectively.

These basic patterns remain when either socioeconomic factors or social support and social stress factors are included in the model. When cultural factors are included in the model, however, the odds ratio for Mexicans is no longer statistically significant while the odds ratio for Puerto Ricans becomes significant and indicates that Puerto Ricans (OR = 0.73) have a lower likelihood of having neither a SUD nor a psychiatric disorder than a dual diagnosis relative to people of European origin.

Despite having a minimal influence on the patterns of racial–ethnic origin- and nativity-based disparities in the likelihood of a dual diagnosis versus neither a SUD nor a psychiatric disorder, many of the socioeconomic, cultural,

Table 2. Odds from Multinomial Regression Models Predicting Comorbidity Status.

	Dual Diagnosis Vs. Neither					Dual Diagnosis Vs. Substance Only					Dual Diagnosis Vs. Psychiatric Only				
	M1	M2	M3	M4	M5	M1	M2	M3	M4	M5	M1	M2	M3	M4	M5
Racial–Ethnic Origin & Nativity															
Africa	1.36***	1.33***	1.52***	1.90***	1.67***	1.24***	1.30***	1.32***	1.56***	1.49***	1.21***	1.14*	1.17*	1.32***	1.08
Asia/Pacific Islands	1.14	1.18	0.97	1.40	1.08	0.68*	0.70*	0.73	0.81	0.84	0.99	1.03	0.74	1.07	0.79
Mexico	1.44***	1.35***	0.90	1.70***	0.89	1.56***	1.56***	1.57***	1.79***	1.64***	1.40***	1.21***	0.81**	1.59***	0.80*
Puerto Rico	1.05	1.02	0.73***	1.19**	0.76**	0.74**	0.73**	0.74*	0.81*	0.79	1.42***	1.28***	0.85*	1.48***	0.83
Other Hispanic	1.12	1.10	0.84	1.20	0.83	0.96	0.96	0.98	0.97	0.97	1.20*	1.16	0.84	1.25*	0.84
Immigrant	2.38***	2.29***	1.64**	1.97***	1.51*	1.13	1.06	1.08	1.05	0.98	1.76***	1.67***	0.95	1.56***	0.98
Socioeconomic Factors															
Less than high school		1.09*			1.09*		1.05			1.07	1.19**			1.19***	
Attended college		0.92**			0.95		0.97			0.98		0.95			0.95
College graduate		0.96			0.93*		1.05			1.02		0.94*			0.90***
Part-time work		0.85***			0.92*		0.89***			0.91*		0.91**			0.96
Not working		0.90***			1.05		0.78***			0.88***		1.04			1.15***
Household income		1.00			0.98***		1.01***			0.99		0.99***			0.98***
Health insurance		0.95			0.76***		0.76***			0.64***		1.08			0.98
Cultural Factors															
Years in the US			0.99		0.99			1.00		1.00			1.00		1.00
English language preference			0.63***		0.67***			0.92		0.95			0.62***		0.68***
Preference for other racial–ethnic groups socially			1.12***		1.13***			0.97		0.95			1.14***		1.17***

Race–ethnic orientation	0.89***		1.01	0.93***		1.01	0.96		1.02
Perceived racial–ethnic discrimination–health care	1.03		1.06**	1.02		1.05*	1.01		1.00
Perceived racial–ethnic discrimination–other	0.75***		0.96*	0.90***		1.03	0.99		1.10***
Social Ties & Stress Factors									
Social network–number of close ties		1.01*	1.01*		1.01**	1.01**		1.00	0.99
Social network–number of instrumental ties		0.99***	1.00**		1.00	1.00		0.99***	1.00*
Social support		1.19***	1.20***		1.09**	1.09**		1.11***	1.13***
Social stress									
Perceived social stress–personal life		0.84***	0.80***		0.80***	0.79***		1.07*	1.02
Perceived social stress–control		0.47***	0.46***		0.57***	0.57***		0.92***	0.89***
Stressful life events		0.71***	0.71***		0.90***	0.90***		0.87***	0.85***

Notes: All models weighted by NESARC sample weights. All models include the sociodemographic and health-related covariates outlined in the text. **p*-value < 0.05; ***p*-value < 0.01; ****p*-value 0.001 (two-tailed test).

social support and stress factors had significant associations in the expected directions. For instance, not working (OR = 0.90) or working part-time (OR = 0.85) relative to working full-time, a higher degree of acculturation as indicated by English language proficiency (OR = 0.63), and higher levels of stress in personal life (OR = 0.84), in control (OR = 0.47), and in the number of stressful life events (OR = 0.71) were all associated with a decreased likelihood of having neither a SUD nor psychiatric disorder relative to having a dual diagnosis.

Dual diagnosis versus SUD only. The second set of five columns of Table 2 report the odds ratios for the series of models introducing successive sets of covariates for the contrast between dual diagnosis (the referent) versus having only a SUD. From Model 1 we see that after controlling for the sociodemographic and health-related covariates, people of African (OR = 1.24) and Mexican origin (OR = 1.56) are more likely to have a SUD than a dual diagnosis relative to people of European origin. In contrast, people from Asian/Pacific Islander origin (OR = 0.68) and people from Puerto Rican origin (OR = 0.74) are less likely to have only a SUD than a dual diagnosis relative to people of European origin. We do not observe a significant association for immigrants.

These patterns largely persist as the socioeconomic, cultural, social support and social stress factors are included in the model. The main exception is that the association for Asian/Pacific Islanders is not statistically significant when either cultural factors or social support and social stress factors are added to the model. In addition, the estimate for Puerto Ricans is not statistically significant in the final model, but the point estimate for the odds ratio is quite similar to the estimates from the other models.

Dual diagnosis versus psychiatric disorder only. Finally, the third set of five columns of Table 2 report the odds ratios for the series of models introducing successive sets of covariates for the contrast between dual diagnosis (the referent) versus having only a psychiatric disorder. From Model 1 we see that people of African (OR = 1.21), Mexican (OR = 1.40), Puerto Rican (OR = 1.42), and other Hispanic (OR = 1.20) origin as well as immigrants (OR = 1.76) all are more likely than people of European origin and nonimmigrants respectively to have a psychiatric disorder rather than a dual diagnosis. These patterns largely remain when either socioeconomic factors or social support and social stress factors are included in the model. The patterns, however, substantially differ when cultural factors – in particular, two measures of acculturation – are included in the model. After adjusting for cultural factors, the positive association for people of African origin remains, but the associations for people of Mexican (OR = 0.81) and people of Puerto Rican (OR = 0.85) origin become negative and the remaining racial–ethnic origin groups along with immigrants are no longer statistically significant. In the final model including all covariates, only people of Mexican origin maintain a significant negative association with dual diagnosis versus only psychiatric disorders.

Do socioeconomic, cultural, and social support/social stress factors account for racial–ethnic origin- and nativity-based disparities? As noted above, it is necessary to examine predicted probabilities in order to determine the extent to which the various factors account for the observed racial–ethnic origin- and nativity-based disparities in dual diagnoses. Fig. 1. illustrates the predicted probabilities based on Models 1 and 5 for each of the four comorbidity statuses for people of different racial–ethnic origins. It is apparent from this figure that adjusting for socioeconomic, cultural, social support and social stress factors does little to alter the predicted probabilities of each racial–ethnic group with respect to having neither a SUD nor psychiatric disorder, only a SUD, only a psychiatric disorder, or a dual diagnosis. In fact, none of the predicted probabilities are significantly different between Models 1 and 5 for any racial–ethnic group across the four comorbidity statuses. The same pattern is found for nativity status (figure not presented). This suggests that despite the few shifts in statistical significance found in the estimates reported in Table 2 other factors underlie racial–ethnic origin- and nativity-based disparities in comorbid conditions.

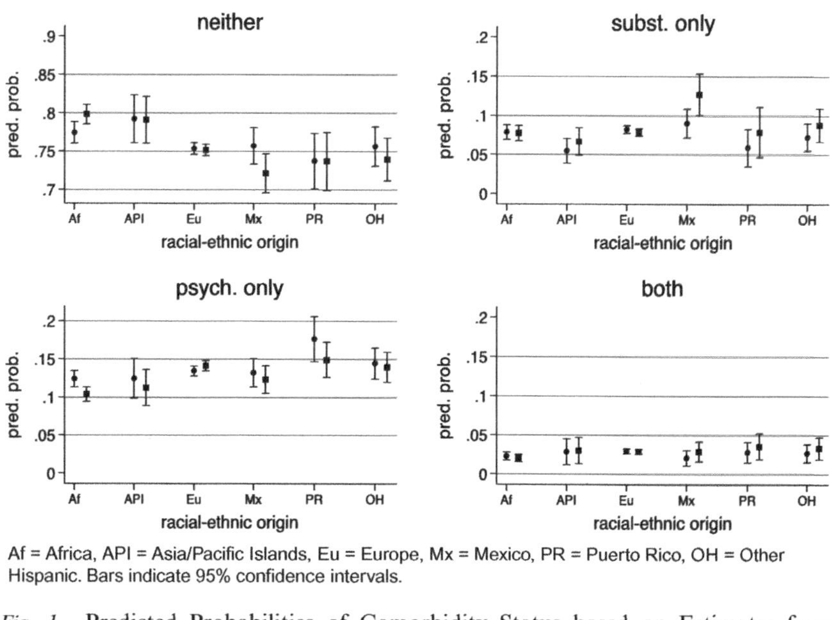

Fig. 1. Predicted Probabilities of Comorbidity Status based on Estimates from Models 1 (Circle) and 5 (Square) – see Table 2. *Notes*: Af = Africa, API = Asia/Pacific Islands, Eu = Europe, Mx = Mexico, PR = Puerto Rico, OH = Other Hispanic. Bars indicate 95% confidence intervals.

DISCUSSION

This study documented significant associations between nativity, race–ethnicity, and dual diagnosis in the US adult population. Immigrants and some racial–ethnic groups (e.g., people of African and Mexican descents) were less likely than US natives and Europeans to have dual diagnosis versus having no SUD or depressive/anxiety disorder. Conversely, immigrants and minorities were more likely than their native and European counterparts to have a depressive/anxiety disorder alone rather than dual diagnosis. There was no nativity-based difference in having a SUD alone versus dual diagnosis, though people of African and Mexican origins were more likely to have this condition compared with Europeans. Thus, the patterns of dual diagnosis appear to vary based on the specific type of comparison.

Our results confirm and extend prior research in regard to the prevalence of dual diagnosis in minority and immigrant populations. A study of dual diagnoses among US Latinos found lower rates among foreign-born than US natives as well as variations by country of origin (Vega et al., 2009). While the earlier study examined lifetime prevalence of dual diagnosis and specific Latino backgrounds, our study was able to address a more recent (past 12 months) diagnosis and included a broader range of racial–ethnic groups. A more comprehensive racial–ethnic comparison was possible because of the NESARC's much larger sample size vis-à-vis other psychiatric surveys (Grant & Dawson, 2006).

Our results also indicated that socioeconomic, cultural, and psychosocial factors did not account for the observed nativity- and origin-based disparities in dual diagnoses. Although the estimated odds ratios shifted a bit with the inclusion of measures of these factors – particularly cultural factors – the predicted probabilities of a dual diagnosis were not significantly different between the baseline model and the final model with all of the socioeconomic, cultural, and psychosocial factors. Little information on this is available. Past research has examined these factors either in SUDs or non-SUD mental disorders. Those studies found little support for the socioeconomic and mixed support for the cultural and psychosocial explanations (Brown, Donato, Laske, & Duncan, 2013; Szaflarski et al., 2016). This prior research and our findings suggest that other factors are at the root of the observed disparities. Future research in this area should seek to identify what else might account for differences in rates of dual diagnoses by nativity and racial–ethnic origin. In addition, the nature of the relationship between SUDs and mental disorders is complex and may vary depending on each particular disorder (Torrens et al., 2006). Future research addressing each disorder separately and comparing effects across different disorders could be helpful.

This study had several limitations. For example, this study did not address other factors shaping the patterns of dual diagnoses among US immigrants, such as age at immigration or historical cohort (Alegria, Shrout, et al., 2007; Alegria, Sribney, Woo, Torres, & Guarnaccia, 2007; Breslau, Borges, Hagar, Tancredi, & Gilman, 2009) or age and order of onset for dual diagnoses (Vega et al., 2009). Social stress indicators were also limited. In particular, this study focused on post-immigration social stress and could not address distress due to stressful experiences preimmigration and during the migration process. Past trauma and other displacement-related factors are known to be associated with poor mental health outcomes (Porter & Haslam, 2005). In addition, there is the potential for misdiagnosis of mental disorders, which increases in dual diagnosis (Schuckit, 2006). Diagnosis can be especially challenging among minority groups because the manifestations of mental disorders, such as idioms of distress and somatization, vary with race, ethnicity, and culture (Kirmayer & Young, 1998; Lin & Cheung, 1999). Further, the survey method and self-reports used in the study can differ from clinical assessments and have its limitations (Schuckit, 2006). Finally, the definition of race–ethnicity was limited in this study. Broad racial–ethnic categories tend to mask cultural heterogeneity of individuals from different countries and cultures. It is also unclear to what extent members of the same ethnic group are similar and different in terms of acculturation modes (Huang et al., 2006).

These limitations notwithstanding, this study provides further insights into social epidemiology of dual diagnoses in US foreign-born and native populations – with attention to racial–ethnic ancestry. The picture is quite complex. More research is needed to disentangle the pathways linking nativity, race–ethnicity, and social factors to the dual diagnosis outcomes and their trajectories over time.

ACKNOWLEDGMENTS

This study was funded by a grant from the National Institute on Drug Abuse (R01-1DA023615). Preliminary analyses for this project were supported through funding from the Peter F. McManus Charitable Trust and a faculty research development grant from the University of Cincinnati Research Council.

REFERENCES

Alegria, M., Canino, G., Stinson, F. S., & Grant, B. F. (2006). Nativity and DSM-IV psychiatric disorders among Puerto Ricans, Cuban Americans, and non-Latino Whites in the United States: Results from the National Epidemiologic Survey on Alcohol and Related Conditions. *Journal of Clinical Psychiatry*, *67*(1), 56–65.

Alegria, M., Mulvaney-Day, N., Torres, M., Polo, A., Cao, Z., & Canino, G. (2007). Prevalence of psychiatric disorders across Latino subgroups in the United States. *American Journal of Public Health*, *97*(1), 68–75.

Alegria, M., Shrout, P. E., Woo, M., Guarnaccia, P., Sribney, W., Vila, D., ... Canino, G. (2007). Understanding differences in past year psychiatric disorders for Latinos living in the US. *Social Science & Medicine*, *65*(2), 214–230.

Alegria, M., Sribney, W., Woo, M., Torres, M., & Guarnaccia, P. (2007). Looking beyond nativity: The relation of age of immigration, length of residence, and birth cohorts to the risk of onset of psychiatric disorders for Latinos. *Research in Human Development*, *4*(1), 19–47.

Amaro, H., Whitaker, R., Coffman, G., & Heeren, T. (1990). Acculturation and marijuana and cocaine use: Findings from HHANES 1982–84. *American Journal of Public Health*, *80*-(suppl.), 54–60.

American Psychiatric Association. (2000). *Diagnostic and statistical manual of mental disorders* (4th rev. ed.). Washington, DC: American Psychiatric Association.

Barry, D. (2001). Development of a new scale for measuring acculturation: The East Asian acculturation measure (EAAM). *Journal of Immigrant Health*, *3*, 193–197.

Barry, D. (2002). An ethnic identity scale for East Asian immigrants. *Journal of Immigrant Health*, *4*, 87–94.

Berry, J. W. (1992). Acculturation and adaptation in a new society. *International Migration*, *30*(s1), 69–85.

Berry, J. W. (2001). A psychology of immigration. *Journal of Social Issues*, *57*(3), 615–631.

Breslau, J., Aguilar-Gaxiola, S., Borges, G., Kendler, K. S., Su, M., & Kessler, R. C. (2007). Risk for psychiatric disorder among immigrants and their US-born descendants: Evidence from the National Comorbidity Survey Replication. *The Journal of Nervous and Mental Disease*, *195*(3), 189–195.

Breslau, J., Borges, G., Hagar, Y., Tancredi, D., & Gilman, S. (2009). Immigration to the USA and risk for mood and anxiety disorders: Variation by origin and age at immigration. *Psychological Medicine*, *39*(7), 1117–1127.

Breslau, J., & Chang, D. F. (2006). Psychiatric disorders among foreign-born and US-born Asian-Americans in a US national survey. *Social Psychiatry and Psychiatric Epidemiology*, *41*(12), 943–950. doi: 10.1007/s00127-006-0119-2

Brown, T. N., Donato, K. M., Laske, M. T., & Duncan, E. M. (2013). Race, nativity, ethnicity, and cultural influences. In C. S. Aneshensel, J. C. Phelan, & A. Bierman (Eds.), *Handbook of the sociology of mental health* (pp. 255–276). New York, NY: Springer.

Camarota, S. A. (2012). *Immigrants in the United States: A profile of America's foreign-born population*. Washington, DC: Center for Immigration Studies.

Cohen, S., Doyle, W. J., Skoner, D. P., Rabin, B. S., & Gwaltney, J. M., Jr. (1997). Social ties and susceptibility to the common cold. *JAMA*, *277*(24), 1940–1944.

Cohen, S., & Hoberman, H. M. (1983). Positive events and social supports as buffers of life change stress. *Journal of Applied Social Psychology*, *13*, 99–125.

Cohen, S., Mermelstein, R., Kamarck, T., & Hoberson, H. M. (1985). Measuring the functional components of social support. In I. G. Sarason & B. R. Sarason (Eds.), *Social support: Theory, research and applications* (pp. 73–94). Newbury, NJ: Sage.

Conway, K. P., Swendsen, J. D., Dierker, L., Canino, G., & Merikangas, K. R. (2007). Psychiatric comorbidity and acculturation stress among Puerto Rican substance abusers. *American Journal of Preventive Medicine*, *32*(6 Suppl), S219–225. doi:10.1016/j.amepre.2007.02.033.

Cooper, M. L., Russell, M., Skinner, J. B., Frone, M. R., & Mudar, P. (1992). Stress and alcohol use: Moderating effects of gender, coping, and alcohol expectancies. *Journal of Abnormal Psychology*, *101*(1), 139–152.

Coronado, G. D., Thompson, B., McLerran, D., Schwartz, S. M., & Koepsell, T. D. (2005). A short acculturation scale for Mexican-American populations. *Ethnicity & Disease*, *15*, 53–62.

Cuellar, I., & Roberts, R. (1997). Relations of depression, acculturation, and socioeconomic status in a Latino sample. *Hispanic Journal of Behavioral Sciences*, *19*(2), 230–238.

Deyo, R. A., Diehl, A. K., Hazoda, H., & Stern, M. P. (1985). A simple language-based acculturation scale for Mexican Americans: Validation and application to health care research. *American Journal of Public Health*, *75*, 51–55.

Escobar, J. I., Hoyos Nervi, C., & Gara, M. A. (2000). Immigration and mental health: Mexican Americans in the United States. *Harvard Review of Psychiatry*, *8*(2), 64–72.

Escobar, J. I., & Vega, W. A. (2006). Cultural issues and psychiatric diagnosis: Providing a general background for considering substance use diagnoses. *Addiction (Abingdon, England)*, *101*(Suppl 1), 40–47.

Gee, G. C., Ryan, A., Laflamme, D. J., & Holt, J. (2006). Self-reported discrimination and mental health status among African descendants, Mexican Americans, and other Latinos in the New Hampshire REACH 2010 Initiative: The added dimension of immigration. *American Journal of Public Health*, *96*(10), 1821–1828.

Gilbert, M. J. (1991). Acculturation and changes in drinking patterns among Mexican-American women. *Alcohol Health & Research World*, *15*, 234–238.

Grant, B. F., & Dawson, D. A. (2006). Introduction to the National Epidemiologic Survey on Alcohol and Related Conditions. *Alcohol Research & Health*, *29*(2), 74–78.

Grant, B. F., Goldstein, R. B., Chou, S. P., Huang, B., Stinson, F. S., Dawson, D. A., ... Compton, W. M. (2009). Sociodemographic and psychopathologic predictors of first incidence of DSM-IV substance use, mood and anxiety disorders: Results from the Wave 2 National Epidemiologic Survey on Alcohol and Related Conditions. *Molecular Psychiatry*, *14*(11), 1051–1066.

Grant, B. F., Kaplan, K., Shepard, J., & Moore, T. (2003). *Source and accuracy statement for Wave 1 of the 2001–2002 National Epidemiologic Survey on Alcohol and Related Conditions*. Bethesda, MD: National Institute on Alcohol Abuse and Alcoholism.

Grant, B. F., Stinson, F. S., Hasin, D. S., Dawson, D. A., Chou, S. P., & Anderson, K. (2004). Immigration and lifetime prevalence of DSM-IV psychiatric disorders among Mexican Americans and non-Hispanic whites in the United States: Results from the National Epidemiologic Survey on Alcohol and Related Conditions. *Archives of General Psychiatry*, *61*(12), 1226–1233.

Hirschfield, R., Hasin, D., Keller, M., Endicott, J., & Wunder, J. (1990). Depression and alcoholism: Comorbidity in a longitudinal survey. In J. Maser & C. Cloninger (Eds.), *Comorbidity of mood and anxiety disorders* (pp. 293–304). Washington, DC: American Psychiatric Press.

Hout, M. (2004). Making the most out of the GSS income measure. GSS Methodological Report #101.

Huang, B., Dawson, D. A., Stinson, F. S., Hasin, D. S., Ruan, W. J., Saha, T. D., ... Grant, B. F. (2006). Prevalence, correlates, and comorbidity of nonmedical prescription drug use and drug use disorders in the United States: Results of the National Epidemiologic Survey on Alcohol and Related Conditions. *The Journal of Clinical Psychiatry*, *67*(7), 1062–1073.

Kessler, R. C., Berglund, P., Demler, O., Jin, R., Koretz, D., Merikangas, K. R., ... National Comorbidity Survey, R. (2003). The epidemiology of major depressive disorder: Results from the National Comorbidity Survey Replication (NCS-R). *JAMA*, *289*(23), 3095–3105. doi:10.1001/jama.289.23.3095

Kessler, R. C., & Neighbors, H. W. (1986). A new perspective on the relationships among race, social class, and psychological distress. *Journal of Health & Social Behavior*, *27*(2), 107–115.

Kirmayer, L. J., & Young, A. S. (1998). Culture and somatization: Clinical, epidemiological, and ethnographic perspectives. *Psychosomatic Medicine*, *60*, 420–430.

Lin, K. M., & Cheung, F. (1999). Mental health issues for Asian Americans. *Psychiatric Services (Washington, D.C.)*, *50*(6), 774–780.

Long, J. S. (1997). *Regression models for categorical and limited dependent variables*. Thousand Oaks, CA: Sage.

Malzberg, B. (1964). Mental disease in native and foreign-born whites in New York State, 1949–1951. *Mental Hygiene*, *48*, 478–499.

Marshall, G. N., Schell, T. L., Elliott, M. N., Berthold, S. M., & Chun, C. A. (2005). Mental health of Cambodian refugees 2 decades after resettlement in the United States. *JAMA*, *294*(5), 571–579.

Miranda, J., Siddique, J., Belin, T. R., & Kohn-Wood, L. P. (2005). Depression prevalence in disadvantaged young black women African and Caribbean immigrants compared to US-born African Americans. *Social Psychiatry & Psychiatry Epidemiology*, *40*(4), 253–258.

Murphy, J. (1990). Diagnostic comorbidity and symptom co-occurrence: The Stirling County Study. In J. Maser & C. Cloninger (Eds.), *Comorbidity of mood and anxiety disorders* (pp. 153–176). Washington, DC: American Psychiatric Press.

Odegaard, O. (1932). *Emigration and insanity: A study of mental disease among the Norwegian-born population of Minnesota*. Copenhagen: Levin & Munksgaards Publishers.

Phinney, J. S. (1990). Ethnic identity in adolescents and adults: Review of research. *Psychological Bulletin*, *108*(3), 499–514.

Porter, M., & Haslam, N. (2005). Predisplacement and postdisplacement factors associated with mental health of refugees and internally displaced persons: A meta-analysis. *JAMA*, *294*(5), 602–612. doi:10.1001/jama.294.5.602

Rebhun, L. A. (1998). Substance use among immigrants to the United States. In S. Loue (Ed.), *Handbook of immigrant health* (pp. 493–519). New York, NY: Plenum Press.

Regier, D. A., Farmer, M. E., Rae, D. S., Locke, B. Z., Keith, S. J., Judd, L. L., & Goodwin, F. K. (1990). Comorbidity of mental disorders with alcohol and other drug abuse: Results from the Epidemiologic Catchment Area (ECA) Study. *JAMA*, *264*(19), 2511–2518.

Ritsner, M., & Ponizovsky, A. (2003). Age differences in stress process of recent immigrants. *Comprehensive Psychiatry*, *44*(2), 135–141.

Rodriguez, R., & DeWolfe, A. (1990). Psychological distress among Mexican–American and Mexican women as related to status on the new immigration law. *Journal of Consulting and Clinical Psychology*, *58*(5), 548–553.

Ruan, W. J., Goldstein, R. B., Chou, S. P., Smith, S. M., Saha, T. D., Pickering, R. P., ... Grant, B. F. (2008). The Alcohol Use Disorder and Associated Disabilities Interview Schedule-IV (AUDADIS-IV): Reliability of new psychiatric diagnostic modules and risk factors in a general population sample. *Drug and Alcohol Dependence*, *92*(1–3), 27–36.

Schuckit, M. A. (2006). Comorbidity between substance use disorders and psychiatric conditions. *Addiction (Abingdon, England)*, *101*(suppl. 1), 76–88. doi:10.1111/j.1360-0443.2006.01592.x

Sellers, R. M., Caldwell, C. H., Schmeelk-Cone, K. H., & Zimmerman, M. A. (2003). Racial identity, racial discrimination, perceived stress, and psychological distress among African American young adults. *Journal of Health & Social Behavior*, *44*(3), 302–317.

Solis, J. M., Marks, G., Garcia, M., & Shelton, D. (1990). Acculturation, access to care, and use of preventive services by Hispanics: Findings from HHANES: 1982–1984. *American Journal of Public Health*, *80*(Suppl)11–19.

Szaflarski, M., Cubbins, L. A., Bauldry, S., Meganathan, K., Klepinger, D. H., & Somoza, E. (2016). Major depressive disorder and dysthymia at the intersection of nativity and racial-ethnic origins. *Journal of Immigrant & Minority Health*, *18*(4), 749–763. doi 10.1007/s10903-015-0293-y

Szaflarski, M., Cubbins, L. A., & Ying, J. (2011). Epidemiology of alcohol abuse among US immigrant populations. *Journal of Immigrant and Minority Health*, *13*(4), 647–658. doi:10.1007/s10903-010-9394-9

Takeuchi, D. T., Alegria, M., Jackson, J. S., & Williams, D. R. (2007). Immigration and mental health: Diverse findings in Asian, black, and Latino populations. *American Journal of Public Health*, *97*(1), 11–12.

Taylor, J., & Turner, R. J. (2002). Perceived discrimination, social stress, and depression in the transition to adulthood: Racial contrasts. *Social Psychology Quarterly*, *65*(3), 213–225.

Torrens, M., Martin-Santos, R., & Samet, S. (2006). Importance of clinical diagnoses for comorbidity studies in substance use disorders. *Neurotoxicity Research*, *10*(3–4), 253–261.

Turner, R. J., & Gil, A. G. (2002). Psychiatric and substance use disorders in South Florida: Racial/ethnic and gender contrasts in a young adult cohort. *Archives of General Psychiatry*, *59*(1), 43–50.

Turner, R. J., & Marino, F. (1994). Social support and social structure: A descriptive epidemiology. *Journal of Health and Social Behavior*, *35*(3), 193–212.

Vega, W. A., Canino, G., Cao, Z., & Alegria, M. (2009). Prevalence and correlates of dual diagnoses in U.S. Latinos. *Drug and Alcohol Dependence*, *100*(1–2), 32–38. doi:10.1016/j.drugalcdep.2008.08.018

Vega, W. A., Kolody, B., Aguilar-Gaxiola, S., & Catalano, R. (1999). Gaps in service utilization by Mexican Americans with mental health problems. *The American Journal of Psychiatry*, *156*(6), 928–934.

Vega, W. A., Sribney, W. M., & Achara-Abrahams, I. (2003). Co-occurring alcohol, drug, and other psychiatric disorders among Mexican-origin people in the United States. *American Journal of Public Health*, *93*(7), 1057–1064.

Volkow, N. D. (2004). The reality of comorbidity: Depression and drug abuse. *Biological Psychiatry*, *56*(10), 714–717. doi:10.1016/j.biopsych.2004.07.007

Wheaton, B. (1999). The nature of stressors. In A. V. Horwitz & T. L. Schied (Eds.), *A handbook of the study of mental health: Social contexts, theories, and symptoms* (pp. 176–197). New York, NY: Cambridge University Press.

Williams, D. R., Haile, R., Gonzalez, H. M., Neighbors, H., Baser, R., & Jackson, J. S. (2007). The mental health of Black Caribbean immigrants: Results from the National Survey of American Life. *American Journal of Public Health*, *97*(1), 52–59.

Williams, D. R., Neighbors, H. W., & Jackson, J. S. (2003). Racial/ethnic discrimination and health: Findings from community studies. *American Journal of Public Health*, *93*(2), 200–208.

Williams, D. R., & Williams-Morris, R. (2000). Racism and mental health: The African American experience. *Ethnicity & Health*, *5*(3–4), 243–268.

Yen, I. H., Ragland, D. R., Greiner, B. A., & Fisher, J. M. (1999a). Racial discrimination and alcohol-related behavior in urban transit operators: Findings from the San Francisco Muni Health and Safety Study. *Public Health Reports*, *114*(5), 448–458.

Yen, I. H., Ragland, D. R., Greiner, B. A., & Fisher, J. M. (1999b). Workplace discrimination and alcohol consumption: Findings from the San Francisco Muni Health and Safety Study. *Ethnicity & Disease*, *9*(1), 70–80.

HYPERTENSION EXPERIENCES OF BLACK MEN: A CRITICAL NARRATIVE STUDY

Rob Haile, Lilian Magalhães and Debbie Laliberte Rudman

ABSTRACT

Although Black individuals are disproportionately affected by hypertension as evidenced by higher prevalence and lower control rates, few studies have investigated this disparity from the lens of those most affected by this condition. This chapter explores how Black men make sense of their hypertension and how they negotiate this condition within their everyday lives, illuminating how racism and power dynamics embedded within their environments affect their experiences living with hypertension.

Critical Race Theory tenets were utilized alongside a narrative design to elicit stories of hypertension experiences of four Black men living in Ontario, Canada. Eight semistructured in-depth interviews were conducted, transcribed, and thematically analyzed to illuminate how participants create meaning in regard to their hypertension.

Participants' experiences with discrimination, isolation, and migration raise awareness of how power relations embedded within social, political, and historical contexts can affect hypertension experiences.

The findings of this study are bounded by its narrative context, and the characteristics of the individuals who shared their experiences.

Health and Health Care Concerns among Women and Racial and Ethnic Minorities
Research in the Sociology of Health Care, Volume 35, 193–209

ISSN: 0275-4959/doi:10.1108/S0275-495920170000035010

This study highlights the importance of how discussions concerning hypertensive minority men should be broadened to include the voices of such men, as well as the structures that discriminate against and oppress minority individuals.

Keywords: Black men; hypertension; Canada; narrative inquiry; qualitative; Critical Race Theory

INTRODUCTION

Studies have shown that hypertension (systolic blood pressure [SBP] $\geq$140 mm Hg or diastolic blood pressure [DBP] $\geq$90 mm Hg) disproportionally affects Black individuals in comparison to other population groups. For example, this group has some of the highest rates of hypertension, coupled with some of the lowest overall hypertension control rates (Hull, Dreyer, Badrick, Chesser, & Yaqoob, 2011; Leenen et al., 2008). However, reasons underlying these differences have yet to be completely understood. Traditionally cited risk factors for hypertension, which focus on individual behaviors and lifestyle choices such as salt rich diets and physical inactivity, do not sufficiently explain reasons for higher prevalence rates in Black populations (Williams, 1992).

Scholars have proposed other explanations, such as the slavery hypertension hypothesis (Kaufman & Hall, 2003), genetic factors (Fox et al., 2011), and socioeconomic factors (Leigh & Du, 2012), to make sense of this populations' susceptibility to hypertension and the challenges they face when managing this condition. In particular, some scholarship has begun to consider links between hypertension and racism. This form of discrimination, which involves hatred or intolerance toward another group of individuals, is rooted in a belief that populations exist in certain hierarchies based on their physical attributes. It has been argued that minorities on the receiving end of such practices are marginalized, and at times, subjected to inequitable access to institutional-level systems – employment, education, and other resources – so that those belonging to the majority can maintain power and privilege (Hoyt, 2012). In turn, sustained experiences of racist practices have also been shown to lead to negative health outcomes. For example, in recent years, studies, largely in the US, have found evidence of relationships between interpersonal racism and ambulatory blood pressure (Brondolo, Love, Pencille, Schoenthaler, & Ogedegbe, 2011), as well as correlations between perceived discrimination and hypertension (Dolezsar, McGrath, Herzig, & Miller, 2014). Further work is needed, however, to fully understand how racism affects health, especially outside of the United States where differences in the composition of Black populations (Milan & Tran,

2004; Rastogi, Johnson, Hoeffel, & Drewery Jr., 2011) and the structure of national health care systems exist.

The present qualitative study explores hypertension from the lens of those affected by this condition. The focus is on examining how four Black men made sense of their diagnosis and negotiated this condition into their everyday lives, drawing on Critical Race Theory (CRT), particular attention was paid to how racism was discussed in relation to experiences of hypertension.

METHODOLOGY

Design

Narrative inquiry was used to illuminate how four Black men constructed stories relating to their hypertension. Informed by a constructivist approach, this form of inquiry elicits stories as a way to understand how individuals make sense of particular experiences and how they negotiate these events into their lives (Sparkes & Smith, 2008). Additionally, this study was situated within a critical theory paradigm and used tenets of CRT. Key tenets, including that racism is ordinarily present in society, those in power have little gain by eradicating racism, and race is not objective rather it is a by-product of social constructions that people use to bestow certain characteristics to certain populations (Delgado & Stefancic, 2001), informed how stories of being "other" were viewed and analyzed. This particular methodology was chosen to enable Black men in Ontario, Canada to present their stories to illuminate alternative views on hypertension, and to challenge the systems that often situate minorities in an inferior position in comparison to their counterparts (Ladson-Billings, 1998).

Participants

As narrative studies aim to elicit depth of stories, as opposed to seeking generalizability, this study involved multiple data collection sessions with four informants (Lieblich, Tuval-Maschiach, & Zilber, 1998). The inclusion criteria consisted of self-reported Black hypertensive men over the age of 18 who were fluent in reading and speaking English. Black individuals were defined as persons who self-identified as being "Black" (Statistics Canada, 2012). Recruitment occurred purposefully via poster advertisements, snowball sampling, and with the help of local organizations and members of the community. The study occurred in Ontario, Canada: a province in which Black residents comprise 4.3% of the total population (Statistics Canada, 2013).

Data Collection

Ethical approval for this study was obtained through Western University's Health Science Research Ethics Board. The first author conducted two semi-structured interviews with each participant. The first interview involved asking two broad initial open-ended questions (Wengraf, 2001), followed by prompt questions to stimulate stories. Prior to the second interview, participants received a summary of the collection of the stories they shared with the lead investigator. This provided participants with a period of reflection, and a means to expand on the initial findings and clarify any misinterpretations in the second interview (Morrow, 2005). As such, the questions for the second interview were not decided upon until after the data from the first interview had been analyzed. In all, the interviews ranged from approximately 30 to 65 minutes.

Data Analysis

All eight interviews were audio recorded and transcribed. A CRT lens was applied during all stages of data analysis to highlight existing power structures and instances where participants' skin color or ethnicity affected their lived experiences. The data were examined using the holistic content approach, such that there was a focus on forming a whole narrative from stories told by each participant prior to considering how various parts of the narrative inter-related across participants via a cross-narrative analysis (Lieblich et al., 1998). It is important to note that even though narrative construction appears to occur in a linear fashion (see Fig. 1, opposite page), the actual process was iterative and flexible to enable multiple layers of analysis to occur over time (Lieblich et al., 1998). Given that the first author is a Black male, he inherently became an insider for this study by conducting research on the very population to which he belonged. As such, he performed ongoing reflexivity during the process of narrative construction and cross-narrative analysis by writing entries into his individual journal, and by engaging in ongoing discussions with the second and third authors.

FINDINGS

The four participants were between the ages of 54 and 78 years. Three participants resided in urban cities (one lived in a rural town), three were migrants, and two were retired. All four had been receiving treatment for their hypertension and described their blood pressure as being under control. Following a brief summary of each participant and the main storylines within their narrative, key findings from the cross-narrative analysis are provided. Quoted texts

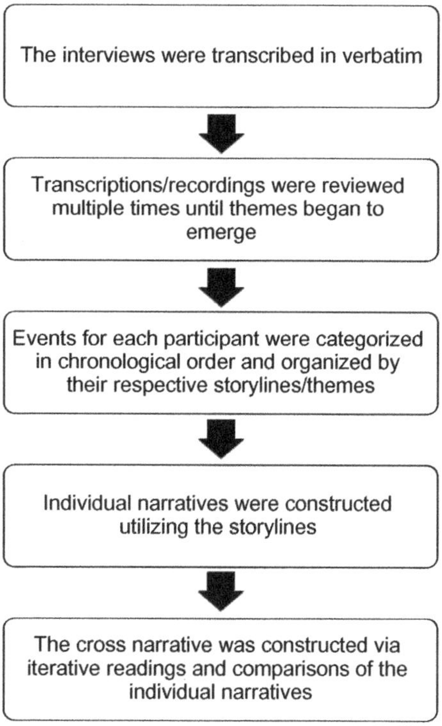

Fig. 1. Steps for Narrative Construction.

found throughout the narratives represent direct quotations and excerpts that were conveyed by participants during their interviews.

Individual Narratives

Participant 1: Joel

Joel was 54 years old at the time of the study, living with his wife and two children in an urban city. He was born and raised in East Africa and migrated to Canada in the 2000s, by way of the United States. Though previously employed as a professor in East Africa, Joel went through various menial jobs in Ontario before earning a "real" living in project management. He remembers being diagnosed with hypertension during a routine check-up, while living in East Africa. He reported that at the time of his diagnosis, "the experience was not traumatic;" he was a teen and thought very little of it. However, over the years Joel experienced side effects that affected his mental, physical and emotional health, and soon it all came to a head when a "traumatizing" experience lead to a second hypertension diagnosis while he was living in the United States. Thereafter Joel began "managing" his condition and a few years later, once his health improved, he migrated to Ontario, Canada with his family. During the time of his interviews, his blood pressure was well controlled, and he felt as though participating in this study and being candid about his experiences could "help other[s]" in similar situations. The storylines that emerged from Joel's narrative include: (a) intersecting personal relationships with hypertension, (b) intersecting migration with hypertension, and (c) living with uncertainty. Through these storylines, Joel discussed the implications of hypertension within his interpersonal life, connected it to the experience of migration and its long-lasting effects, and emphasized a pervasive sense of uncertainty tied to the diagnosis.

Participant 2: David

David was a 67-year-old retiree residing with his wife and daughter in an urban city. He was born and raised in West Africa, and completed his university degree in the Sciences before migrating to Canada in the 1970s. Shortly after his arrival, he registered in classes at a local university in the hopes of pursuing a "career in medicine." However, the combination of being "financially" strapped, and not having the proper documentation led David toward a different path. Instead, he enrolled in an allied health professional program, and subsequently began practicing as a clinician in Ontario. After 10 years of working at a hospital, David "contracted an [infectious disease] from a patient." Following this incident, he had a stroke and was later diagnosed with diabetes. Then several years later, after attending frequent check-ups with his physician, David was diagnosed with hypertension. During the interviews, David reported that his health had since stabilized and that he felt "pretty good" about his health. The storylines that materialized from David's narrative include: (a) feeling normal, (b) negotiations of diabetes and hypertension: awareness, acceptance and action, and (c) fitting in: experiences in Canada versus Africa. Throughout his narrative, David reflected on his multiple health conditions as he highlighted distinctions between the physiological side effects of his hypertension and diabetes, and emphasized how migration and stress affected his overall well-being.

Participant 3: James

James, a widower of 2 years, was in his late 70s, living alone in a rural retirement community. His children, who were adults with families of their own, lived in a nearby city and visited often. He was born and raised in a small segregated town in Nova Scotia and served in the military for three years, before moving to Ontario in his early 20s. He spent the majority of his working life employed in the manufacturing industry. A few years prior to his retirement, "approximately 20 to 25 years ago," James was diagnosed with hypertension.

Several years later, he was diagnosed with diabetes. Subsequent to each diagnosis, he was prescribed medication to manage either condition. While his hypertension was said to be under "control" during the time of the interviews, James was scheduled to meet with a nephrologist a few weeks after the second interview to investigate whether his escalating "diabetic readings" were affecting his kidneys. In hindsight, James felt as though his contribution to this study made him think about his health in ways he did not consider prior to his participation. The storylines that transpired from James' narrative include: (a) early experiences in Eastern Canada, (b) hypertension diagnosis and physician relationship, and (c) spirituality in everyday life. Throughout his narrative, James implicitly discussed the effects of segregation in his early years, and emphasized how his commitment to his faith played an influential role in how he made sense of his being throughout the course of his life.

Participant 4: Michael

Michael was a divorcee in his early sixties residing in an urban city, and had three adult children. He was born in the Caribbean's, and migrated to Ontario with his family at the age of six. His father, "an activist," played an influential role in his upbringing, as he faced several challenges growing up in a largely segregated city. Over the years, he succeeded in overcoming these barriers by "mitigating the circumstances" and remaining "in control" of whatever situation was at-hand. However, while in his 40s, Michael's health deteriorated; he contracted an autoimmune disease and was forced to relocate his family, as his job was not "conducive" to his health. Furthermore, several years later, after many visits with his family physician, he was diagnosed with hypertension. The diagnosis was initially tough on Michael because he felt as though he lost "control." Nevertheless, Michael eventually accepted his condition after his physician eased his concerns about his daily medication requirements. The storylines that emerged from Michael's narrative include: (a) racial discrimination and segregation: fighting back and attempting to get in control, (b) health struggles and the need for lifestyle changes, and (c) the diagnosis: a sense of defeat and regaining control. Through these storylines, Michael recounted his early struggles with racism, connected it to his experiences managing hypertension, and highlighted the implications that his condition had on his cultural identity.

Cross-Narratives

The five cross-narrative themes that emerged through analysis included: Connection to homeland: negotiating lifestyle changes in relation to maintaining cultural identity; Racism: stress and its enduring effects; Perceptions of high blood pressure: making sense of the diagnosis; Universal health care:

patient–physician relationships and medication as the primary source of control; and Reluctance to talk about health: constraints of masculinity.

Connections to Homeland: Negotiating Lifestyle Changes in Relation to Maintaining Cultural Identity

Three migrant participants (Joel, David, and Michael) experienced geographical and cultural transitions from their respective homeland to Canada, and all had attempted to remain connected to their cultural roots. Participants spoke of the stress that accompanied their transitions, and the sometimes-conflicting goals of maintaining their cultural identity and changing their lifestyles to manage their hypertension and/or settle into their new environments. For instance, Michael was often conflicted by the dietary restrictions his condition imposed on his lifestyle as his identity was very much attached to his community and the foods they ate. As he described:

> In [our] community, there are certain types of food [we] eat. Like for example, I'm cooking some goat, some ox tail, and jerk chicken and [...] at the end of the day, that's the diet! It's very rich, okay!? You know, you can't just say, 'let's cook some low fat curry goat or some low fat ox tail!'

Joel struggled to adjust to his new environment after migrating to Ontario. His hypertension "intensified" as he encountered difficulties finding relevant employment and acclimating to the colder temperatures. In an attempt to ease his, and others' transitions, he mimicked the "community-type life" found back in Africa by organizing a local community group. Ultimately, this group played a key role for Joel and many newcomers, as they were able to lean on each other for support during times of need. David, on the other hand, said the very thought of preserving his West African ancestry enabled him to "counter balance" his daily Canadian experience. In keeping to his roots, he maintained close contact with those in West Africa via recurrent travels to his homeland, and by sending money back home to support his family and friends.

Racism: Stress and Its Enduring Effects

Participants occasionally spoke about the isolation and stress caused by the discrimination they faced while living in Canada. Such stories of experiencing racism seemed to be one way that they were attempting to make sense of how they came to be hypertensive. Michael most explicitly attended to racism, within his narrative including many stories with direct reference to racism and how these instances affected him during his formative years. Here, he recalls the isolation he experienced from his peers during his childhood:

> Even though I [would have] loved to [have spent time] around White people to learn about their culture and to learn about them, because I didn't grow up here, [...] I couldn't, because [I was not] allowed in. [I was] discriminated against.

Joel, David, and James all implicitly referenced instances in which they were affected by racial discrimination. For Joel, it came in the form of his stories regarding his early years in Canada searching for a job to support his family. Though he was a university graduate, and previously employed as a professor in East Africa, Joel spent his initial years in Canada working as a gas station attendant. Here, he connects his accompanying stress with his health:

> If you're hypertensive, and you don't have a job, I'm telling you, you just feel it. Nobody can tell you the symptoms; you [just] know it. Your temper will always be high, and your heart will [always] be pumping really hard.

Kept ever more silent was the notion of discrimination found within David and James' narratives, respectively. David's talk of stress in Canada was to some extent a result of his inability to connect with others while living in Ontario. He further discussed how life in West Africa was more "relaxed," because amongst other things he was able to "associate with more people" despite having lived in Canada for many decades. James, on the other hand, was more apt to dismiss talks of discrimination even though he appeared to discuss events that constituted this type of mentality or behavior. For instance, he mentioned that during his childhood he and his family lived in a racially segregated area of a town, and further alluded to acts of discrimination when he declared his family was unable to work at places like "grocery stores and banks." After further probing, however, James admitted that "if [he] was really sincere, [racism] might have been there, but [he] didn't look at it that way."

Perceptions of High Blood Pressure: Making Sense of the Diagnosis

The distinct ways that participants interpreted their hypertension, especially in regard to their diagnostic experience, was evident throughout the interviews. Two of the participants, David and James, offered little detail in regard to this event and spoke of no troubles accepting their condition. Conversely, Joel and Michael not only shared greater details about their diagnostic experiences, but also articulated initial periods of neglect or struggles to accept their hypertension.

> I felt like the medication won. [...] I felt defeated. I thought I could control [the hypertension] by myself, because everything I ever came up against, I had control. [...] With the blood pressure, I thought I could do it. I did everything there was, [like] the exercising and the dieting. [...] But at that point, I finally had to accept that it was inevitable. [...] I eventually bowed down to accept [my diagnosis]. (Michael, 60)

Participants also discussed issues of heredity in relation to having a genetic predisposition to chronic conditions such as hypertension. For example, James, Michael and Joel conveyed their belief that little could have been done to prevent their hypertension since the condition was highly prevalent in their families and the greater Black population. Joel alluded to the hereditary nature of his hypertension by asserting that his condition was most likely not a by-product of other predisposing factors, but rather "was probably something that [he] was born with." Here, he describes how this revelation affects him:

> My hypertension is physiological. It is has nothing to do with my diet, because I got it while I was still young. It does appear that it is physiological. So I get helpless, because there is nothing that I can do. Whatever I do can just help to control it, but it will always be there. [...] I'm going to have [to take] medication almost throughout [my entire life]. So it's just a control measure. I can't eliminate it.

Universal Health Care: Patient–Physician Relationships and Medication as the Primary Source of Control

All the men in this study equated their satisfaction with their doctors in regard to them monitoring their health on a consistent basis. Michael and David each highlighted the time spent with their physicians during their appointments as a catalyst for the positive bilateral relations they had with one another. For instance, David declared that his specialist always gave him "more time to discuss issues" relevant to his health, while Michael stated that the extra time he spent with his physician enabled them to "work together" to improve his overall health. James also enjoyed a great relationship with his physician. However, in stark contrast to the other participants, he deferred to his doctor for all of his medical decisions. He describes:

> I don't ask questions. I never ask questions. He's smarter than I [am]. He knows what's up. [...] If he says, 'take this pill, because you need it.' I'll say, 'that's fine I'll take it', because I need it.

Furthermore, across the narratives it was evident that the use of pharmacological interventions carried a greater weight in how participants went about managing hypertension, even though most of the participants described engaging in physical activity or maintaining a healthy diet. At the same time, however, medication was discussed in different ways. For example, for James, taking medication was simply an act carried out to comply with his physicians' demands; that is, he described taking his "pills" as something his "doctor [told] him to do," and so he did it without question. Eventually, it became "automatic," almost "like taking a drink of water." Though David, too, similarly expressed his medication intake was "very much like a routine" and that he carried it out to comply with his physician's recommendations, he also expressed feelings of resentment and confinement when describing this daily practice:

> You feel enslaved. [...] Your life seems to revolve around medication. Your activit[ies], time, budget, and your whole life. [...] It's just like drinking water, and eating a meal.

Reluctance to Talk about Health: Constraints of Masculinity

In spite of the participants representing different backgrounds, a common theme prevalent in their descriptions of their respective communities was a sense of struggle for other Black men to speak openly about their health concerns with others. The men suggest cultural differences and perceptions of masculinity prevent Black men from engaging in these forms of discussions. Joel posited that Black men "rarely [...] [felt] free to discuss their health," because they had to "act strong" to avoid scaring their families. While similarly, Michael spoke of how "pride" and a "macho" feeling existed amongst this community of men. He further declared that talking openly about their health not only showed "weakness," but also went against the concept that "Black men [...] never [get] sick." Interestingly, however, all four participants declared their receptiveness to speaking candidly about their health with others, because in doing so, they believed their stories have the potential to aid others who are experiencing similar illnesses under similar circumstances. Here, James explains the benefits to sharing his experiences:

> I don't think there is no harm in it. You know you might help someone else along the way. [...] I think it's great. Things [might] come out now, things I didn't think about before. I think it's a good idea really.

DISCUSSION

This study highlighted how Black men in Ontario, Canada made sense of their hypertension, and how they negotiated this condition into their everyday lives. Drawing upon a CRT perspective, five themes were identified across participants' narratives. Men in this study relayed stories from their past to shape their narratives and thereby convey understandings of their conditions in the present and the future. In doing so, participants drew upon dominant biomedical understandings of hypertension to make sense of the causality of their conditions, while also placing their diagnoses and their ability to manage their blood pressure in other contextual factors such as experiencing racism or stress.

Scholars of CRT contend that while racism ordinarily exists in society, storytelling provides a way to elucidate how Black individuals are oppressed and often affected by axes of domination (Delgado & Stefancic, 2001; Parker & Lynn, 2002). In this study, stories of racism were fore fronted within participants' narratives related to being a migrant, not just in relation to challenges faced with obtaining employment commensurate with their experiences but also in everyday attempts to integrate into their educational or social environments. While exposure to racism can lead to elevated rates of blood pressure (Brondolo et al., 2011; Dolezsar et al., 2014), it cannot be definitively concluded that discrimination directly contributed to participants' hypertension given the narrative approach used. However, the narratives raise awareness of how racism was embedded in participants' lives, and in particular, shows how the men storied this form of intolerance in implicit ways, perhaps parallel to the so-called "silent" nature of hypertension. Employing a critical analytical approach, it became evident that certain situations, involving facing systemic barriers, social exclusion, and interpersonal challenges, were manifestations of racial discrimination. Research from Sue (2013) has shown that dialogues concerning race can place visible minorities in compromising positions, as they oftentimes conform to societal pressures that dictate they follow a "politeness protocol" (p. 666). As a result, the manner in which the men in this study highlight racism offers insight into how their lives were shaped by the strategies they appeared to use to suppress these difficult experiences.

A notable observation across the narratives was the potentially restrictive influences of notions of masculinity on the willingness and opportunities for Black men to engage in open dialogues about their health with others in their families and community. This finding parallels literature that has documented that adherence to traditional notions of masculinity amongst males negatively affects their health (Santana, Raj, Decker, La Marche, & Silverman, 2006), and that a common treatment barrier for Black men is their reluctance to discuss their health with others (Friedman, Thomas, Owens, & Hébert, 2012). Yet, in contrast to their generalizations about this population, the men in this study expressed comfort when discussing aspects of their personal health with the interviewer, as well as relayed discussions they had with others. The interviewer's insider status could very well have created the necessary space for participants to reflect on their experiences, given that individuals often feel as though they have an enhanced level of trust and experience more openness with researchers to whom they share a likeness with (Dwyer & Buckle, 2009).

Despite the common themes prevalent throughout the narratives, participants still expressed unique experiences regarding their diagnosis and their negotiations of this condition into their everyday lives. Such differences highlight the importance of not homogenizing "Black men." For example, the participants' diagnostic experiences were diverse; two participants expressed vivid and emotional memories about this particular period in time, whereas the other two men conveyed very little feelings and thoughts about this occasion. Furthermore, the participants also had different experiences when it came to discussing the physical manifestations of having hypertension. David and James were adamant their hypertension yielded no observable side effects, whereas Joel identified symptoms being associated with his hypertension. Though evidence concerning the symptomatic nature of hypertension has been put forth (Bokhour et al., 2012), it continues to be thought of as an essentially symptom-less condition (World Health Organization, 2013). The findings from this study suggest that listening to the stories of those who are not part of the majority can inform care providers, educators, and researches alike how "symptoms" are expressed differently. Schoenberg and Drew (2002) highlight that a dichotomy exists amongst patients who attribute symptoms to hypertension versus health professionals who prescribe to commonly held notions of this condition's asymptomatic nature. Under these circumstances, the authors argue that patients' lay beliefs are invalidated as being "inferior" to the "expert" opinions of medical professionals and scientists (p. 469). This underlines the critical power imbalance that exists between hypertensive individuals and their respective physicians, and points to how a "hierarchy of knowledge" can ultimately silence individual hypertension experiences in favor of traditionally held objective notions associated with this condition (Schoenberg & Drew, 2002, p. 469).

Many Canadians often fail to receive pertinent lifestyle recommendations from their physicians to treat their blood pressure (Walker et al., 2011), and previous research has problematized Black men as noncompliant. Contrastingly, men in this study not only indicated they had received such information, but also depicted themselves as having attempted to integrate these recommendations into their daily life. At the same time, the findings, display particular challenges faced in such attempts, such as the tension between maintaining low salt diets and the desire to maintain a diet reflective of one's cultural identity.

In addition, medication was a central object within the participant's narratives, with all participants indicating that they had to come to rely upon their medication to control their blood pressure. For James, implementing this form of treatment into his daily routine was simple. In comparison, though, the other participants each had difficulties with either accepting or maintaining medication as a form of treatment for their hypertension. Commonly, research investigations have indicated that hypertensive individuals that encounter such difficulties with their medications (i.e., side effects and fear of addiction) oftentimes altered their use of this form of treatment (Beune, Haafkens, Agyemang, Schuster, & Willems, 2008; Lee, Mokhtar, Krauss, & Ong, 2014). Yet, unlike these findings, Joel, David, and Michael described that they continued taking their medications despite facing initial or continuous challenges with their pharmacological interventions. Perhaps this unyielding dedication may have been a result of participants entrusting their physicians and their recommendations to continue medicating, or perhaps the nature of the health care context facilitated their ongoing commitment to their drugs given that coverage for pharmaceuticals were likely provided by Canada's universal health care system. Whatever the case may be, understanding how individuals narrate their relationship to their medication can reveal complex meanings that can help to understand participants' medication behaviors.

Researchers have identified that a collaborative patient–physician relationship aids medication adherence (Schoenthaler, Allegrante, Chaplin, & Ogedegbe, 2012) and the hypertension management process as a whole (Flynn et al., 2013). Within this study, most of the participants portrayed themselves as active agents within their relationships with physicians, and connected their successful control of blood pressure at least partly to a satisfactory, positive relationship with physicians. However, James' story reveals that not all individuals seeks to position themselves as active agents in their relationships with physicians, in that he positioned himself as both preferring to defer medical decisions to his physicians as adherent to his medications. Since the men in this study adhered to their medication despite having different care preferences, this finding cautions against any homogenous understandings of patient needs. Given that Black populations are commonly classified into a homogenous population (Statistics Canada, 2012), even though they migrate from different countries, speak different languages, and maintain different cultures and traditions, this finding is of great significance because it speaks to the importance of varied experiences. Therefore, simply prescribing hypertension programs (Savoca et al., 2013) and treatments (Dasgupta et al., 2014) based on the color of one's black skin overlooks the many differences that individuals belonging to this population possess, and ultimately fails to address the broad spectrum of determinants that affects this population's well-being.

According to the Ottawa Charter for Health Promotion, health promotion is defined as "the process of enabling people to increase control over their health and its determinants, and thereby improve their health" (World Health Organization, 2005, 168). In light of this definition, the findings from this study suggest that discussions concerning health promotion amongst this community of men be equally inclusive of constructs existing at the individual, community, and organizational levels. It can be argued that neglecting any of these constructs fosters a disempowering environment, as it fails to tackle important concerns that affect these individuals' well-being. For instance, by only addressing typical biomedical views that attribute the source and maintenance of this condition to the individual alone, one loses sight of the greater processes (i.e., the social struggles created by racist interactions) that affect these men and the larger visible minority population as a whole. Thus, from a health promotion perspective, this study advocates for investigators, health professionals, and educators to broaden their discussions to be inclusive of the structures that place visible minorities in an inferior position in comparison to their White counterparts when implementing health initiatives or conducting research with this population.

Additionally, pharmacological treatments are considered an important therapy for hypertensive individuals. The men in this study ascribed different meanings to their medication; it shaped how they made sense of their hypertension, and how they subsequently negotiated this condition into their everyday lives. Future research directed at examining how hypertensive individuals make sense of their medication can illuminate whether or not its sometimes disempowering properties affects their blood pressure or even other aspects of their health. Moreover, since participants in this study felt as though the greater proportion of Black men shied away from discussions about health, research focusing on creating empowering environments for this population to discuss their well-being with others may provide useful tools to care providers working with this population.

The findings of the narrative study are bounded within the particular context of the study as well as the particular characteristics of the four participants. For example, all participants were all older Black men who understood their blood pressure as well controlled. Therefore, given that hypertension oftentimes goes unnoticed, and happens to develop at younger age for Black populations (Leenen et al., 2008), future studies concerning these groups of men may provide other useful interpretations of hypertension experiences. Since the men in this study were also of different nationalities, research focusing on the hypertension experiences of Black populations consisting of the same nationality may contribute further insight into specific ethnic disparities that may exist in and amongst different Black populations. In addition, the application of other methodological approaches, such as critical ethnography or participatory methodologies, could add further insight into the ways in which various contextual elements influence how Black men come to understand and negotiate hypertension.

CONCLUSION

The purpose of this investigation was to explore how Black men in Ontario, Canada made sense of their hypertension diagnosis, and how they negotiated this condition into their everyday lives. By situating this study within a CRT framework, we aimed to examine how stories concerning participants' hypertension, and other aspects of their lives, were shaped by power relations embedded within their social, political, and historical contexts. This approach illuminated insights into Black Canadian men's thoughts and understandings, and their experiences that otherwise have been predominately projected through biomedical views.

Though some of the findings concerning this particular group of men's hypertension experiences were demonstrated in previous research, it is important to note that this study contributes to new understandings about how notions of ethnicity and health intersect in Canada. This investigation not only demonstrated how racism affected each of the participants, but also challenged mainstream perceptions of race and the standardization of Black populations into one ethnicity.

ACKNOWLEDGMENTS

This research fulfilled Rob Haile's thesis requirements of the Master of Science in Health and Rehabilitation Sciences program at Western University.

REFERENCES

Beune, E. J., Haafkens, J. A., Agyemang, C., Schuster, J. S., & Willems, D. L. (2008). How Ghanaian, African-Surinamese and Dutch patients perceive and manage antihypertensive drug treatment: A qualitative study. *Journal of Hypertension*, *26*(4), 648–656.

Bokhour, B. G., Cohn, E. S., Cortés, D. E., Solomon, J. L., Fix, G. M., Elwy, A. R., ... Kressin, N. R. (2012). The role of patients' explanatory models and daily-lived experience in hypertension self-management. *Journal of General Internal Medicine*, *27*(12), 1626–1634.

Brondolo, E., Love, E. E., Pencille, M., Schoenthaler, A., & Ogedegbe, G. (2011). Racism and hypertension: A review of the empirical evidence and implications for clinical practice. *American Journal of Hypertension*, *24*(5), 518–529.

Dasgupta, K., Quinn, R. R., Zarnke, K. B., Rabi, D. M., Ravani, P., Daskalopoulou, S. S., ... Tremblay, G. (2014). The 2014 Canadian hypertension education program recommendations for blood pressure measurement, diagnosis, assessment of risk, prevention, and treatment of hypertension. *Canadian Journal of Cardiology*, *30*(5), 485–501.

Delgado, R., & Stefancic, J. (2001). *Critical race theory: An introduction*. New York, NY: NYU Press.

Dolezsar, C. M., McGrath, J. J., Herzig, A. J., & Miller, S. B. (2014). Perceived racial discrimination and hypertension: A comprehensive systematic review. *Health Psychology*, *33*(1), 20.

Dwyer, S. C., & Buckle, J. L. (2009). The space between: On being an insider-outsider in qualitative research. *International Journal of Qualitative Methods*, *8*(1), 54–63.

Flynn, S. J., Ameling, J. M., Hill-Briggs, F., Wolff, J. L., Bone, L. R., Levine, D. M., ... Boulware, L. E. (2013). Facilitators and barriers to hypertension self-management in urban African Americans: Perspectives of patients and family members. *Patient Preference and Adherence*, *7*, 741.

Fox, E. R., Young, J. H., Li, Y., Dreisbach, A. W., Keating, B. J., Musani, S. K., ... Pihur, V. (2011). Association of genetic variation with systolic and diastolic blood pressure among African Americans: The candidate gene association resource study. *Human Molecular Genetics*, *20*(11), 2273–2284.

Friedman, D. B., Thomas, T. L., Owens, O. L., & Hébert, J. R. (2012). It takes two to talk about prostate cancer: A qualitative assessment of African American men's and women's cancer communication practices and recommendations. *American Journal of Men's Health*, *6*(6), 472–484.

Hoyt, C. (2012). The pedagogy of the meaning of racism: Reconciling a discordant discourse. *Social work*, *57*(3), 225–234.

Hull, S., Dreyer, G., Badrick, E., Chesser, A., & Yaqoob, M. M. (2011). The relationship of ethnicity to the prevalence and management of hypertension and associated chronic kidney disease. *BMC Nephrology*, *12*(1), 41–50.

Kaufman, J. S., & Hall, S. A. (2003). The slavery hypertension hypothesis: Dissemination and appeal of a modern race theory. *Epidemiology*, *14*(1), 111–118.

Ladson-Billings, G. (1998). Just what is critical race theory and what's it doing in a nice field like education?. *International Journal of Qualitative Studies in Education*, *11*(1), 7–24.

Lee, K., Mokhtar, H. H., Krauss, S. E., & Ong, B. K. (2014). Hypertensive patients' preferences for complementary and alternative medicine and the influence of these preferences on the adherence to prescribed medication. *Complementary Therapies in Clinical Practice*, *20*(2), 99–105.

Leenen, F. H. H., Dumais, J., McInnis, N. H., Turton, P., Stratychuk, L., Nemeth, K., Lum-Kwong, M. M., & Fodor, G. (2008). Results of the Ontario survey on the prevalence and control of hypertension. *Journal of Canadian Medical Association*, *178*(11), 1441–1449.

Leigh, J. P., & Du, J. (2012). Are low wages risk factors for hypertension? *The European Journal of Public Health*, *22*(6), 854–859.

Lieblich, A., Tuval-Maschiach, R., & Zilber, T. (1998). *Narrative research: Reading analysis and interpretation*. Thousand Oaks, CA: Sage.

Milan, A., & Tran, K. (2004). Blacks in Canada: A long history. *Canadian Social Trends*, *72*, 2–7.

Morrow, S. L. (2005). Quality and trustworthiness in qualitative research in counseling psychology. *Journal of Counseling Psychology*, *52*(2), 250–260.

Parker, L., & Lynn, M. (2002). What's race got to do with it? Critical race theory's conflicts with and connections to qualitative research methodology and epistemology. *Qualitative Inquiry*, *8*(1), 7–22.

Rastogi, S., Johnson, T. D., Hoeffel, E. M., & Drewery Jr, M. P. (2011). *The Black population: 2010*. Retrieved from United States Census Bureau website: http://www.census.gov/prod/cen2010/briefs/c2010br-06.pdf.

Santana, M. C., Raj, A., Decker, M. R., La Marche, A., & Silverman, J. G. (2006). Masculine gender roles associated with increased sexual risk and intimate partner violence perpetration among young adult men. *Journal of Urban Health*, *83*(4), 575–585.

Savoca, M., Oakley, M., Austin, A., Wideman, L., Martinek, T., & Carter, K. (2013). Heart of hypertension project: Development of a community-based prevention program for young African American men. *Progress in Community Health Partnerships: Research, Education, and Action*, *7*(2), 163–169.

Schoenberg, N. E., & Drew, E. M. (2002). Articulating silences: Experiential and biomedical constructions of hypertension symptomatology. *Medical Anthropology Quarterly*, *16*(4), 458–475.

Schoenthaler, A., Allegrante, J. P., Chaplin, W., & Ogedegbe, G. (2012). The effect of patient–provider communication on medication adherence in hypertensive Black patients: Does race concordance matter?. *Annals of Behavioral Medicine*, *43*(3), 372–382.

Sparkes, A. C., & Smith, B. (2008). Narrative constructionist inquiry. In J. A. Holsteim & J. F. Gubrium (Eds.), *Handbook of constructions research* (pp. 295–314). New York, NY: The Guilford Press.

Statistics Canada. (2012). *Classification of visible minority*. Ottawa. Modified on April 22, 2015. Retrieved from http://www.statcan.gc.ca/concepts/definitions/minority01-minorite01a-eng.htm. Accessed on June 17, 2015.

Statistics Canada. (2013). *National household survey (NHS) profile*. 2011 National Household Survey. Statistics Canada Catalogue no. 99-004-XWE, Ottawa. Released September 11, 2013. Retrieved from http://www12.statcan.gc.ca/nhs-enm/2011/dp-pd/prof/index.cfm?Lang=E. Accessed on June 17, 2015.

Sue, D. W. (2013). Race talk: The psychology of racial dialogues. *American Psychologist*, *68*(8), 663.

Walker, R. L., Gee, M. E., Bancej, C., Nolan, R. O., Kaczorowski, J., Joffres, M., ... Campbell, N. R. (2011). Health behaviour advice from health professionals to Canadian adults with hypertension: Results from a national survey. *Canadian Journal of Cardiology*, *27*(4), 446–454.

Wengraf, T. (2001). *Qualitative research interviewing: Biographic narrative and semi-structured methods*. Thousand Oaks, CA: Sage.

Williams, D. R. (1992). Black-white differences in blood pressure: The role of social factors. *Ethnicity and Disease*, *2*, 126–141.

World Health Organization. (2005). The Bangkok Charter for health promotion in a globalized world. *Health Promotion Journal of Australia*, *16*(3), 168–171.

World Health Organization. (2013). *A global brief on hypertension: Silent killer, global public health crisis: World Health Day 2013*. Geneva: World Health Organization.

INFLUENCE OF HEALTHCARE UTILIZATION AND SOCIAL CHARACTERISTICS ON HEALTH OUTCOMES AMONG ELDERLY ASIAN AMERICANS: A STRUCTURAL EQUATION ANALYSIS

Jacob Chao-Lun Huang

ABSTRACT

Since health behaviors of elderly Asian Americans are often underreported, the study, based on the health behavioral model (Andersen's model), was to examine if there is a reciprocal relationship between healthcare utilization and health outcomes, and how social characteristics play their role in this relationship between US-born and foreign-born elderly Asian Americans.

Using structural equation modeling, this research examined the proposed hypotheses which consisted of direct and indirect effects among health outcomes, healthcare utilization and social characteristics, as well as the

Health and Health Care Concerns among Women and Racial and Ethnic Minorities
Research in the Sociology of Health Care, Volume 35, 211–230

ISSN: 0275-4959/doi:10.1108/S0275-495920170000035011

disparities of the effects between US-born and foreign-born elderly Asian Americans (65+). A sample size of elderly Asian Americans was divided into a US-born group (N=1,305) and a foreign-born group (N=4,902) from the National Health Interview Survey (NHIS) 1998–2012. Health outcomes consisted of current health status and health change. Healthcare utilization included general doctor visit, ER, and mental health professional visit. Social characteristics of population included predisposing characteristics (such as age, sex, marital status, and region of residency) and enabling resources (such as education, family size, and family income).

Results from the study indicated that first, there was a reciprocal relationship between health outcomes and healthcare utilization for both groups. Second, predisposing characteristics had a direct effect on health outcomes, and enabling resources had an indirect effect on health outcomes via healthcare utilization. In addition, living in the West had both direct and indirect effects on health outcomes. Third, regarding disparities of the effects between both groups, the US-born elderly are more likely to attain health benefits from healthcare utilization and their social characteristics than the foreign-born. As a result, the interactive relationship between health outcomes, healthcare utilization, and social characteristics, as well as disparities of healthcare outcomes through health utilization and social characteristics for elderly Asian Americans is highlighted.

First, due to the design of NHIS, this research was limited to fully present the needs and more characteristics of elderly Asian Americans. This shows the great need for a large scale, representative study for health behaviors of elderly Asian Americans. Second, in the dataset, the study was limited to explore health behaviors of elderly Asian Americans into each Asian ethnic subgroup. Since the culture of Asian Americans is heterogeneous, it is recommended that future research can explore differences and commonalities of the health behaviors between Asian subgroups. Third, based on the health behavioral model and the design of the dataset, this study was limited to illustrate variations of life experiences between both groups. These differences regarding their needs and desires for healthcare services and health outcomes can become an important foundation for service providers and policy makers to provide appropriate services that improve the quality of the later lives of elderly Asian Americans.

First, the study applied the health behavioral model and proved that the effect of healthcare utilization and social characteristics on health outcomes is greater for the US-born elderly Asian Americans than for the foreign-born. Second, this study confirmed that the healthcare services in US society are still beneficial for the health outcomes of elderly Asian Americans. Third, the study found that when family is used to explain the social behaviors of elderly Asian Americans, researchers need to be more careful to identify various family factors in accordance to its dynamics, such as interpersonal relationship, material supply, and emotional support.

Keywords: Healthcare utilization; Health Behavioral Model; Andersen's model; elderly Asian Americans; structural equation modeling

INTRODUCTION

Despite the elderly being seen as the population that most frequently accesses health services in US society, the health utilization of elderly Asian Americans is often underrepresented. Since aging is associated with increased health risks of functional limitation, chronic diseases as well as potential social disengagement, the effectiveness of healthcare services for health can diverge between US-born and foreign-born elderly Asian Americans.

Compared to other racial minorities in US society, Asian Americans, including their elderly population, are often characterized by their unique immigration experience. This socially constructed perception assumes: First, health of elderly Asian Americans is influenced by culture of origin factors, such as healthy diet habits and lifestyle. This is used to explain why elderly Asian Americans are generally healthy, especially immigrants who are healthier than native/US born (Gomez, Kelsey, Glaser, Lee, & Sidney, 2004; Guo, 2000). On the other hand, the immigration experience affects cultural competency and social assimilation in the US healthcare system due to a lack of English proficiency and knowledge of medication and treatment. That means that elderly immigrant Asian Americans are limited in their ability to access institutional healthcare services for maintaining their health (Choi, 2000; Frisbie, Cho, & Hummer, 2001). Moreover, immigrant elderly are more likely to face these obstacles than those who are US born (Choi, 2000; Gryn & Gambino, 2012; Mui, 2003; Mui, Nguyen, Kang, & Domanski, 2006; Reeves & Bennett, 2004; Vincent & Velkoff, 2010). The divergence between US-born and foreign-born elderly Asian Americans causes a knowledge gap in understanding the effects of health utilization on health between these two groups.

There are three factors that contribute to this knowledge gap. First, many health studies of elderly Asian Americans are either relatively small scaled or regionally conducted. Without a nationwide or a large scaled survey, the results are limited in their ability to depict the general health conditions of this population (Zhang, Snowden, & Su, 1998). Therefore, due to the fragmented information, elderly Asian Americans may receive inadequate services in the US healthcare system (Choi, 2000).

Second, although some research employing qualitative methods is able to explore some underreported factors about health status (Mui, 2003; Mui et al.,

2006), such as family dynamics, researchers tend to study in the foreign-born group who usually are seen as the voiceless in the society. The US-born group that is supposed to be an important reference group in this topic can be easily ignored.

Third, despite the variation in social and cultural characteristics, US-born and foreign-born elderly Asian Americans are often viewed monolithically and treated as one group. Since approximately eighty percent of elderly Asian Americans are foreign-born immigrants, this approach may cause an ecological fallacy in that a higher percentage of foreign-born elderly might determine statistical significance than the US-born group (Gryn & Gambino, 2012). Therefore, the effects of healthcare utilization on health for the US-born elderly might be easily underreported.

Keeping in mind that the culture of origin, in terms of place of birth, is a key indicator for distinguishing the disparities between these two groups (Mui, 2003; Mui et al., 2006), this study aims to reduce the knowledge gap identified above by examining the relationship between health behaviors in the institutional health services and health outcomes among US-born and foreign elderly born Asian Americans. By utilizing a nationwide health survey, we believe the results are found here valuable in helping healthcare professionals, aging service facilitators, and social gerontologists to provide more appropriate and sustainable services for elderly Asian Americans.

PATTERNS OF HEALTHCARE UTILIZATION AND HEALTH OUTCOMES

Regarding the relationship between health behaviors, healthcare utilization, and health outcomes, Andersen's (1968) early works on individuals' ability to access healthcare services as influenced by family composition, social structure, and health beliefs form the conceptual basis for this study. In his conceptual framework, age, sex, family size, ethnicity, and social class are significant indicators of family composition. Family composition illustrates factors related to how individuals are able to use relevant resources, including healthcare services, in society. This original theoretical framework, called the health behavioral model or Andersen's model, viewed social characteristics as determinants in the relationship between healthcare utilization and health outcomes.

Andersen and Newman (1973) indicated that predisposing components (including socio-demographic characteristics and personal health belief) and enabling components (including resources obtained from family and community) can affect the perceived need for accessing institutional health services. That means that the use of healthcare services is not based merely upon health conditions, but also upon the perceived need of the service. In addition, this model is lacking because the relationship between institutional health service utilization and health outcomes is rarely discussed. In contrast, inspired by Andersen's early model, Evans and Stoddart (1990) pointed out that use of formal healthcare services and health outcomes are indeed correlated. With better health, healthcare services are less needed; however, when healthcare services are in high demand, worse health status is expected. In this relationship, perceived health status is key for perceiving a need for healthcare services. On the other hand, use of healthcare services may become an indicator for examining how perceived health status is influenced by a person's social characteristics. Their finding illustrates that there is a dynamic interrelationship between use of healthcare services and health outcomes.

In fact, social characteristics, in terms of daily health practices, such as diet, exercise, and self-care, should not been seen as direct determinants of health outcomes. Instead, these characteristics can be used to examine patterns of healthcare utilization. When healthcare utilization and health outcomes are correlated, social characteristics can affect individuals' ability to access healthcare services, and that in turn can affect health outcomes.

In regard to health outcomes, health status can only indicate current health conditions; however, perceived health change after using healthcare services is another important indicator to examine the effectiveness of healthcare services. Aday et al. (1993) indicated that the effectiveness of healthcare services should be examined through the relationship between health status as well as use of healthcare services. According to the input and output relationship, their model is based upon an assumption that use of healthcare services should be beneficial for health outcomes in terms of both current health status and health change.

Andersen (1995, 2002) revised his prior research and finalized the most recent version of the health behavioral model (see Fig. 1). This model is composed of four components, environment, population characteristics, health behavior, and outcomes. Here it is theorized that health outcomes are affected by environment, predisposing characteristics of population characteristics, as well as health behavior. Health behavior is affected by health outcomes and need of population characteristics. Enabling resources of population characteristics is affected by health outcomes and health behavior. In this model,

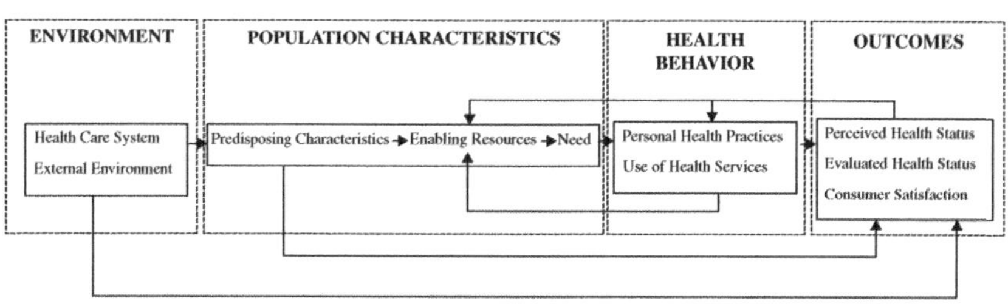

Fig. 1. The Emerging Model of the Health Behavioral Model. *Source*: Anderson (1995, p.8).

relationships between health outcomes, use of health services, and population characteristics are more clearly demonstrated. First, predisposing characteristics of population characteristics can directly indicate health outcomes and health outcomes can also indicate enabling resources of population characteristics. That means that some social demographic characteristics, such as age, gender, marital status, and so on, as predisposing conditions, can be used to predict health outcomes. At the same time, health outcomes can be used as indicators for levels of enabling resources in the healthcare system, such as income. Second, health outcomes can be directly affected by health behaviors in terms of use of healthcare services. Again, at the same time, health outcomes can also affect health behaviors. The relationship between health outcomes and health behaviors is interrelated. Third, population characteristics in terms of predisposing characteristics, enabling resources, and need can affect health behaviors which further impact health outcomes.

When examining the effectiveness of healthcare services, many studies have partially applied this model in order to discover the health outcomes and predisposing social characteristics in various types of healthcare services (Andersen et al., 2002; Bradley et al., 2002; Phillips, Morrison, Andersen, & Aday, 1998). However, Babitsch, Gohl, and von Lengerke (2012) noted that many prior studies that employed the health behavioral model often misplaced use of healthcare services, perceived health status, and evaluated health status, using them as dependent variables instead of the perceived need.

As a result, it is imperative to determine, not only the direction in the relationships between population characteristics, health behavior, and health outcomes, but also to indicate which category has the most impact on the relationships. In addition, prior research was limited in its ability to demonstrate cause and effect relationships as well as the strength of these relationships with the indicator variables that were used. Without employing advanced statistical techniques, the complexity of the conceptual model may not be fully presented. Therefore, to adequately operationalize the variables by adopting advanced statistical analysis is strongly expected (Babitsch et al., 2012).

RESEARCH HYPOTHESIS

Discussions of health and healthcare utilization between US-born and foreign-born Asian Americans diverge. Some researchers noted that immigrant elderly Asian Americans are generally healthier than the US-born due to their lifestyle factors such as a healthy diet (Gomez et al., 2004); meanwhile, other researchers indicated that healthcare utilization seen as a social behavior is beneficial for health outcomes of US-born elderly Asian Americans more than the foreign-born due to having a higher level of cultural and social assimilation in the health system (Choi, 2000; Frisbie et al., 2001; Gryn & Gambino, 2012; Guo,

2000; Mui, 2003; Mui et al., 2006; Reeves & Bennett, 2004; Vincent & Velkoff, 2010). Based on recent research and the health behavioral model, we thus hypothesize that the impact of healthcare utilization on health outcomes for the US-born is positive and greater than for the foreign-born elderly Asian Americans (H_1). On the other hand, regarding the need for healthcare services, with better health status, we also hypothesize that less healthcare utilization is needed for both groups (H_2)

Moreover, social characteristics in terms of predisposing characteristics and enabling resources, which are associated with the ability to access relevant resources, affect health outcomes. Predisposing characteristics such as age, sex, marital status and region of residency can be directly used to predict the tendency of health outcomes. Therefore, we make the following predictions for both groups. With increased age, health outcomes are expected to decline (H_3). Elderly males are more likely to face health risks than elderly females (H_4). Married elderly have better health outcomes than those who are not married (H_5). Considering the region of aging services and resources provided, the elderly living in the West are healthier than those living in other regions (H_6).

Enabling resources, such as education, family size, income, and so on, can affect health outcomes via healthcare utilization. Therefore, the following hypotheses are also for groups. With increased education, better health outcomes are expected by utilizing healthcare services (H_7). With increased size of family, better health outcomes are expected by utilizing healthcare services (H_8). Finally, with increased income, better health outcomes are expected by utilizing healthcare services for both groups (H_9).

DATA

Population

The participants were respondents who self-reported an Asian with an age of 65 or above in the National Health Interview Survey (NHIS) of 1998–2012. NHIS, constructed by the U.S. Census Bureau, the Centers for Disease Control (CDC), and Prevention's National Center for Health Statistics, is used to monitor health status and changes for the general US population. Since the questionnaires and sample design are revised, modified, and updated every 10–15 years, this study used the data from 1998 to 2012, so that the results would be consistently represented. In addition, the dataset is a cross sectional survey, meaning that samples collected in each year can be different. However, in order to overcome the limitation that US-born elderly Asian Americans were often underreported statistically, in this case, samples across years were combined for comparable analysis for both groups.

In the sampling process, 6,261 elderly Asian Americans were selected. The sample was then divided into two groups, 1,359 US born and 4,902 foreign born. In this study, approximately 78.3% of Asian American elderly are foreign born and nearly 21.7% are US born.

Variables and Measurement

Informed by the conceptual framework, there are three categories in this study: health outcomes, healthcare utilization, and social characteristics. First, for the measurement of health outcomes as an unmeasured latent variable, self-reported health status, and health status change compared to last year, are both included. Both of these variables are ordinal variables. Self-reported health status refers to how a respondent self-reported their current health status on a scale from 1 (poor) to 5 (excellent). Health status change indicates how the respondent perceived their health status change compared to last year on a scale from 1 (worse) to 3 (better).

In addition, healthcare utilization as another latent variable has three main indicators. The first indicator is to ask if the respondent has seen/talked to a general doctor in the past 12 months. The second indicator is whether the respondent has seen/talked to any mental health professional in the past 12 months. The last indicator variable is whether the respondent has had any surgery in the past 12 months. The indicator variables of healthcare utilization are dichotomous (0 = no and 1 = yes).

Social characteristic variables, in terms of predisposing characteristics and enabling resources, are considered determinants of health outcomes and healthcare utilization ability. As mentioned above, predisposing characteristics include age, sex, marital status, and region of residency. Age is an interval variable (65–99). Sex is a dichotomous nominal variable with female as the reference category (0 = female, 1 = male). Current marital status is a dichotomous nominal variable with not married as the reference category (0 = not married, 1 = married). Region of residency was also a dichotomous nominal variable and non-West was the reference category (0 = non-West, 1 = West). Enabling resources include education, family size, and combined family income. Education is an ordinal variable scaled from 1 (lower than high school) to 4 (college graduate or higher). Family size is an interval variable scaled from 1 to 30. Combined family income is an ordinal variable on a scale from 1 ($0-$4,999) to 11 ($75,000 and above).

Data Analysis Procedures

Structural equation modeling (SEM) using LISREL 8.70 was used to examine the fit of the hypothesized conceptual model. SEM is the appropriate method because it can evaluate the fit and operate measurement and structural models simultaneously. First, measurement model based on confirmatory factor analysis is to test the degree of indicator variables that can be captured into the essence of unmeasured latent variable(s). Second, the structural model is similar to path analysis in that it presents a causal analysis among variables. When a SEM model is created, the structural coefficients, and the measurement coefficients between all variables, are estimated simultaneously (Meyers, Gamst, & Guarino, 2006). In an established causal model, direct, indirect, as well as total, effects among variables can be presented with statistical significance (Kelloway, 1998).

Furthermore, in a SEM model, all variables can be categorized as endogenous or exogenous variables. Endogenous variables can be predictors and dependent variables at the same time. In this research, two endogenous variables were identified. First, health outcomes as a latent variable was composed of current health status and health status change compared to last year. Second, healthcare utilization was another latent variable which included seen/talked to a general doctor in the past 12 months, seen/talked to a mental health professional in the past 12 months, and having any surgery in the past 12 months. In order to ensure that all these indicators can be appropriately included the latent variable, the factor loading is expected to reach .3 or above.

Each exogenous variable is considered an independent indicator to the endogenous variables. In this research, the social characteristics of the sample, such as sex, marital status, region of residency, education, family size, and combined family income are used to predict health outcomes and healthcare utilization.

For operating a SEM, there are some requirements that researchers should follow. First, in regard to the sample size, the minimum requirement is 200 cases or more, and each parameter must have at least five cases or observations (Kelloway, 1998). Since the initial sample size for the US-born group is 1,359 and the foreign-born group is 4,902, and each parameter needs to have more than five cases, the minimum requirements are therefore met.

Second, based on the maximum likelihood of estimation, both chi-square and p-value are commonly used to evaluate whether the model is a good fit. However, the chi-square value is greatly affected by the sample size. That means that with an increased sample size, the chi-square value is more likely to be generated with statistical bias. Therefore, in order to reduce statistical bias from data with a large sample size, the comparative fit index (CFI) and the root mean square error of approximation (RMSEA) are needed to evaluate the fit of the model. CFI that ranges from 0 to 1 is used to test if the proposed model is a baseline or null model. When the value is close to 0, which means that none of the variables are correlated, and that the latent constructs are meaningless. On the other hand, when the CFI value is closer to 1.0, the model is approaching a good fitting model. RMSEA is used to evaluate the proposed model. When the RMSEA value ranges from .01 to .1, the proposed model can be seen as a good fit to the data (Kelloway, 1998, p. 27).

In order to reduce possible errors of estimation due to the amount of missing values, this research applied single imputation, in which the substituted values for the missing values of measurements of healthcare utilization (such as seen/talked to a general doctor in the past 12 months, seen/talked to a mental health professional in the past 12 months, and having surgery in the past 12 months), are replaced by the predicted value through regression analyses (Allison, 2001). Despite the increased sample size, we found that there is no statistically significant difference between the missing and non-missing groups in regard to the variables selected for this research.

RESULTS

Participants

Table 1 presents the descriptive statistics for the social characteristics variables used in this study. The average age for US-born elderly Asian Americans was 75.74, which was slightly higher than 72.81 for the foreign-born elderly Asian Americans. Regarding the gender distribution, approximate 44.3% of the US-born elderly were males compared to 43.2% of the foreign-born elderly. 56.8% of US-born elderly Asian Americans were married compared to 65.2% of the foreign-born elderly. For region of residency, 81% of the US-born group was living in the West compared to 59.3% of the foreign-born group.

Table 1. Means and Standard Deviations (S.D.) of Social Characteristics Used in the Analysis, US-Born (N = 1,359) and Foreign-born (*N* = 4,902) Elderly Asian Americans.

Variables	Frequency		Mean		S.D.	
	US born	*Foreign born*	*US born*	*Foreign born*	*US born*	*Foreign born*
Social Characteristics						
Age	1,359	4,902	75.74	72.81	6.646	6.141
Sex (Male)	602	2,119	.443	.432	.497	.495
Marital Status (Married)	768	3,173	.568	.652	.496	.477
Region of Residency (the West)	1,106	2,905	.814	.593	.389	.491
Education	1,320	4,540	2.387	2.168	.870	1.122
Family Size	1,359	4,902	2.225	3.113	1.261	1.982
Combined Family Income	1,359	4,902	7.405	6.961	2.845	3.320

Source: The 1998–2012 NHIS.

The average family size of the US-born elderly was 2.2 which was somewhat lower than 3.1 for the foreign-born elderly. Educational attainment in both groups was very similar (US born: 2.387, foreign born: 2.168), indicating that both groups had at an average level of education of at a least high school education. For combined family income, the US-born group fell into the range of $35,000–49,999 per year (US born: 7.4) and the foreign-born group fell into the range of $ 25,000–34,999 per year (foreign born: 6.96). That means that the US-born elderly Asian Americans had a higher combined family income than the foreign born.

Factor Loadings of the Latent Variables

In Table 2, the factor loadings of health outcomes and healthcare utilization among US-born elderly Asian Americans are presented. For the latent variable of health outcomes, both indicators' scores were above .30. This means that both health status and health status changes were appropriate measures of health outcomes in the model. For the latent variable of healthcare utilization, only seeing/talking to a general doctor was above .30. That means that in the US-born group, seeing/talking to a general doctor was the only appropriate measure of healthcare utilization. The factor loadings for seeing/talking to a mental health professional and having surgery were below .30. That means that they were not quite suitable measures of healthcare utilization. However, in this case, for the purposes of fair comparison with the foreign-born group, these variables were still kept in order to construct a compatible model.

In Table 3, the factor loadings of health outcomes and healthcare utilization among foreign-born elderly Asian Americans are presented. For health outcomes, both indicators' factor loadings were above .30. For healthcare utilization, the three indicators' factor loadings were also above .30. That means that

Table 2. Factor Loadings for the Latent Variables for US-Born Elderly Asian Americans ($N = 1{,}359$).

	Unstandardized	(SE)	Standardized	S.D.
Health outcomes				
Health status	.31	.90	.41	.84
Health status change	.16*	.10	.73	.47
Healthcare Utilization				
Seen/talked to a general doctor	.31	.05	.82	.32
Seen/talked to a mental health professional	−.05**	.02	−.31	.90
Having surgery	−.05**	.06	−.20	.96

Source: The 1998–2012 NHIS.
$^{*}p \leq 0.05$, $^{**}p \leq 0.01$, $^{***}p \leq 0.001$ (one-tailed test).

Table 3. Factor Loadings for the Latent Variables for Foreign-Born Elderly Asian Americans ($N = 4{,}902$).

	Unstandardized	(SE)	Standardized	S.D.
Health outcomes				
Health status	.80	.69	.72	.48
Health status change	.18**	.26	.33	.89
Healthcare Utilization				
Seen/talked to a general doctor	.34	.04	.85	.27
Seen/talked to a mental health professional	.04**	.01	.40	.84
Had surgery	.12**	.04	.53	.72

Source: The 1998–2012 NHIS.
$^{*}p \leq 0.05$, $^{**}p \leq 0.01$, $^{***}p \leq 0.001$ (one-tailed test).

seeing/talking to a general doctor, seeing/talking to a mental health professional, and having any surgery are appropriate measures of healthcare utilization in the SEM model.

SEM Models for US-Born and Foreign-Born Elderly Asian Americans

US-Born Elderly Asian Americans

Fig. 2 shows the best model of SEM for the US-born group. In the model, RMSEA was .053 and CFI was .90. Both values noted that statistically the model was a good fitting model. Since the model was a good fit, path coefficients among the predictor variables to health status for the US-born group were considered significant indicators. In the model, there was a reciprocal relationship between health outcomes and healthcare utilization. On one hand, healthcare utilization had a positive effect on health outcomes; on the other hand, health outcomes had a negative effect on healthcare utilization. That means that for US-born elderly Asian Americans, the better their health outcomes were, the less healthcare services were used (−.84). In addition, when the elderly were more likely to use healthcare services, their health outcomes were expected to benefit (.84).

Regarding the standardized effects of the socio-demographic characteristics on health outcomes (see Table 4), age (−.27), being male (−.04), and living in the West (−.04) had a direct negative effect on health outcomes, respectively. However, being married (.19) had a direct positive effect on health outcomes. That means that age, being male, and living in the West were negative factors to health outcomes, while being married was a positive factor to health outcomes.

In addition, as having an indirect effect on health outcomes via healthcare utilization, living in the West, education, family size and combined family

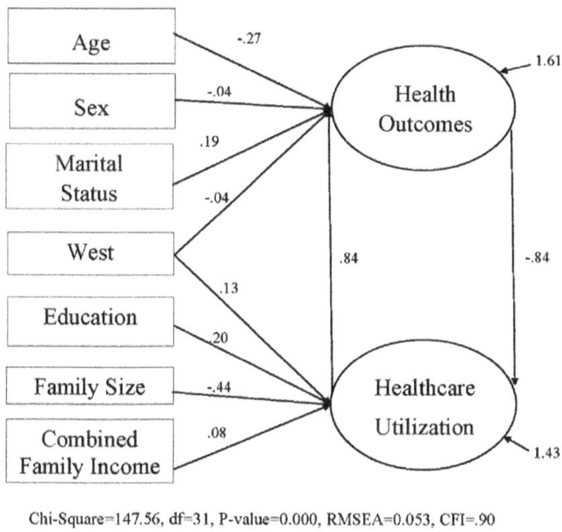

Fig. 2. Healthcare Utilization and Health Outcomes for US-Born Elderly Asian Americans.

Table 4. Decomposition of the Effects of Predictor Variables for Elderly Asian Americans during 1998–2012.

	Direct Effect		Indirect Effect		Total Effect	
	US born	Foreign born	US born	Foreign born	US born	Foreign born
Predictor on healthcare Utilization						
Health Outcomes	–.84	–.41	NA	NA	–.84	–.41
Predictors on health Outcomes						
Healthcare Utilization	.84	.31	NA	NA	.84	.31
Social Characteristics						
Age	–.27	–.29	NS	NS	–.27	–.29
Sex (male)	–.04	.03	NS	NS	–.04	.03
Married	.19	.11	NS	NS	.19	.11
West	–.04	–.09	.11	–.03	.07	–.12
Education	NS	NS	.17	.03	.17	.03
Family Size	NS	NS	–.37	–.09	–.37	–.09
Combined family income	NS	NS	.07	–.01	.07	–.01

Source: The 1998–2012 NHIS.
Note: NA, Not applicable; NS, Not Significant.

income were confirmed. Living in the West had a positive indirect effect on health outcomes via healthcare utilization is positive (.11). Education (.17) and combined family income (.07), respectively, had a slightly positive indirect effect on health outcomes via healthcare utilization. However, family size (−.37) had a negative indirect effect on health outcomes via healthcare utilization.

Foreign-Born Elderly Asian Americans

In the foreign-born group, in Fig. 3, RMSEA (.053) and CFI (.94) also show that the SEM model was a good fitting model. At the same time, the model also indicated that there was a reciprocal relationship between health outcomes and healthcare utilization. Like the US-born group, for foreign-born elderly Asian Americans, when their health outcomes were toward a positive direction, they are less likely to use healthcare services (−.41); while the more they used healthcare services, their health outcomes were also expected to improve (.31).

Age (−.29), being male (.03), married (.11), and living in the West (−.09) had a direct effect on health outcomes, respectively. Age and living in the West had a negative effect on health outcomes. Being male and married have a positive effect on health outcomes. Considering their separate indirect effects on health outcomes via healthcare utilization, living in the West, education, family size and combined family income had an indirect effect. Living in the West (−.03), family size (−.09), and combined family income (−.01), respectively, had an indirect effect on health outcomes via healthcare utilization. Education had a slightly positive indirect effect on health outcomes through healthcare utilization (.03).

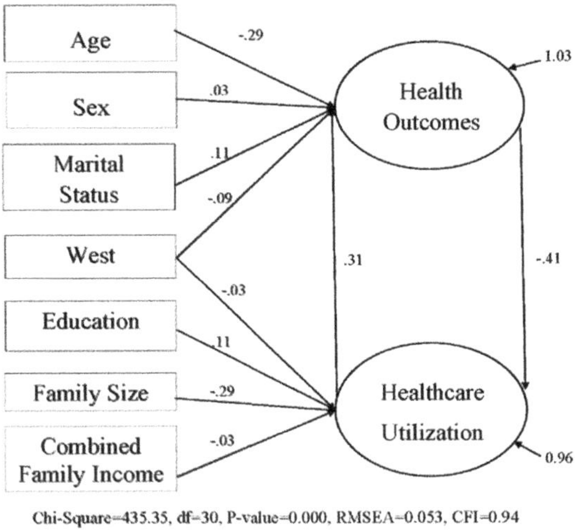

Fig. 3. Healthcare Utilization and Health Outcomes for Foreign-Born Elderly Asian Americans.

US-Born Group versus Foreign-Born Group
When comparing with both groups, as shown in Table 4, healthcare utilization and being married, respectively, had a greater direct positive effect on health outcomes in the US-born group than in the foreign-born group. Moreover, education had a greater positive indirect effect on health outcomes through healthcare utilization for the US born rather than for the foreign born.

Considering the negative effects on health outcomes, age and living in the West, were direct negative effect on health outcomes. In both groups, family size had an indirect negative factor to health outcomes. Last, being male, living in the West, and family income, respectively, had opposite effects on health outcomes between the US-born and the foreign-born groups. However, more research is needed in the future to further discuss the nuances of these variations.

DISCUSSION AND CONCLUSION

Results from this study revealed that there was a reciprocal relationship between health outcomes and healthcare utilization. First, healthcare utilization on health outcomes was effective for elderly Asian Americans. In this relationship, healthcare utilization for the US-born group had a greater positive effect on health outcomes than for the foreign-born group (US born: .84 vs. foreign born: .31). The first hypothesis (H_1) was therefore confirmed. As mentioned above, US-born elderly Asian Americans can receive greater health benefits from accessing healthcare services than can those foreign born due to their greater social and cultural competency in the healthcare system, such as language proficiency and cultural acculturation (Choi, 2000; Frisbie et al., 2001; Gryn & Gambino, 2012; Guo, 2000; Mui, 2003; Mui et al., 2006; Reeves & Bennett, 2004; Vincent & Velkoff, 2010). However, due to the limited design of the dataset, this study was unable to directly discover what kind of specific factors served as obstacles for foreign-born elderly Asian Americans to use healthcare services.

The results also confirmed the second hypothesis (H_2). With better health outcomes, elderly Asian Americans were less likely to use healthcare services (US born: −.84 vs. foreign born: −.41). The result showed that with better health outcomes, healthcare utilization was less. Therefore, for elderly Asian Americans, effective health management for the prevention of health risks can reduce expenditures of healthcare services. Many studies have indicated how elderly Asian Americans, especially the foreign born, maintain their health in good condition by using non-medical ways, such as a healthy diet and daily exercises (Frisbie et al., 2001; Gomez et al., 2004; Guo, 2000). Once aging service facilitators implement the approaches of preventive healthcare into services for elderly Asian Americans, the demand and expenditures of healthcare services will be expected to decline.

In the health behavioral model, Anderson (1995) indicated that the need and the ability for healthcare services is somehow determined by the social characteristics of population in terms of predisposing characteristics and enabling resources. Predisposing characteristics, such as age, sex, marital status, and region of residency, can directly influence health outcomes. The results confirmed that with increased age, health outcomes declined (US born: −.29 vs. foreign born: −.27). The third hypothesis (H_3) was therefore confirmed. The health outcomes of males were worse than those of females in the US-born group (−.04); however, in the foreign-born group, the health outcomes of males were better than those of females (.03). Since there was an opposite effect of sex on health outcomes between the two groups, the forth hypothesis (H_4) was thus rejected. Regarding marital status, married elderly Asian Americans had greater positive health outcomes than those who were not married (US born: .19 vs. foreign born: .11). Thus is the fifth hypothesis (H_5) was confirmed. Since marriage is an important source of social support (Mui & Kang, 2006), elderly Asian Americans can receive more health benefits from being married. For region of residency, both US born and foreign born elderly living in the West had worse health outcomes than those living in other regions (US born: −.04 vs. foreign born: −.09). Nevertheless, for the US born group, impact of living in the West on health outcomes was indirectly positive through healthcare utilization (.11). For the foreign-born group, there was no positive indirect effect of living in the West on health outcomes (−.03). The sixth hypothesis (H_6) was rejected. The result implies that healthcare utilization for US-born elderly Asian Americans living in the West is more beneficial for their health outcomes than for the foreign born living in the same region. That could be because the US-born elderly have a better knowledge of accessing relevant healthcare resources to improve their health outcomes than do those that are foreign born since that tend to be more dependent on non-institutional health services, such as remedies and informal prescriptions. In order to better explore and explain the possible factors within this relationship, more research with an appropriate design is needed in the future.

In addition, enabling resources, such as education, family size, and family income, refer to the resources that the population can use to access healthcare services, which in turn, can improve their health outcomes. For education, an indirect positive effect between education and health outcomes via healthcare utilization in both groups was supported (US born: .17 vs. foreign born: .03). Therefore, the seventh hypothesis (H_7) was confirmed. Since the effect of education was stronger for the health of the US-born group that could be that the US-born group was likely to benefit more from increased education than the health of the foreign-born group. The result can be used to explain that education for the US-born elderly is more beneficial for health outcomes via healthcare utilization than for the foreign-born elderly.

Family size was expected to be another indirect factor in supporting elderly Asian Americans to access healthcare services and in turn, improve their health outcomes. Even though previous research pointed out that family is a factor that offers great support for Asian Americans' health (Bajekal, Blane, Grewal, Karlsen, & Nazroo, 2004; Park, 2011; Ta, Holck, & Gee, 2010; Wong, Yoo, & Stewart, 2005), the result from this study indicated that for elderly Asian American, family size did not improve their health outcomes by accessing healthcare services (US born: −.37 vs. foreign born: −.09). Therefore, the eighth hypothesis (H_8) was rejected. Juang and Alvarez (2010) noted that conflicts and struggles within a family can be harmful for health status. Since there may be a possible interaction of family size and family conflict on health outcomes for the elderly, more research in the future needs to examine this.

Last, in both groups, family income as an indirect factor of improving health outcomes via healthcare utilization only applied to the US-born group, not to the foreign-born group (US born: .07 vs. foreign born: −.01). Although Kakai, Maskarinec, Shumay, Tatsumura, and Tasaki (2003) noted that family income can help Asian Americans have better health outcomes, the result of this study only showed that the US born could receive health benefits from family income which enable access to healthcare services. As a result, the ninth hypothesis (H_9) was partially accepted.

Study Strengths and Limitations

There are several important strengths of this study. Inspired by the health behavioral model (Andersen, 2002), this study sought to illustrate how the causal relationships among health outcomes, healthcare utilization, and social characteristics of population varies between US-born and foreign-born elderly Asian Americans. Previous research indicated that considering different levels of the adherence of their original culture, US-born and foreign-born elderly Asian Americans' behaviors of accessing healthcare services that affect their health outcomes are at different levels (Choi, 2000; Guo, 2000; Mui, 2003; Mui et al., 2006). Based on this acknowledgement, this study tested the proposed hypotheses and demonstrated causal relationships between the three major categories mentioned above. Most importantly, the study examined if the effect of healthcare utilization and social characteristics on health outcomes are greater for the US-born elderly Asian Americans than for the foreign born.

Since Evans and Stoddart (1990) were limited in their ability to fully demonstrate the causal relationships among all variables, this study not only supported that there is a correlation between health outcomes and healthcare utilization, but also noted that the relationship is actually a reciprocal relationship for elderly Asian Americans. For this reason, the causal relationships in the health behavioral model can be further confirmed because health outcomes are a common significant indicator of the effectiveness of healthcare utilization (Aday et al., 1993). Although there were some variations of how healthcare utilization affected health outcomes of both groups, generally, this study proved that the healthcare services in US society are still beneficial for the health outcomes of elderly Asian Americans.

In addition, some prior research examined how predisposing characteristics directly affect health outcomes and how enabling resources can indirectly affect health outcomes via healthcare utilization (Aday et al., 1993; Andersen & Newman, 1973). In this study, it was not surprising to find that predisposing characteristics, such as age, marital status, and region of residency, directly affect health outcomes. However, enabling resources, especially family size, and family income did not indirectly affect health outcomes via healthcare utilization in both groups. In other words, there were variations of family-related factors, such as marital status, family size, and combined family income, on health outcomes between both groups. That means that when family is used to explain the social behaviors of elderly Asian Americans, researchers need to be more careful to identify family factors in accordance to its dynamics, such as interpersonal relationship, material supply, emotional support, and so on. Otherwise, family can be used to overgeneralize factors to the social behaviors of elderly Asian Americans.

Moreover, study limitations and recommendations for future research can be identified. First, since Asian Americans were often underrepresented in many nationwide health surveys, including the NHIS, this study was unable to fully present the needs and characteristics of elderly Asian Americans. Therefore, this shows the great need for a large scale, representative study for health behaviors of elderly Asian Americans.

Second, since this study was limited by the design of NHIS, elderly Asian Americans are the main research subject instead of Asian subgroups. The concept of Asian cannot fully represent its heterogeneous subcultures. Each Asian subgroup has developed its own specific social and historical motivations for immigration, such as fleeing wars, international trade, education, and so on. Based on the demonstration of health behaviors among elderly Asian Americans found in this study, it is recommended that future research that explore differences and commonalities related to the health behaviors among Asian subgroups.

Furthermore, based on the health behavioral model and the design of the dataset, this study was limited in its ability to modify the model by including other indicators which could also be used to present variations of life experiences between both groups. Since US-born and foreign-born elderly Asian Americans have developed life experiences in US society differently, future research should specifically present their needs and desires for healthcare services and health outcomes. These differences can become an important foundation for service providers and policy makers to provide appropriate services that improve the quality of the later lives of elderly Asian Americans.

REFERENCES

Aday, L., Begley, C., Lairson, D., Slater, C., Richard, A., & Montoya, I. (1993). *Evaluating the Medical Care System: Effectiveness, Efficiency, and Equity*. Ann Arbor, MI: Health Administration Press.

Allison, P., (2001). *Missing data*. Thousand Oaks, CA: Sage Publications.

Andersen, R. (1968). *Families' Use of Health Services: A Behavioral Model of Predisposing, Enabling, and Need Components [Dissertation]*. West Lafayette: Purdue University. Available from http://docs.lib.purdue.edu/dissertations/AAI6902884/

Andersen, R. (2002). Expanding the Andersen model: The role of psychosocial factors in Long-Term care use. *Health Services Research*, *37*(5), 1221–1242.

Andersen, R., & Newman, J. (1973). Societal and individual determinants of medical care utilization in the United States. *Milbank Quarterly*, *51*(1), 95–124.

Andersen, R., Yu, H., Wyn, R., Davidson, P., Brown, E., & Teleki, S. (2002). Access to medical care for low-income persons: How do communities make a difference? *Medical Care Research and Review: MCRR*, *59*(4), 384–411.

Andersen, R. (1995). Revisiting the behavioral model and access to medical care: Does it matter? *Journal of Health and Social Behavior*, *36*, 1–10.

Babitsch, B., Gohl, D., & von Lengerke, T. (2012). Re-revisiting Andersen's behavioral model of health services use: A systematic review of studies from 1998–2011. *GMS Psycho-Social-Medicine*, *9*, Doc 11. doi:10.3205/psm000089.

Bajekal, M., Blane, D., Grewal, I., Karlsen, S., & Nazroo, J. (2004). Ethnic differences in influences on quality of life at older ages: A quantitative analysis. *Ageing and Society*, *24*(5), 709–728.

Bradley, E., McGraw, S., Curry, L., Buckser, A., King, K., Kasl, S., & Andersen, R. (2002). Expanding the Andersen model: The role of psychosocial factors in long-term care use. *Health Services Research*, *37*(5): 1221–1242.

Choi, N. (2000). Diversity within diversity: Research and social work practice issues with Asian American elders. *Journal of Human Behavior in the Social Environment*, *3*(3–4), 301–319.

Evans, R., & Stoddart, G. (1990). Producing health, consuming health care. *Social Science & Medicine*, *31*(12), 1347–1363.

Frisbie, W., Cho, Y., & Hummer, R. (2001). Immigration and the health of Asian and Pacific islander adults in the United States. *American Journal of Epidemiology*, *153*(4), 372–380.

Gomez, S., Kelsey, J., Glaser, S., Lee, M., & Sidney, S. (2004). Immigration and acculturation in relation to health and health-related risk factors among specific Asian subgroups in a health maintenance organization. *American Journal of Public Health*, *94* (11), 1977–1984.

Gryn, T., & Gambino, C. (2012). *The Foreign Born from Asia: 2011*. Washington, DC.: U.S. Department of Commerce, Economics and Statistics Administration, U.S. Census Bureau.

Guo, Z. (2000). *Ginseng and Aspirin: Health Care Alternatives for Aging Chinese in New York*. Ithaca, NY: Cornell University Press.

Juang, L., & Alvarez, A. (2010). Discrimination and adjustment among Chinese American adolescents: Family conflict and family cohesion as vulnerability and protective factors. *American Journal of Public Health*, *100*(12), 2403–2409.

Kakai, H., Maskarinec, G., Shumay, D., Tatsumura, Y., & Tasaki, K. (2003). Ethnic differences in choices of health information by cancer patients using complementary and alternative medicine: An exploratory study with correspondence analysis. *Social Science & Medicine*, *56*(4), 851–862.

Kelloway, E. (1998). *Using LISREL for Structural Equation Modeling: A Researcher's Guide*. Thousand Oaks, CA: Sage Publications.

Meyers, L. Gamst, G., & Guarino, A. (2006). *Applied Multivariate Research: Design and Interpretation*. Thousand Oaks, CA: Sage Publications.

Mui, A. (2003). Physical health, mental health, and quality of life. *Asian American elders in New York City: A Study of Health, Social Networks, Quality of Life and Quality of Care* (pp. 30–46). New York, NY: The Asian American Federation of New York.

Mui, A., & Kang, S. (2006). Acculturation stress and depression among Asian immigrant elders. *Social Work*, *51*(3), 243–255.

Mui, A., Nguyen, D., Kang, D., & Domanski, M. (2006). Demographic profiles of Asian immigrant elderly residing in metropolitan ethnic enclave communities. *Journal of Ethnic & Cultural Diversity in Social Work*, *15*(1/2), 193–214.

Park, K. (2011). Asian medicine and holistic aging. *Pastoral Psychology*, *60*(1), 73–83.

Phillips, K., Morrison, K., Andersen, R., & Aday, L. (1998). Understanding the context of healthcare utilization: Assessing environmental and provider-related variables in the behavioral model of utilization. *Health Services Research*, *33*(3 Pt 1), 571–596.

Reeves, T., & Bennett, C. (2004). *We the people: Asians in the United States*. Washington, DC: US Department of Commerce, Economic and Statistics Administration, US Census Bureau.

Ta, V., Holck, P., & Gee, G. (2010). Generational status and family cohesion effects on the receipt of mental health services among Asian Americans: Findings from the national Latino and Asian American study. *American Journal of Public Health*, *100*(1), 115–121. doi:10.2105/AJPH.2009.160762

Vincent, G., & Velkoff, V. (2010). *The next four decades: The older population in the United States: 2010 to 2050*. Washington, DC: US Department of Commerce, Economics and Statistics Administration, US Census Bureau.

Wong, S., Yoo, G., & Stewart, A. (2005). Examining the types of social support and the actual sources of support in older Chinese and Korean immigrants. *The International Journal of Aging and Human Development*, *61*(2), 105–121.

Zhang, A., Snowden, L., & Sue, S. (1998). Differences between Asian and white Americans' help seeking and utilization patterns in the Los Angeles area. *Journal of Community Psychology*, *26*(4), 317–326.

BEHAVIORAL FUNCTIONING AMONG MEXICAN-ORIGIN CHILDREN: THE ROLES OF PARENTAL LEGAL STATUS AND THE NEIGHBORHOOD CONTEXT

Aggie J. Noah and Nancy S. Landale

ABSTRACT

Research on behavioral functioning among Mexican-origin children primarily uses an individual-centered approach that ignores the residential context. In addition, most studies have been unable to consider an important measure of inequality for this population, legal status; and mental health of children with undocumented parents is underexplored. We address these gaps by investigating the influence of parental legal status and neighborhood characteristics on Mexican-origin children's behavioral functioning using a multilevel approach.

We use data from the Los Angeles Family and Neighborhood Study and 2000 decennial census. Our primary focus is variation in internalizing and externalizing behavior problems among Mexican-origin youth ($N = 2{,}535$) with mothers who are undocumented, documented or naturalized citizens, or US-born using multilevel models.

The multilevel results show the importance of considering parental legal status. Mexican children of unauthorized mothers are more likely to exhibit

Health and Health Care Concerns among Women and Racial and Ethnic Minorities
Research in the Sociology of Health Care, Volume 35, 231–248

ISSN: 0275-4959/doi:10.1108/S0275-495920170000035012

internalizing and externalizing problems than all other groups of Mexican children. Furthermore, neighborhood-concentrated disadvantage is significantly associated with internalizing behavior problems, and neighborhood-concentrated affluence is significantly associated with externalizing behavior problems. In short, the results demonstrate the importance of considering both parental legal status and neighborhood contexts for understanding behavior problems of Mexican-origin children.

Our findings suggest that Mexican children's mental health outcomes – measured by internalizing and externalizing behavior problems – vary significantly by parental legal status and neighborhood contexts. This study provides important nuances for public policy for health care prevention and interventions.

Keywords: Legal status; immigrant; behavior problems; neighborhoods

INTRODUCTION

Nearly 10–20% of children experience one or more mental health problems during childhood (World Health Organization, 2001), and mental health problems have been linked to significant reductions in children's quality of life (U. S. Public Health Service, 2000). Children's mental health problems are often conceptualized as falling into two overarching but conceptually intertwined domains (Cosgrove et al., 2011): *internalizing behavior problems* (e.g., depression, anxiety, and somatic problems) that reflect inwardly expressed psychological distress, and *externalizing behavior problems* (e.g., aggression and antisocial behavior) that reflect outwardly directed psychological distress (Xue, Leventhal, Brooks-Gunn, & Earls, 2005). These behavior problems can negatively affect multiple domains of individuals' lives, including school performance and relationships with family and friends. Moreover, individuals with childhood behavior problems are more prone to developing mental disorders in adulthood (Campbell, 1995). Understanding the multiple factors influencing childhood mental health problems is thus important in guiding public policy aimed at prevention and intervention to reduce the likelihood of long-term mental health problems.

Behavior problems in childhood vary by race/ethnicity, class, and gender (Landale, Hardie, Oropesa, & Hillemeier, 2015; Pachter, Auinger, Palmer, & Weitzman, 2006); and understanding why some groups have higher risks of behavior problems is important for reducing mental health disparities. Identifying factors influencing behavior problems among Mexican-origin children is particularly important for several reasons. First, Mexican-origin children represent a large and growing share of US children, particularly children of immigrants (Landale, Thomas, & Van Hook, 2011). Second, children's behavior problems vary by ethnicity, parental nativity, and parental legal status. For example, Mexican-origin children have higher risks of behavior problems than non-Hispanic children (Flores, 2013). Furthermore, Mexican children of immigrants exhibit lower risks of behavior problems than Mexican children of US-born parents (Roosa et al., 2005), and children of undocumented migrants exhibit higher risks of behavior problems than children of documented or naturalized citizens (Landale et al., 2015). Third, Mexican-origin children are disproportionately exposed to contextual-level risk factors because they are more likely to live in disadvantaged neighborhoods than children of most other racial or ethnic groups (Bennett & Lu, 2000; Brooks-Gunn, Duncan, Klebanov, & Sealand, 1993; Deng et al., 2006). Finally, Mexican-origin children have several family-level protective factors that may interact with the neighborhood context to influence behavior problems (Landale, Oropesa, & Noah, 2014; Nair, White, Roosa, & Zeiders, 2013; White & Roosa, 2012).

Most studies of racial/ethnic disparities in behavioral functioning have focused on black and white children or included Latino children as a panethnic group (Pachter et al., 2006), despite the long-standing call for disaggregating Latino subgroups (Bean & Tienda, 1988) and recent interest in heterogeneity within the Mexican-origin population (White, Deardorff, & Gonzales, 2012; White, Roosa, & Zeiders, 2012). We focus on behavior problems among Mexican-origin children relative to children in other racial and ethnic groups, and extend the literature by highlighting two important factors that are often overlooked: parental legal status and neighborhood characteristics. Building on a new study finding that having undocumented parents is associated with significantly higher risks of internalizing and externalizing behavior problems (Landale et al., 2015), we investigate whether the influence of parental legal status remains when controlling for key aspects of children's larger neighborhood contexts.

BACKGROUND

Studies of behavior problems among Mexican-origin children have predominantly emphasized the roles of nativity and acculturation. Previous studies have found that foreign-born Mexican-origin children have a lower risk of behavior problems than their US-born counterparts (Deng et al., 2006; Flores, 2013). In addition, parents' nativity matters: Mexican children of immigrants have a lower risk of behavior problems than Mexican children of US-born parents (Roosa et al., 2005). Similarly, studies have found that higher levels of acculturation are associated with an increased risk of behavior problems (Dinh, Roosa, Tein, & Lopez, 2002; Sullivan et al., 2007).

This individual-centered emphasis on nativity and acculturation ignores important structural and contextual factors that may influence behavioral functioning among Mexican-origin children. Multiple dimensions of inequality at both the individual and contextual levels intersect to influence the outcomes of individuals (Viruell-Fuentes, Miranda, & Abdulrahim, 2012) and these dimensions of inequality – specifically, parental legal status and neighborhood context – must be explicitly accounted for in examining behavior problems among Mexican-origin children (Glick, 2010).

Parental Legal Status and Behavior Problems

In 2011, the United States held an estimated 11.1 million undocumented immigrants, a great majority of whom were from Mexico (Passel & Cohn, 2012). With a large proportion of undocumented migrants in the total immigrant population, legal status has emerged as a critical factor for understanding immigrant incorporation and well-being (Donato & Armenta, 2011; Glick, 2010; Landale et al., 2015; Massey & Bartley, 2005). Studies investigating the influence of legal status on individuals and families are scarce because of data limitations (Bachmeier, Van Hook, & Bean, 2014; Landale et al., 2015), but several studies have documented difficulties associated with undocumented legal status, including living with the threat of deportation, limited access to resources, and marginalization (Yoshikawa & Kholoptseva, 2013). Consequently, undocumented legal status can negatively affect individuals through heightened and chronic stress. Because immigrants in the United States – especially Mexicans – are heterogeneous with respect to legal status, incorporating legal status can help us better understand the different pathways of incorporation.

The reach of parental legal status potentially extends beyond immigrant parents to their children (Landale et al., 2015; Yoshikawa & Kalil, 2011; Yoshikawa & Kholoptseva, 2013). Legal status can affect postmigration contexts, such as neighborhoods. Neighborhood characteristics and interactions, in turn, can shape the everyday experiences of immigrants and their children, thereby influencing children's health and development (Yoshikawa & Kalil, 2011). For example, Landale et al. (2015) found that children of undocumented Mexican migrants have significantly higher risks of internalizing and externalizing behavior problems than their counterparts whose mothers are documented or naturalized citizens. The study, however, considered only one characteristic of neighborhood contexts (i.e., perceived child-centered closure and social control), and the authors recommended further research on the role of neighborhood contexts in conjunction with parental legal status. Thus, we investigate how neighborhood contexts affect the behavioral functioning of Mexican-origin children with different parental legal statuses.

Neighborhood Contexts and Behavior Problems

Since the early 2000s, studies have increasingly incorporated a broader ecological perspective by considering neighborhood factors. Drawing from Bronfenbrenner's ecological framework (1986), which focuses on the multiple contexts in which individuals are embedded, neighborhood characteristics represent important distal factors impacting more proximal individual- and family-level factors. Individuals' behavior problems are the product of individual characteristics and family characteristics, but these attributes can interact with neighborhood characteristics to affect behavior problems. Incorporating neighborhood factors in addition to individual and family factors is important not only conceptually but also empirically in order to avoid specification errors, either from omitted variables bias that exaggerates the effects of included variables or from possible interactions between family and neighborhood characteristics (Burton & Jarrett, 2000; Leventhal & Brooks-Gunn, 2000).

The importance of incorporating neighborhood contexts in the study of children's behavior problems is reflected in the number of multilevel studies in recent decades. These studies have documented that several characteristics of neighborhoods are associated with behavior problems in childhood, including structural characteristics, such as *concentrated disadvantage* (Browning, Soller, Gardner, & Brooks-Gunn, 2013; Caughy, Murray Nettles, & O'Campo, 2008; Lara-Cinisomo, Xue, & Brooks-Gunn, 2013), *concentrated affluence* (Beyers, Bates, Pettit, & Dodge, 2003), and *racial and ethnic composition* (e.g., percentage black and immigrant concentration) (Wickrama & Bryant, 2003); social processes, such as *collective efficacy* (i.e., a form of social organization that combines social cohesion and informal social control) (Katz, Esparza, Carter, Grant, & Meyerson, 2012; Sampson, Raudenbush, & Earls, 1997; Xue et al., 2005); and perceived neighborhood characteristics, such as *perceived safety* and *neighborhood danger* (Callahan, Scaramella, Laird, & Sohr-Preston, 2011). Individual and family characteristics interact with neighborhood characteristics to affect behavior problems through multiple interconnected mechanisms (Foster & Brooks-Gunn, 2013).

Incorporating neighborhood characteristics into research on behavior problems among Mexican-origin children is important for several reasons. First, the characteristics of the neighborhoods in which Mexican children reside may be qualitatively distinct from those of other racial and ethnic groups. For example, high levels of racial segregation can have detrimental effects on behavior problems for African American children (Aneshensel & Sucoff, 1996; Leventhal & Brooks-Gunn, 2000), but ethnic segregation may have salubrious effects on behavior problems for Mexican-origin children if segregation produces concentrated social and structural resources within ethnic enclaves. The evidence suggests that levels of collective efficacy and cultural cohesion are higher in predominantly Mexican and Latino neighborhoods than in non-Latino neighborhoods, even when neighborhoods are socioeconomically disadvantaged (Gonzales et al., 2011; Nair et al., 2013). Second, because of the unique individual and family characteristics of Mexican-origin children, neighborhood characteristics that are pertinent to children's behavior problems may affect these children differently than children of other racial and ethnic groups. For example, Mexican children of recent immigrants may be less aware of some aspects of neighborhood contexts (e.g., the US racial climate) and therefore may be less susceptible to them (Krieger, 2012). Similarly, Mexican children of undocumented immigrant parents may be less likely to spend time outside of their homes owing to fear of deportation, and lower exposure to the neighborhood may translate into little or no neighborhood effects on their behavior problems.

We investigate whether and how neighborhood characteristics are associated with behavior problems among Mexican-origin children with different parental legal statuses. Following the *cultural ecological framework*, which emphasizes that "culture is not only a function of a shared cultural identity (i.e., ethnic group membership), but also is determined by factors such as family socioeconomic status (SES), immigration status, and the types of communities in which individuals settle" (Gonzales et al., 2011, p. 99), we ask, How do parental legal status and neighborhood characteristics conjointly influence behavior problems among Mexican-origin children? We hypothesize that neighborhood characteristics are associated with internalizing and externalizing behaviors among Mexican youths with diverse parental legal statuses through both direct and moderating influences.

METHODS

Individual-level data come from the first wave of the Los Angeles Family and Neighborhood Survey (L.A.FANS), which was conducted in 2000–2002. The L.A.FANS contains a representative sample of all residents in Los Angeles County and is based on stratified random sampling of neighborhoods and households (Sastry, Ghosh-Dastidar, Adams, & Pebley, 2006). In each household, one adult was randomly selected to answer an adult survey questionnaire. In households with children, one child was also randomly selected. A primary caregiver provided information on the selected child and a randomly selected sibling (under age 18) via the child questionnaire. Our analytic sample includes focal children and siblings who were matched to a primary caretaker who completed an adult questionnaire, a parent questionnaire, and a primary caregiver questionnaire ($N = 3{,}122$). We excluded children who were under the age of 3 ($N = 514$) and children whose information on the sample stratification indicator was missing ($N = 66$). In addition, we excluded children of undocumented white and Asian parents ($N = 7$) because their sample sizes are too small. Our final sample includes 2,535 children. The contextual-level data on census tracts are from the 2000 US decennial census (U.S. Census Bureau, 2000).

Measures

Behavioral Functioning

Children's behavioral functioning was measured with the internalizing and externalizing subscales of the Behavior Problems Index (Parcel & Menaghan, 1998). The questions used to construct these measures ask parents whether specific behaviors are often, sometimes, or never true of their child. The *internalizing scale* was drawn from 11 questions indicating sad or withdrawn behaviors, and the *externalizing scale* was drawn from 17 questions indicating aggressive behaviors. The L.A.FANS coded these questions so that higher scores indicate more frequent problematic behaviors; when responses are summed for each subscale, higher numbers indicate more behavior problems (Landale et al., 2015). The internalizing behavior problem scale ranges from 0 to 22, and the externalizing behavior problem scale ranges from 0 to 33.

Parental Legal Status

Parental legal status was estimated from a series of questions asking foreign-born mothers whether they (a) were naturalized citizens, (b) had a "green card" or legal permanent residence, (c) had refugee, asylee, or temporary protected status, or (d) had a valid visa for temporary residence in the United States. Using the residual method, foreign-born mothers who did not have one of these statuses were coded as undocumented immigrants. Bachmeier et al. (2014) demonstrated that the estimates and profile of undocumented immigrants from these procedures in the L.A.FANS are consistent with estimates drawn from other sources. Using information on parental legal status, race/ethnicity, and nativity, we created 12 categories: Mexican undocumented migrant (the reference group), Mexican naturalized or documented immigrant, Mexican US-born, other Latino undocumented, other Latino naturalized or documented, other Latino US-born, white naturalized or documented, white US-born, black naturalized or documented, black US-born, Asian naturalized or documented, and Asian US-born.

Other Child and Family Characteristics

Two child characteristics included in the models are *gender* (coded 1 if female and 0 if male) and *age* (a continuous variable ranging from 3 to 17 years). Five maternal and family characteristics are included. *Mother's education* is coded as 1 if she had less than a high school education (0 otherwise). *Maternal depression* is a dichotomous variable constructed from the Composite International Diagnostic Interview Short-Form (CIDI-SF) depression inventory. The CIDI-SF indicates the probability that a respondent would meet the criteria for major depression if she were given the full CIDI interview. Maternal depression was coded as 1 if the mother's probability of depression was greater than 0.5. In addition to maternal characteristics, we included a dichotomous variable for *single parent* to measure family structure and two family characteristic variables. *Family poverty* is a dichotomous variable derived from the federal poverty thresholds (coded as 1 if family income was below the 2001 poverty threshold). *Family routine* was constructed from questions about the number of days per week that four activities occurred at a regular time: children's breakfast, family dinner, household chores, and children's bedtime.

Neighborhood Structural Characteristics

We considered four structural characteristics of neighborhoods. *Concentrated disadvantage* and *concentrated affluence* measure the socioeconomic characteristics of neighborhoods (Browning et al., 2013; Sampson et al., 1997). We used a factor analysis of 10 variables obtained from the 2000 census and confirmed the emergence of two factors, which we then used to create regression-weighted scales measuring the socioeconomic characteristics of the neighborhood. *Concentrated disadvantage* includes the percentages of individuals below the poverty line, on public assistance, unemployed, less than age 18, and black; and the percentage of households that are female-headed. *Concentrated affluence* includes the log of per capital income; the percentage of individuals with at least a bachelor's degree; the percentage in professional, administrative, or managerial positions; and the percentage of families with an annual income greater than $75,000. *Immigrant concentration* is measured from the percentage Latino and the percentage foreign-born. *Residential stability* is measured from the percentage living in the same location in 1995 and the percentage of owner-occupied housing.

Neighborhood Social Characteristic

Collective efficacy refers to the combination of trust and cohesion among neighborhood residents that allows for social control (Sampson et al., 1997). Following previous research (Sampson et al., 1997), our measure of collective efficacy is based on the mothers' level of agreement with statements about whether (a) the neighborhood is close-knit, (b) people are willing to help neighbors, (c) neighbors generally get along, (d) people in the neighborhood share the same values, (e) people in the neighborhood can be trusted, (f) neighbors would intervene if children were hanging out, (g) neighbors would intervene if children were spray-painting graffiti on a building, and (h) neighbors would intervene if children were showing disrespect to an adult. Each question was measured on a scale ranging from 1 to 5, and some questions were reverse-coded so that higher values represent greater collective efficacy. We used a regression-weighted method to create the scale (Sampson, Morenoff, & Gannon-Rowley, 2002; Sampson et al., 1997).

Analytic Strategy

Although the contextual data had no missing values, a small percentage of individual-level data had missing values (1.1%). We used the mean imputation method to account for missing data (Allison, 2002). We estimated a series of multilevel logistic regression models. Because the underlying assumption of complete independence among individual observations in ordinary least squares estimates is not applicable to our hypotheses, we used hierarchical linear models to incorporate a different error term in the model intercept (Raudenbush & Bryk, 2002). We first assessed whether multilevel modeling is an appropriate analytic strategy by testing null models with no explanatory variables. The null models have statistically significant variance of the intercept, which indicates that multilevel modeling is appropriate for this study.

RESULTS

Descriptive Statistics

Table 1 includes the weighted descriptive statistics for all measures included in the analyses by the mothers' race/ethnicity. Mexican-origin children have the highest mean score (3.5) for the internalizing index, and white children have the lowest mean score (2.1). In contrast, Mexican-origin children are somewhat similar to white children in terms of externalizing behavior (6.8 and 6.2, respectively), and black children have the highest mean score (7.4). However, Mexican children have significantly higher mean scores on the externalizing index than other Latino children (6.0) and Asian children (5.1).

Maternal and family characteristics differ significantly by race/ethnicity. Mother's immigration status varies substantially, with nearly 30% of Mexican-origin children but only 16% of other Latino children having undocumented mothers. Overall, compared with white children and black children, Mexican-origin, other Latino, and Asian children are substantially more likely to have foreign-born mothers. Mexican-origin children are more likely to have a mother with less than a high school education (61%) than are children of any other race/ethnicity. They are also more likely than other children to live in a poor family (51%), although other Latino children are also very likely to be poor (48%). High shares of Mexican-origin children (40%) and other Latino children (52%) live in single-parent households, although the percentages are significantly lower than that for black children (83%). Despite the

Table 1. Descriptive Statistics by Race and Ethnicity.

	Total	Mexican	Other Latino	White	Black	Asian
Behavior Problems Index						
Internalizing index	2.95	3.51	3.37	2.11	2.79	2.17
Externalizing index	6.45	6.85	5.99	6.25	7.41	5.13
Child Characteristics						
Female (%)	49.56	50.38	50.38	47.88	48.97	49.53
Age	9.67	9.36	9.47	10.10	9.91	10.02
Mother/Family Characteristics						
Mother's Immigration Status						
Undocumented (%)	13.59	29.42	16.00	0.00	0.00	0.00
Naturalized or documented (%)	42.52	48.84	63.50	17.53	8.78	76.55
US-born (%)	43.89	23.74	20.51	82.47	91.22	23.45
Mother's low education (%)	35.95	60.96	43.46	6.86	19.19	9.33
Poor family (%)	41.90	50.56	47.83	29.98	37.54	31.19
Single parent (%)	41.54	39.59	51.70	29.03	82.73	24.58
Maternal depression (%)	14.05	12.43	19.77	15.63	16.96	6.69
Family routine	20.16	20.20	20.05	20.43	19.20	20.45
Neighborhood Characteristics						
Concentrated disadvantage	0.49	0.76	0.68	−0.09	1.06	−0.04
Concentrated affluence	−0.45	−0.85	−0.75	0.28	−0.60	0.33
Immigrant concentration	0.86	1.38	1.39	−0.04	0.67	0.34
Residential stability	−0.18	−0.38	−0.46	0.25	−0.34	0.15
Collective efficacy	26.78	26.50	26.51	27.53	26.31	27.01
Unweighted *N*	2535	1217	397	506	212	213

Source: Los Angeles Family and Neighborhood Survey; 2000 Census.
Note: Analysis is based on weighted data.

socioeconomic disadvantage of Mexican-origin families, Mexican-origin children are less likely to have a depressed mother (12%) than children in all other racial/ethnic groups except Asians (7%). The presence of family routines does not differ by race/ethnicity.

Black children and Mexican-origin children are more likely to reside in neighborhoods with high concentrated disadvantage and low concentrated affluence, whereas white children and Asian children are more likely to reside in neighborhoods with low concentrated disadvantage and high concentrated affluence. Mexican-origin children and other Latino children live in neighborhoods that are similar. Both groups reside in neighborhoods with high immigrant concentrations, relative to children of any other race/ethnicity. Interestingly, neighborhood immigrant concentration is relatively low for both

Asian and white children. Thus, black children reside in neighborhoods with higher immigrant concentrations than Asian children. Levels of collective efficacy are similar across racial/ethnic groups.

Hierarchical Linear Model Results

The results in Table 2 demonstrate the associations between neighborhood characteristics and internalizing behavior problems for children of all racial/ethnic and legal status groups. Overall, the intercept-only null models (i.e., variance components intercepts) show that a large proportion of the variance in internalizing behavior (nearly 17%) is between neighborhoods. However, the variance components decrease when we control for several maternal and family characteristics, demonstrating the importance of accounting for both family and neighborhood contexts. The variance component intercepts for all models are statistically significant, confirming that using the multilevel models is appropriate (Raudenbush & Bryk, 2002).

Because the results for individual-level variables are consistent across models, we discuss the results from the full model (Model 3). Mexican children of undocumented mothers have significantly higher rates of internalizing behavior problems than all other children except other Latino children with undocumented mothers and black children of naturalized or documented mothers. These relationships hold when we control for child, mother, and family characteristics. Children with a mother who did not complete high school, those in a single-parent household, and children with depressed mothers have higher rates of internalizing behavior problems than others. In contrast, living in a family that maintains a daily routine is associated with lower levels of internalizing behavior problems.

As is shown in Table 3, Mexican children of undocumented mothers also have significantly higher rates of externalizing behavior problems than all other children. Importantly, Mexican children with undocumented mothers are more likely to have externalizing problems than their coethnic counterparts with naturalized/documented or US-born mothers. This pattern holds across all three models. In addition, female children and older children are less likely than male children or younger children to exhibit externalizing problems. Among the maternal and family characteristics, family structure, maternal depression, and family routines are significantly associated with externalizing behavior in the full model.

Although the intercept-only null models demonstrate that neighborhood characteristics can explain a large proportion of the variance in Mexican-origin children's internalizing and externalizing behaviors, neighborhood characteristics have relatively weak associations with behavior problems compared with parental legal status. Concentrated disadvantage is significantly associated with

Table 2. HLM Analysis of Children's Internalizing Behavior Problems.

Variable	Model 1	Model 2	Model 3
Ethnicity/Mother's Immigration Status ($N = 2{,}535$)			
Mexican undocumented	(Ref)	(Ref)	(Ref)
Mexican naturalized/documented	−0.93***	−0.92***	−0.89***
Mexican US born	−2.00***	−2.00***	−1.91***
Other Latino undocumented	−0.34	−0.34	−0.45
Other Latino naturalized/documented	−0.65*	−0.65*	−0.64*
Other Latino US born	−1.97***	−1.97***	−1.88***
White naturalized/documented	−2.13***	−2.13***	−1.86***
White US born	−1.66***	−1.66***	−1.51***
Black naturalized/documented	−0.92	−0.92	−1.12
Black US born	−1.55***	−1.55***	−1.65***
Asian naturalized/documented	−1.57***	−1.57***	−1.17***
Asian US born	−2.18***	−2.18***	−2.00***
Child Characteristics			
Female (%)		0.03	0.04
Age		−0.01	−0.03+
Mother/Family Characteristics			
Mother's low education (%)			0.43*
Poor family (%)			0.22
Single parent (%)			0.32*
Maternal depression (%)			1.53***
Family routine			−0.04***
Neighborhood Characteristics ($N = 90$)			
Concentrated disadvantage	0.21*	0.25*	0.18+
Concentrated affluence	−0.25+	−0.19	−0.17
Immigrant concentration	0.16	0.25+	0.12
Residential stability	0.3	0.04	0.03
Collective efficacy	−0.01	−0.01	−0.01
Variance Components	0.168	0.167	0.135

Source: Los Angeles Family and Neighborhood Survey; 2000 Census.
Note: Analysis is based on weighted data.
$+p < 0.10$, $^{*}p < 0.05$, $^{**}p < 0.01$, $^{***}p < 0.001$ (two-tailed tests).

higher rates of internalizing behavior, but the association is attenuated when mother and family characteristics are controlled. This direct association between neighborhood concentrated disadvantage and internalizing behavior problems indicates that children residing in more disadvantaged neighborhoods are about 20% more likely to exhibit internalizing behavior problems. In

Table 3. HLM Analysis of Children's Externalizing Behavior Problems.

Variable	Model 1	Model 2	Model 3
Ethnicity/Mother's Immigration Status ($N = 2{,}535$)			
Mexican undocumented	(Ref)	(Ref)	(Ref)
Mexican naturalized/documented	−1.40***	−1.32***	−1.37***
Mexican US born	−1.23**	−1.23**	−1.36**
Other Latino undocumented	−1.20	−1.28 +	−1.56*
Other Latino naturalized/documented	−1.36**	−1.32**	−1.43**
Other Latino US born	−1.59*	−1.50*	−1.57*
White naturalized/documented	−2.44**	−2.31**	−1.90**
White US born	−0.13	−0.08	−0.01
Black naturalized/documented	−1.31	−1.34	−1.98 +
Black US born	−0.33	−0.38	−0.14
Asian naturalized/documented	−2.42***	−2.39***	−1.85***
Asian US born	−0.40	−0.34	−0.22
Child Characteristics			
Female (%)		−0.78***	−0.77***
Age		−0.06*	−0.11***
Mother/Family Characteristics			
Mother's low education (%)			0.55
Poor family (%)			0.07
Single parent (%)			0.71*
Maternal depression (%)			2.51***
Family routine			−0.13***
Neighborhood Characteristics ($N = 90$)			
Concentrated disadvantage	−0.15	−0.15	−0.15
Concentrated affluence	−0.97***	−0.97***	−0.80***
Immigrant concentration	−0.18	−0.18	−0.19
Residential stability	−0.15	−0.15	−0.13
Collective efficacy	−0.05 +	−0.05*	−0.05 +
Variance Components	0.271	0.262	0.172

Source: Los Angeles Family and Neighborhood Survey; 2000 Census.
Note: Analysis is based on weighted data.
$+ p < 0.10$, $*p < 0.05$, $**p < 0.01$, $***p < 0.001$ (two-tailed tests).

contrast, concentrated affluence is significantly associated with lower rates of externalizing behavior. Children living in neighborhoods with higher levels of neighborhood affluence are less likely to exhibit externalizing behavior problems than those in less advantaged neighborhoods. Collective efficacy is also significantly associated with lower rates of externalizing behavior problems.

In addition to testing the direct association between neighborhood characteristics and internalizing and externalizing behavior problems, we tested whether neighborhood characteristics moderate the associations between parental legal status and behavior problems. We tested two-way cross-level interactions for both internalizing and externalizing behavior problems, following the recommendations from previous studies (Aguinis, Gottfredson, & Culpepper, 2013); no significant interactions emerged for either outcome. We also tested three-way interactions to determine whether moderating associations may be contingent on gender, but we did not find any significant interactions.

DISCUSSION AND CONCLUSION

Mental health problems have been identified as a major negative influence on the current and future well-being of children in the United States (U.S. Public Health Service, 2000). Often conceptualized as internalizing and externalizing behavior problems, mental health problems vary by race/ethnicity and are products of distal and proximal factors at multiple levels (Bronfenbrenner, 1986). In this study, we moved beyond the individual-centered approach to incorporate an important dimension of structural inequality: neighborhood characteristics. Using a cultural ecological framework that highlights the roles of nativity, legal status, and the context of reception in immigrant outcomes, we investigated whether and how neighborhood characteristics are associated with behavior problems among Mexican-origin children with different parental legal statuses.

Similar to previous research (Landale et al., 2015), we found that Mexican children of undocumented mothers have significantly higher rates of internalizing and externalizing behavior problems than do Mexican children of documented mothers. The former group is more likely to have a mother with less than high school education, to live in poverty, and to live in a single-parent household than the latter. Thus, differences in children's behavior problems are in part compositional. Furthermore, higher rates of behavior problems for Mexican children of undocumented mothers may be partially attributable to family disadvantages that we have not been able to consider here rather than to parental legal status per se. Determination of the causal relationship between parental legal status and children's behavior problems must be left to future studies using a longitudinal approach.

Our results demonstrate that extending the individual-centered approach is important for understanding children's behavior problems. Specifically, the intercept-only null models show that neighborhood characteristics explain a relatively large proportion of the variance in children's internalizing and externalizing behaviors even after we control for key individual and family characteristics. This is a particularly important finding: it suggests that an individual-centered approach that ignores the neighborhood context may cause serious specification errors from omitted variables bias, exaggerating the effects of included variables (Burton & Jarrett, 2000; Leventhal & Brooks-Gunn, 2000). Results for the direct association of neighborhood characteristics with behavior problems suggest that different neighborhood characteristics matter for internalizing and externalizing behavior problems. A high level of neighborhood concentrated disadvantage is significantly associated with higher rates of internalizing behavior problems (Browning et al., 2013; Caughy et al. 2008; Lara-Cinisomo et al., 2013). In contrast, neighborhood concentrated affluence is significantly associated with lower rates of externalizing behavior (Beyers et al., 2003).

Our study has some limitations. Because the data utilized in this study are cross-sectional, a causal relationship between neighborhood characteristics and behavior problems could not be established. Future studies should utilize longitudinal data and methods to better assess causality and to elucidate specific mechanisms through which neighborhoods matter for children's behavioral functioning. Additionally, several individual-level measures that may be associated with behavior problems among Mexican-origin children were not considered here because of data constraints. For example, peer networks (e.g., the number of delinquent peers in children's peer networks) may play an important role in understanding the mechanisms through which neighborhood characteristics influence behavior problems, especially among adolescents. Future studies should investigate how the attributes of peer networks are associated with neighborhood characteristics and behavior problems among Mexican-origin children.

The results of our study contribute to the literature on Mexican-origin youth in three ways. First, our study confirms that parental legal status plays an important role in the outcomes of children of immigrants even when we take neighborhood contexts into account. Our results demonstrate the importance of incorporating parental legal status, in addition to nativity and acculturation, in examining outcomes for Mexican-origin children. A great deal of heterogeneity can be found within children of immigrants by parental legal status, and future studies should be more cautious about the differences among children of immigrants. Second, our results show that it is important to move beyond the individual-centered approach to consider the characteristics of children's residential contexts. Finally, in highlighting the importance of parental legal status and place in Mexican-origin children's behavior problems, our results have implications for designing more effective public policies.

ACKNOWLEDGMENTS

We would like to acknowledge assistance from the Eunice Kennedy Shriver National Institute of Child Health and Human Development (NICHD) (R24

HD041025-11). We would also like to acknowledge funding from the NICHD Predoctoral Training Program (T-32HD007514).

REFERENCES

Aguinis, H., Gottfredson, R. K., & Culpepper, S. A. (2013). Best-practice recommendations for estimating cross-level interaction effects using multilevel modeling. *Journal of Management*, *39*, 1490–1528.

Allison, P. D. (2002). *Missing data series: Quantitative applications in the social sciences*. Thousand Oaks, CA: Sage.

Aneshensel, C. S., & Sucoff, C. A. (1996). The neighborhood context of adolescent mental health. *Journal of Health & Social Behavior*, *37*(4), 293–310.

Bachmeier, J. D., Van Hook, J., & Bean, F. D. (2014). Can we measure immigrants' legal status? Lessons from two US surveys. *International Migration Review*, *48*(2), 538–566.

Bean, F. D., & Tienda, M. (1988). *The Hispanic population of the United States*. New York, NY: Russell Sage Foundation.

Bennett, N. G., & Lu, H.-H. (2000). *Child poverty in the states: Levels and trends from 1979 to 1998*. New York, NY: National Center for Children in Poverty.

Beyers, J. M., Bates, J. E., Pettit, G. S., & Dodge, K. A. (2003). Neighborhood structure, parenting processes, and the development of youths' externalizing behaviors: A multilevel analysis. *American Journal of Community Psychology*, *31*(1–2), 35–53.

Bronfenbrenner, U. (1986). Ecology of the family as a context for human development. research perspectives. *Developmental Psychology*, *22*(6), 723–742.

Brooks-Gunn, J., Duncan, G. J., Klebanov, P. K., & Sealand, N. (1993). do neighborhoods influence child and adolescent development? *American Journal of Sociology*, *99*(2), 353.

Browning, C. R., Soller, B., Gardner, M., & Brooks-Gunn, J. (2013). "Feeling disorder" as a comparative and contingent process: Gender, neighborhood conditions, and adolescent mental health. *Journal of Health & Social Behavior*, *54*(3), 296–314. doi:10.1177/0022146513498510

Burton, L. M., & Jarrett, R. L. (2000). In the mix, yet on the margins: The place of families in urban neighborhood and child development research. *Journal of Marriage & Family*, *62*(4), 1114–1135. doi:10.1111/j.1741-3737.2000.01114.x

Callahan, K. L., Scaramella, L. V., Laird, R. D., & Sohr-Preston, S. L. (2011). Neighborhood disadvantage as a moderator of the association between harsh parenting and toddler-aged children's internalizing and externalizing problems. *Journal of Family Psychology*, *25*(1), 68–76.

Campbell, S. B. (1995). Behavior problems in preschool children: A review of recent research. *Journal of child Psychology and Psychiatry*, *36*(1), 113–149.

Caughy, M. O. B., Murray Nettles, S., & O'Campo, P. J. (2008). The effect of residential neighborhood on child behavior problems in first grade. *American Journal of Community Psychology*, *42*(1/2), 39–50. doi:10.1007/s10464-008-9185-9

Cosgrove, V. E., Rhee, S. H., Gelhorn, H. L., Boeldt, D., Corley, R. C., Ehringer, M. A., ... Hewitt, J. K. (2011). Structure and etiology of co-occurring internalizing and externalizing disorders in adolescents. *Journal of Abnormal Child Psychology*, *39*(1), 109–123.

Deng, S., Lopez, V., Roosa, M. W., Ryu, E., Burrell, G. L., Tein, J. Y., & Crowder, S. (2006). Family processes mediating the relationship of neighborhood disadvantage to early adolescent internalizing problems. *Journal of Early Adolescence*, *26*(2), 206–231.

Dinh, K. T., Roosa, M. W., Tein, J. Y., & Lopez, V. A. (2002). The relationship between acculturation and problem behavior proneness in a hispanic youth sample: A longitudinal mediation model. *Journal of Abnormal Child Psychology*, *30*(3), 295–309.

Donato, K. M., & Armenta, A. (2011). What we know about unauthorized migration. *Annual Review of Sociology*, *37*, 529–543.

Flores, Y. G. (2013). *Chicana and Chicano mental health*. Tucson, AZ: University of Arizona Press.

Foster, H., & Brooks-Gunn, J. (2013). Neighborhood Influences on antisocial behavior during childhood and adolescence. In C. L. Gibson & M. D. Krohn (Eds.), *Handbook of life-course criminology* (pp. 69–90). New York, NY: Springer.

Glick, J. E. (2010). Connecting complex processes: A decade of research on immigrant families. *Journal of Marriage and Family*, *72*(3), 498–515.

Gonzales, N. A., Coxe, S., Roosa, M. W., White, R. M. B., Knight, G. P., Zeiders, K. H., & Saenz, D. (2011). Economic hardship, neighborhood context, and parenting: Prospective effects on Mexican-American adolescent's mental health. *American Journal of Community Psychology*, *47*(1/2), 98–113. doi:10.1007/s10464-010-9366-1

Katz, B. N., Esparza, P., Carter, J. S., Grant, K. E., & Meyerson, D. A. (2012). Intervening processes in the relationship between neighborhood characteristics and psychological symptoms in urban youth. *Journal of Early Adolescence*, *32*(5), 650–680.

Krieger, N. (2012). Methods for the scientific study of discrimination and health: An ecosocial approach. *American Journal of Public Health*, *102*(5), 936–944.

Landale, N. S., Hardie, J. H., Oropesa, R. S., & Hillemeier, M. M. (2015). Behavioral functioning among Mexican-origin children: Does parental legal status matter? *Journal of Health & Social Behavior*, *56*(1), 2–18.

Landale, N. S., Oropesa, R., & Noah, A. J. (2014). Immigration and the family circumstances of Mexican-origin children: A binational longitudinal analysis. *Journal of Marriage and Family*, *76*(1), 24–36.

Landale, N. S., Thomas, K. J., & Van Hook, J. (2011). The living arrangements of children of immigrants. *The Future of Children*, *21*(1), 43.

Lara-Cinisomo, S., Xue, Y., & Brooks-Gunn, J. (2013). Latino youth's internalising behaviours: Links to immigrant status and neighbourhood characteristics. *Ethnicity and Health*, *18*(3), 315–335.

Leventhal, T., & Brooks-Gunn, J. (2000). The neighborhoods they live in: The effects of neighborhood residence on child and adolescent outcomes. *Psychological Bulletin*, *126*(2), 309–337.

Massey, D. S., & Bartley, K. (2005). The changing legal status distribution of immigrants: A caution. *International Migration Review*, *39*(2), 469–484.

Nair, R. L., White, R. M. B., Roosa, M. W., & Zeiders, K. H. (2013). Cultural stressors and mental health symptoms among Mexican Americans: A prospective study examining the impact of the family and neighborhood context. *Journal of Youth and Adolescence*, *42*(10), 1611–1623.

Pachter, L. M., Auinger, P., Palmer, R., & Weitzman, M. (2006). Do parenting and the home environment, maternal depression, neighborhood, and chronic poverty affect child behavioral problems differently in different racial-ethnic groups? *Pediatrics*, *117*(4), 1329–1338.

Parcel, T. L., & Menaghan, E. G. (1998). Measuring behavior problems in a large cross-sectional survey: Reliability and validity for children of the NLS youth. Retrieved from http://www.nlsinfo.org/site/childya/nlsdocs/otherdocs/other/ParcelMenaghanBPI1988.pdf. Accessed on September 19, 2014.

Passel, J., & Cohn, D. (2012). *Unauthorized immigrants: 11.1 million in 2011*. Washington, DC: Pew Hispanic Center.

Raudenbush, S. W., & Bryk, A. S. (2002). *Hierarchical linear models: Applications and data analysis methods* (Vol. 2). Thousand Oaks, CA: Sage Publications.

Roosa, M. W., Deng, S., Ryu, E., Lockhart Burrell, G., Tein, J.-Y., Jones, S., ... Crowder, S. (2005). Family and child characteristics linking neighborhood context and child externalizing behavior. *Journal of Marriage and Family*, *67*(2), 515–529.

Sampson, R. J., Morenoff, J. D., & Gannon-Rowley, T. (2002). Assessing "neighborhood effects": Social processes and new directions in research. *Annual Review of Sociology*, *28*, 443–478.

Sampson, R. J., Raudenbush, S. W., & Earls, F. (1997). Neighborhoods and violent crime: A multilevel study of collective efficacy. *Science*, *277*(5328), 918–924.

Sastry, N., Ghosh-Dastidar, B., Adams, J., & Pebley, A. R. (2006). The design of a multilevel survey of children, families, and communities: The Los Angeles family and neighborhood survey. *Social Science Research*, *35*(4), 1000–1024. doi:10.1016/j.ssresearch.2005.08.002

Sullivan, S., Schwartz, S. J., Prado, G., Shi, H., Pantin, H., & Szapocznik, J. (2007). A bidimensional model of acculturation for examining differences in family functioning and behavior problems in hispanic immigrant adolescents. *Journal of Early Adolescence*, *27*(4), 405–430.

U.S. Census Bureau. (2000). *2000 Census*.

U.S. Public Health Service. (2000). *Report of the surgeon general's conference on children's mental health: A national action agenda*. Washington, DC: Department of Health and Human Services.

Viruell-Fuentes, E. A., Miranda, P. Y., & Abdulrahim, S. (2012). More than culture: Structural racism, intersectionality theory, and immigrant health. *Social Science & Medicine*, *75*(12), 2099–2106.

White, R. M. B., Deardorff, J., & Gonzales, N. A. (2012). Contextual amplification or attenuation of pubertal timing effects on depressive symptoms among Mexican American girls. *Journal of Adolescent Health*, *50*(6), 565–571.

White, R. M. B., & Roosa, M. W. (2012). Neighborhood contexts, fathers, and Mexican American young adolescents' internalizing symptoms. *Journal of Marriage and Family*, *74*(1), 152–166.

White, R. M. B., Roosa, M. W., & Zeiders, K. H. (2012). Neighborhood and family intersections: Prospective implications for Mexican American adolescents' mental health. *Journal of Family Psychology*, *26*(5), 793–804.

Wickrama, K. A. S., & Bryant, C. M. (2003). Community context of social resources and adolescent mental health. *Journal of Marriage and Family*, *65*(4), 850–866.

World Health Organization. (2001). *The World health report 2001: Mental health: New understanding, new hope*. Geneva, Switzerland: WHO.

Xue, Y., Leventhal, T., Brooks-Gunn, J., & Earls, F. J. (2005). Neighborhood residence and mental health problems of 5- to 11-year-olds. *Archives of General Psychiatry*, *62*(5), 554–563.

Yoshikawa, H., & Kalil, A. (2011). The effects of parental undocumented status on the developmental contexts of young children in immigrant families. *Child Development Perspectives*, *5*(4), 291–297.

Yoshikawa, H., & Kholoptseva, J. (2013). *Unauthorized immigrant parents and their children's development: A summary of the evidence*. Washington, DC: Migration Policy Institute.

DO YOU WANT TO SEE A DOCTOR FOR THAT? CONTEXTUALIZING RACIAL AND ETHNIC DIFFERENCES IN CARE-SEEKING

Emily Walton and Denise L. Anthony

ABSTRACT

Racial and ethnic minorities utilize less healthcare than their similarly situated white counterparts in the United States, resulting in speculation that these actions may stem in part from less desire for care. In order to adequately understand the role of care-seeking for racial and ethnic disparities in healthcare, we must fully and systematically consider the complex set of social factors that influence healthcare seeking and use.

Data for this study come from a 2005 national survey of community-dwelling Medicare beneficiaries (N = 2,138). We examine racial and ethnic variation in intentions to seek care, grounding our analyses in the behavioral model of healthcare utilization. Our analysis consists of a series of nested multivariate logistic regression models that follow the sequencing of the behavioral model while including additional social factors.

We find that Latino, Black, and Native American older adults express greater preferences for seeking healthcare compared to whites. Worrying about one's health, having skepticism toward doctors in general, and living in a small city rather than a Metropolitan Area, but not health need, socioeconomic status, or healthcare system characteristics, explain some of the racial

Health and Health Care Concerns among Women and Racial and Ethnic Minorities
Research in the Sociology of Health Care, Volume 35, 249–278

ISSN: 0275-4959/doi:10.1108/S0275-495920170000035013

and ethnic variation in care-seeking preferences. Overall, we show that even after comprehensively accounting for factors known to influence disparities in utilization, elderly racial and ethnic minorities express greater desire to seek care than whites.

We suggest that future research examine social factors such as unmeasured wealth differences, cultural frameworks, and role identities in healthcare interactions in order to understand differences in care-seeking and, importantly, the relationship between care-seeking and disparities in utilization.

This study represents a systematic analysis of the ways individual, social, and structural context may account for racial and ethnic differences in seeking medical care. We build on healthcare seeking literature by including more comprehensive measures of social relationships, healthcare and system-level characteristics, and exploring a wide variety of health beliefs and expectations. Further, our study investigates care seeking among multiple understudied racial and ethnic groups. We find that racial and ethnic minorities are more likely to say they would seek healthcare than whites, suggesting that guidelines promoting the elicitation and understanding of patient preferences in the context of the clinical interaction is an important step toward reducing utilization disparities. These findings also underscore the notion that health policy should go further to address the broader social factors relating to care-seeking in the first place.

Keywords: Race and ethnicity; care-seeking; health care utilization; health care disparities

Health and healthcare disparities play a large role in racial and ethnic inequality in American society. While we know that access to and use of medical services are important to health outcomes, we also know that racial and ethnic minorities use less healthcare than whites (Smedley, Stith, & Nelson, 2003), including both preventive services (Armstrong, Micco, Carney, Stopfer, & Putt, 2005; Hebert, Frick, Kane, & Marshall McBean, 2005; Schenck, Klabunde, & Davis, 2006) and intensive medical interventions (Epstein et al., 2003; Skinner, Weinstein, Sporer, & Wennberg, 2003). Structural factors, such as the distribution of insurance, health system characteristics, and socioeconomic status differentials are associated with racial and ethnic disparities in healthcare utilization (Fiscella, Franks, Gold, & Clancy, 2000; LaVeist, Keith, & Gutierrez, 1995; Smedley et al., 2003). In addition to these structural factors, sociologists and social epidemiologists have examined the ways that social context – that is, "pervasive social influences beyond the characteristics of an illness"

(Boyer & Lutfey, 2019, p. S81) – can both facilitate and inhibit care seeking (Mojtabai, Olfson, & Mechanic, 2002; Pescosolido, 1992; Pescosolido, Wright, Alegría, & Vera, 1998). For example, health beliefs, expectations about treatment effectiveness, and predispositions to seek care sometimes vary across race and ethnicity (Armstrong et al., 2005; Hebert et al., 2005; Schenck et al., 2006; Schnittker, 2003; Schnittker, Freese, & Powell, 2000).

This line of reasoning suggests that differences in utilization may exist in part because racial and ethnic minorities seek care differently than whites. For example, African Americans are less likely to have a usual source of care than are whites, which may cause them to seek care less regularly (Lillie-Blanton, Martinez, & Salganicoff, 2001; Phillips, Mayer, & Aday, 2000). Some evidence demonstrates that racial and ethnic minorities are more likely to refuse recommended services (Sedlis et al., 1997), and less likely to seek testing and medical intervention than whites (Ayanian, Cleary, Weissman, & Epstein, 1999; Martins, Ukoumunne, Banks, Raine, & Hamilton, 2015). In contrast, others find evidence that minorities are no less predisposed to seek care (Schnittker, Pescosolido, & Croghan, 2005) and, if anything, express preferences for seeking more care than whites (Barnato, Anthony, Skinner, Gallagher, & Fisher, 2009; Diala et al., 2001; Schnittker et al., 2005). For example, Schnittker et al. (2005) found few racial differences in expressed likelihood of seeking care in response to hypothetical health needs as defined in the SF-12, a set of generic measures of health "needs" (Ware, Keller, & Kosinski, 1998), and in two cases African Americans were more likely than whites to say they would seek care. Similarly, Barnato et al. (2009) find that racial and ethnic minority elders are more likely to want end-of-life care and treatment interventions even after adjusting for a variety of sociocultural factors.

Despite conflicting evidence about racial and ethnic differences in care-seeking and continued debate about the role of patient preferences, health beliefs, and expectations in care seeking (Pescosolido & Boyer, 1999), medical practice guidelines incorporate patient preferences into recommendations. In fact, the idea comprises part of the recent interest in "shared decision making" as a way to reduce health disparities (Katz, 2001), by encouraging clinicians and patients to establish a partnership as they share preferences and negotiate treatment decisions together (Elwyn et al., 2012; Kaplan, 1999). Yet, sociological work suggests that care-seeking is "a socially embedded process, tied not only to the decision-making of individuals...but also to the communities in which they live and the people who surround them in their daily lives and in the treatment system" (Pescosolido & Boyer, 1999, p. 404). Though various models of healthcare seeking have been proposed that take into account a comprehensive range of "socially embedded" factors (Pescosolido & Boyer, 1999) including socioeconomic and demographic factors, health system characteristics, health beliefs, and social relationships, few have been able to empirically examine all within one model across multiple racial and ethnic groups. Indeed, Schnittker et al. (2005) call for more rigorous comparative research on healthcare seeking to explore a wider variety of preferences, beliefs and expectations, and to expand to multiple racial and ethnic groups beyond African Americans and whites.

We take up this call in this study, and address some of the limitations of prior research by using data from a nationally representative sample of Medicare beneficiaries that over-samples minority populations to examine racial and ethnic differences in predispositions for seeking care. A sample of elderly (over 65 years of age) Medicare beneficiaries is an advantage in that it is a population with high levels of need for and use of healthcare services, but without variation in health insurance status. Our study also advances the field because it includes a set of explanatory variables situated in the Behavioral Model of healthcare (Aday & Andersen, 1974), arguably the most comprehensive model available to understand factors related to the use of health services. The Behavioral Model is innovative because it includes not just measures of health need, but also recognizes that individuals are embedded in social and economic contexts that influence the healthcare they receive, thus the model also includes multiple measures of predisposing and enabling factors related to the use of healthcare. While the Behavioral Model was developed initially in a sociological context, it has been used almost exclusively by health economists, health services, and healthcare utilization researchers (Andersen, 1995). Our study answers the call to build on the Behavioral Model (Pescosolido & Kronenfeld, 1995) by including alternative measures of social relationships (Umberson, Crosnoe, & Reczek, 2010) and health beliefs (Schnittker et al., 2005), as well as healthcare and system-level characteristics (Andersen, 1995).

BACKGROUND

Race and Ethnic Differences in Care Seeking

Compared to their white counterparts, racial and ethnic minorities in the United States experience illness earlier in life (Bibbins-Domingo et al., 2009; Geronimus, Hicken, Keene, & Bound, 2006), have more severe expressions of disease (Cronin et al., 2012), and die at younger ages (Levine et al., 2001; Williams, 2012). Decades of sociological and demographic research have demonstrated that inequalities in social factors – such as socioeconomic resources (Hayward, Crimmins, Miles, & Yang, 2000), structural and interpersonal discrimination (Gee & Ford, 2011; Williams & Mohammed, 2009), and stress exposure (Sternthal, Slopen, & Williams, 2011) – contribute to racial and ethnic disparities in disease burden throughout the life course (Shuey & Willson, 2008).

Individuals from different racial and ethnic groups may exhibit dissimilar preferences for medical treatments and seeking healthcare, but as we discuss earlier, the findings are inconsistent. While most empirical investigations of care-seeking focus on Black/white disparities, we broaden our examination of racial and ethnic minorities to include African Americans, Latinos, Native Americans, and whites. Based on theoretical and empirically demonstrated factors, we expect that these groups may differ from each other in their predispositions for seeking healthcare for a number of reasons. First, there are group differences in mistrust of the healthcare system; in particular, a legacy of distrust exists among African Americans due to a history of unethical experimentation by medical researchers, such as in the (in)famous Tuskegee Syphilis Study (Freimuth et al., 2001). Second, there may also be group specific differences in English language proficiency that influence preferences for healthcare; limited English proficiency may be a particularly salient issue among Latinos, contributing to worse overall health status and lower access to healthcare (DuBard & Gizlice, 2008). Third, Native Americans occupy a distinctive position relative to other racial and ethnic minority groups in their interaction with the healthcare system; as citizens of sovereign, yet dependent, tribal nations, Native Americans often encounter cultural and power asymmetries in healthcare interactions that reflect their complicated history with colonialism and the US government (Gone, 2007). Finally, relative to individuals belonging to racial and ethnic minority groups, whites are more likely to be both culturally aligned to the healthcare system (Shim, 2010) and racially aligned with their particular providers (LaVeist, Nuru-Jeter, & Jones, 2003). We do not posit directions of difference, but argue that these global experiences with the healthcare system and specific interactions with providers may influence group-level differences in, and preferences for, seeking care.

The Behavioral Model

Our investigation is grounded in the idea that racial and ethnic differences in care-seeking are related to a broad set of social factors that also affect healthcare utilization. Like utilization, care-seeking is interdependent with the individual, social and healthcare context in which an individual lives, therefore factors that account for differences in utilization may also largely account for any differences in care-seeking. To investigate care-seeking, we use the framework of the Behavioral Model of healthcare utilization (Aday & Andersen, 1974; Andersen, 1995), which incorporates individual demographic characteristics, as well as social factors pertaining to health need, predisposing, and enabling characteristics. We also build on the original behavioral model by including measures of social relationships, health beliefs, healthcare, and system-level characteristics, proposing that this comprehensive set of factors will explain variation in care-seeking preferences, such that any racial and ethnic differences will disappear once the Behavioral Model variables are incorporated.

Demographic Characteristics

Our models must account for basic demographic characteristics, such as gender and age, which are clearly related to healthcare utilization. Overall, women use more healthcare than men (Bertakis, Azari, Helms, Callahan, & Robbins, 2000), a reflection of both sex differences and gender influences (Anspach, 2010). As people age, they are disproportionate users of healthcare compared to their younger counterparts; this increase is largely due to greater health need but may also reflect overuse (Korenstein, Falk, Howell, Bishop, & Keyhani, 2012). Yet, there is also evidence of underuse of necessary care among elderly African Americans (Asch, Sloss, Hogan, Brook, & Kravitz, 2000). We are particularly interested in understanding the ways racial and ethnic differences in care-seeking may play a part in these disparities in healthcare that emerge or are maintained in older adulthood.

Health Need Characteristics

Theoretically, if one is or perceives oneself to be sick, then one will seek healthcare. Given the higher morbidity and mortality rates among many racial and ethnic minorities (Bibbins-Domingo et al., 2009; Cronin et al., 2012; Levine et al., 2001), we should expect much higher rates of healthcare utilization. Adjusting for health need, however, does not eliminate the healthcare utilization disparity among African Americans and Latinos compared to whites (Fiscella, Franks, Doescher, & Saver, 2002), indicating that the perceived or objective need for healthcare is but one of many factors predicting utilization. Indeed, nearly 50 years ago, medical sociologists showed that physical symptoms or pain appeared to explain little about whether or when patients actually seek care (Suchman, 1965; Zola, 1973 [1967]). We therefore include health need as a dimension of care seeking, but focus the bulk of our substantive inquiry on other socially determined factors.

Predisposing Characteristics

Socioeconomic Status (SES). A substantial proportion of socioeconomic effects on healthcare utilization occur because of lack of health insurance, a serious barrier to accessing care that is also related to race and ethnicity (LaVeist et al., 1995), but the effects of having low income often remain even after accounting for insurance status (Lum & Chang, 1998). Even among older adults covered by Medicare, for example, researchers observe racial and ethnic disparities in healthcare utilization (Dunlop, Manheim, Song, & Chang, 2002). Because our study focuses on universally insured Medicare beneficiaries, we emphasize feelings of financial strain when seeking healthcare, which has been shown to account for some of the racial disparities in healthcare use among Medicare beneficiaries (Gornick, 2003).

Educational attainment, another integral component of SES, consistently demonstrates robust positive associations with health (Adler & Newman, 2002; Lynch, 2003) and is differentially distributed among racial and ethnic groups in the United States (United States Census Bureau, 2013). LaVeist et al. (1995) find that increasing education influences healthcare utilization more strongly among African Americans compared to whites. While the association between education and health status has been well-documented, the overall association of education with healthcare seeking or utilization is not consistent (de Boer, Wijker, & de Haes, 1997; Mutchler & Burr, 1991; Schnittker et al., 2000).

Social Factors

Social Relationships. The social factors we consider include both the absence and presence of social relationships. Socially isolated individuals are at a greater risk of poor health (Seeman, 1996), and may be unable to utilize health services because they are unaware of available resources (Bauer, Rodriguez, Quiroga, & Flores-Ortiz, 2000; Coulton & Frost, 1982). The presence and quality of social relationships, both intimate ties and attachments to organizations, can influence health through social control over health-related habits and behaviors, including seeking care (Umberson et al., 2010). Maintaining connections with family and friends may increase social support related to care-seeking and utilization, such as instrumental assistance with attending medical appointments and adherence to treatment regimens (DiMatteo, 2004). In addition, influence from family members may be associated with differences in preferences for care seeking (Griffith, Allen, & Gunter, 2011). Social relationships with organizations, particularly religious involvement, could affect care seeking by providing contact with larger social networks of like-minded individuals who can assist with instrumental tasks or by fostering a sense of community that motivate individuals to take care of their health needs (Ellison & Levin, 1998).

Health Beliefs and Attitudes. A growing line of scholarship has examined the role of skepticism toward medical care in producing differences in care-seeking. Skepticism is doubt about the ability of conventional medical care to improve health status and is associated with uniformly lower utilization (Fiscella, Franks, & Clancy, 1998). Pescosolido et al. (2001) show that there is growing skepticism toward physicians among Americans' in general, and racial and ethnic minorities generally place even less value on healthcare than do whites (Born, Greiner, Sylvia, Butler, & Ahluwalia, 2004; Schnittker, 2004). These differences may not be due to intrinsic negative attitudes or ideologies about medical practice, but rather to systematic differences in clinical experiences with providers (Diala et al., 2000; Schnittker et al., 2005), or beliefs about the efficacy of medications and treatment (Barnato et al., 2009; Schnittker, 2003).

Health-related worry represents another attitudinal dimension of care-seeking. Research has shown that those who are more worried about their health in general are more likely to use healthcare (Wolinsky & Johnson, 1991). In some regards, health-related worry is protective of health in that it is associated with an increase in preventive health behavior (McCaul, Schroeder, & Reid, 1996). On the other hand, much of the research on health-related worry is concerned with its association with the overuse of healthcare, particularly among racial and ethnic minorities (Mangione-Smith et al., 2004). There do appear to be race differences in the effects of health-related worry; while it is an important motivator of preventive health behaviors such as increasing exercise and improving eating habits among Blacks, it is not related to the initiation of healthy behaviors among whites (Ransford, 1986).

Enabling Characteristics

Micro-Level Patient-Provider Relationship. Having a "usual source of care" and having "unmet need for care" are important factors related to healthcare seeking, access and use. Individuals who have established a regular, ongoing relationship with either a health service facility or an individual provider are more likely to seek and use healthcare regardless of health insurance (DeVoe, Fryer, Phillips, & Green, 2003). However, whites are significantly more likely to have a usual source of care than all other racial and ethnic groups, particularly Latinos (Phillips et al., 2000). A related concept is unmet need for care, broadly defined as the difference between the health services that are deemed necessary and those that are actually received (Levesque et al., 2008). Individuals may report unmet need for care because of access, financial, or insurance barriers (Diamant et al., 2004), and unmet need is disproportionately distributed among Blacks and Latinos (Ngui & Flores, 2007). Failing to receive healthcare when it is needed may lead to the exacerbation of health problems, requiring more invasive and expensive care later (Long, King, & Coughlin, 2005). Finally, overall quality of care is associated with utilization, but racial and ethnic minorities are more likely to receive and perceive lower quality care (Baicker, Chandra, Skinner, & Wennberg, 2004; Sorkin, Ngo-Metzger, & Alba, 2010), leading to the speculation that they may also seek care less often because of resignation to the perceived status quo (Katz, 2001).

Macro-Structural Healthcare Context. Care-seeking may also be affected by physician supply and the geographic context of the overall healthcare system. Though we might expect that a greater concentration of physicians in a local area to be associated with better quality of care and superior health outcomes, this is often not the case (Goodman & Grumbach, 2008; Nyweide, Anthony, Chang, & Goodman, 2011). While objective indicators demonstrate that rural residents experience fewer options for primary care, longer wait times for routine care, longer travel distances for services, and higher rates of physician turnover compared to urban residents, rural residents tend to subjectively evaluate their access to healthcare more positively than their urban counterparts (Haggerty et al., 2007). Beyond rural/urban differences, the socioeconomically and racially stratified nature of our cities affects access to and use of healthcare. Because we lack national coordination of healthcare in the United States, the result is often a patchwork of healthcare facilities and services driven by mechanisms at the local level (Archibald & Rankin, 2013; Robert, 1999). The clustering of African Americans and Latinos in socioeconomically deprived neighborhoods with weak or nonexistent healthcare infrastructure (Williams & Collins, 2001), then, is related to less healthcare among members of these groups (Gaskin, Dinwiddie, Chan, & McCleary, 2012).

THE CURRENT STUDY

Racial and ethnic minorities utilize less healthcare than their similarly situated white counterparts in the United States, resulting in speculation that these actions may stem in part from less desire for care. In order to adequately understand the role of care-seeking for racial and ethnic disparities in healthcare, we must be sure to fully and systematically consider the complex set of social factors that influence healthcare seeking and use. Previous studies on predispositions for seeking care have suffered from data limitations and lack of an integrative framework for evaluating the multiple social determinants of care seeking. Using a nationally representative survey of Medicare beneficiaries, we ground our analyses in the behavioral model of healthcare utilization (Aday & Andersen, 1974), which considers health-related need, predisposing and enabling characteristics, and in addition examine social factors, like social relationships and health attitudes, that matter for care-seeking. We ask how well this model accounts for racial and ethnic variation in stated preferences for seeking care with the following research questions:

1. What is the nature of racial and ethnic differences in care-seeking preferences?
2. Do social determinants of care-seeking (defined as need, predisposing, and enabling characteristics, plus social relationships and health beliefs/attitudes) account for apparent racial and ethnic differences in stated intentions to seek care?

DATA AND METHODS

Data for this study come from a national survey of community-dwelling Medicare beneficiaries conducted in 2005, the Causes and Consequences of Health Care Intensity Patient Survey. Medicare beneficiaries are an important population for examining racial and ethnic differences in preferences for care because they use a large proportion of the total healthcare in the US and there is excellent representation among many racial and ethnic groups in this population. Survey respondents are drawn from the eligible pool of community-dwelling Medicare beneficiaries from 2003 – a complete random sample and an oversample of African Americans ($N = 2{,}847$). A more complete description of the survey methods can be found elsewhere (Barnato et al., 2009). In the current study, we limit the survey sample to individuals who identify with the racial and ethnic groups included in our study and had complete responses on all of our study variables, resulting in a final sample of $n = 2{,}138$ individuals.

Measures

Outcome Variables. We analyze two outcome variables representing respondents' stated preferences for visiting a doctor and seeing a specialist in the scenario of a lingering cough after an episode of the flu. We chose the condition of cough because it corresponds to basic care seeking; use of a minor health condition can more likely capture underlying predispositions for care-seeking, rather than patient's knowledge about the effectiveness or the perception of risk related to medical treatment for a more serious condition. Preferences for *seeking a doctor visit* come from the question, "Suppose you had the flu and after the other symptoms were gone, you still had a severe cough. If the cough lasted 2 days after your flu seemed to be over, would you be more likely to go see a doctor or wait longer to see if the cough went away?", and were coded as 1 = prefer to visit and 0 = prefer to wait. Preferences for *seeking a specialist referral* come from the question, "If s/he said you probably did not need to see a lung specialist, but you could if you wanted to, would you be more likely to go see a specialist or not to see the specialist?" and were coded as 1 = seek specialist referral and 0 = prefer not to seek a specialist referral.

Race and Ethnicity. We assessed race and ethnicity based on two separate survey questions. Latino ethnicity is determined from the question, "Are you of Hispanic or Latino origin or descent?" Another question measured race, "[In addition to being Hispanic or Latino] What is your race? Please choose one or more of the following: [white, Black, Asian, Native Hawaiian/Pacific Islander, American Indian/Alaska Native (heretofore Native American), and Other (specify)]" We excluded individuals identifying as Asian, Native Hawaiian/Pacific Islander, and Other from our analyses due to small sample sizes. For the other categories, we used the following priority scheme to categorize each individual into one racial or ethnic group. First, if a respondent identified as Black, they were categorized as Black, regardless of other categories chosen. We made this decision based on the social salience of blackness in the United States' racial context and the historically significant rule of hypodescent, or the automatic assignment of a mixed-race person to the Black category (Hollinger, 2003). Following the argument that Latinos in the United States are also subject to strong pan-ethnic racialization (Rumbaut, 2009), if an individual identified as Latino and any other race aside from Black, we categorized them as Latino. Similarly, if a respondent identified as Native American and white, we categorized them as Native American. Finally, individuals identifying as only white and non-Hispanic were categorized as white.

Health Need and Demographics. Self-rated health comes from the question, "In general, how would you rate your overall health?" Responses were collapsed into a dichotomous variable, where 1 = excellent, very good, or good health, and 0 = fair or poor health (reference category). Self-rated mental health comes from the question, "In general, how would you rate your overall mental or emotional health?" Responses were collapsed into a dichotomous variable, where 1 = excellent, very good, or good mental health, and 0 = fair or poor mental health (reference category). We also include a variable representing whether the respondent *has a medical condition*, coming from a combination of two questions, "Do you have any physical or medical conditions that often cause you pain or discomfort?" and, "Do any of your doctors know about this?" Responses were combined and coded as 1 = has a doctor-confirmed medical condition, and 0 = does not have a medical condition (reference category). Finally, we also control for *survey mode* in this section by including dummy variables referring to completion of the survey by telephone or mail (reference category). We dichotomize the *age* variable into 0 = 65–74 years old (reference category), and 1 = 75 years or older. We dichotomize *gender* into 1 = male and 0 = female (reference category).

Predisposing Characteristics. The *importance of finances in medical care decisions* comes from the question, "How important are financial issues for you when you decide whether or not to get any medical care?" We collapse the categorical responses into a dichotomous variable representing 1 = finances are very important, important, or somewhat important, and 0 = finances are not important (reference category). We represent the respondent's highest level of *educational attainment* in categories, where 1 = 0–11 years, 2 = 12 years (reference category), 3 = 13–15 years, and 4 = 16 or more years.

Social Factors. We measure *daily family or friend contact* from a combination of two questions assessing the frequency of personal contact with friends and family members who do not live with the respondent. Each question's response categories include daily, weekly, monthly, less often, and never; we collapsed the responses from these two questions into a dichotomous variable representing 1 = daily contact with either family or friend, and 0 = less than daily contact with family or friend (reference category). Finally, the variable representing *at least weekly church or social activities* comes from a combination of two questions. The first asks, "About how often do you attend church, synagogue, or mosque?" and the second asks, "About how often do you attend social or community groups or activities?" We combine the questions and collapse the response categories to create a dichotomous variable representing 1 = at least weekly attendance at church or social activities, and 0 = less than weekly attendance (reference category). The variable called *worries about health* represents responses to the question, "Are you someone who worries about health more than other people your age?" We dichotomized the responses into 1 = worries about health and 0 = doesn't worry about health (reference category). *Avoids the doctor* represents responses to the question, "Are you someone who tries to avoid going to the doctor?" It is coded as 1 = avoids the doctor, and 0 = does not avoid the doctor (reference category).

Enabling Characteristics. The variable *usual source of care* comes from the question, "Your personal doctor is the one you would see if you need a check-up, want advice about a health problem, or get sick or hurt. Do you have a personal doctor?" We coded the responses as 1 = has a usual source of care, and 0 = does not have a usual source of care (reference category). We measured *quality of care* from a question asking respondents to rate their healthcare from the last 12 months from all doctors and other healthcare providers on a scale from 0 (worse possible care) to 10 (best possible care). We dichotomized responses into 1 = high quality (rating of 8–10), 0 = low quality (rating of 0–7). Finally, *unmet desire for care* represented responses to two questions, "In the last 12 months, was there any medical care, tests, or treatment you wanted, but didn't get?" and, "In the last 12 months, was there ever a time when you wanted to see a specialist and didn't?" If the respondent answered yes to either question, they were coded as 1 = unmet desire for care, and if they did not, they were coded as 0 = no unmet desire for care (reference category). We include measures of *geographic area* based on the Census Rural-Urban Commuting Area (RUCA) codes, coding the respondent's area as 1 = Metropolitan area (core urban area of at least 50,000 residents), 2 = Micropolitan area (core urban area with 10,000–49,999 residents), 3 = Small town (2,500–9,999 residents), and 4 = Isolated rural (fewer than 2,500 residents). Finally, we categorize the *number of primary care providers* (PCPs) per capita in the respondent's Health Services Area into four categories based on national percentiles, with 1 = lower than 10th percentile, 2 = between 10th and 50th percentile, 3 = between 50th and 90th percentile, and 4 = greater than 90th percentile.

Analytic Plan

Table 1 provides descriptive statistics for the total sample, and stratifies by race and ethnicity. Tables 2 and 3 report the results from a series of regressions on

Table 1. Descriptive Statistics by Race and Ethnicity.

	Total ($N = 2138$)		Black ($n = 320$)		Latino ($n = 85$)		Native ($n = 65$)		White ($n = 1668$)	
	n	%	*n*	%	*n*	%	*n*	%	*n*	%
Care-Seeking Preferences										
Seek doctor visit for cough	650	30%	142	44%	45	53%	23	35%	440	26%
Seek specialist referral for cough	764	36%	155	48%	48	56%	31	48%	530	32%
Demographic Characteristics										
Male	910	43%	113	35%	36	42%	23	35%	739	44%
Age 75+ years	1032	48%	134	42%	39	46%	21	32%	699	42%
Health Need Characteristics										
Good SRH	1539	72%	192	60%	60	71%	45	69%	1243	75%
Good SRMH	1847	86%	253	79%	67	79%	54	83%	1474	88%
Has Medical Condition	1205	56%	197	62%	41	48%	35	54%	932	56%
Predisposing Characteristics										
Finances important for medical decisions	1608	75%	265	83%	68	80%	58	89%	1218	73%
Education 0–11 years	455	21%	120	38%	36	42%	24	37%	275	16%
Education 12 years	756	35%	84	26%	21	25%	20	31%	632	38%
Education 13–15 years	510	24%	70	22%	15	18%	15	23%	410	25%
Education 16 years	417	20%	46	14%	13	15%	6	9%	352	21%
Social Factors										
Lives alone	670	31%	114	36%	21	25%	19	29%	517	31%
Daily family or friend contact	1374	64%	212	66%	49	58%	48	74%	1065	64%
At least weekly church or social activities	1459	68%	239	75%	52	61%	43	66%	1126	68%

Table 1. *(Continued)*

	Total ($N = 2138$)		Black ($n = 320$)		Latino ($n = 85$)		Native ($n = 65$)		White ($n = 1668$)	
	n	%	*n*	%	*n*	%	*n*	%	*n*	%
Health Beliefs and Attitudes										
Worries about health	261	12%	65	20%	28	33%	11	17%	157	9%
Avoids the doctor	791	37%	108	34%	25	29%	31	48%	628	38%
Enabling Characteristics										
Micro-Level Patient-Provider Relationship										
Has a usual source of care	2042	96%	301	94%	79	93%	57	88%	1606	96%
High quality of care	1739	81%	248	78%	71	84%	53	82%	1368	82%
Unmet desire for care	209	10%	39	12%	13	15%	5	8%	152	9%
Macro-Structural Healthcare Context										
Metropolitan area	1289	60%	248	78%	65	76%	34	52%	942	56%
Micropolitan area	248	12%	20	6%	3	4%	10	15%	216	13%
Small town	236	11%	19	6%	6	7%	6	9%	205	12%
Isolated rural	365	17%	33	10%	11	13%	15	23%	306	18%
PCP density ≤ 10th percentile	382	18%	47	15%	24	28%	19	29%	292	18%
PCP density > 10th and < 50th percentile	735	34%	113	35%	26	31%	22	34%	574	34%
PCP density > 50th and < 90th percentile	801	37%	121	38%	25	29%	22	34%	633	38%
PCP density > 90th percentile	220	10%	39	12%	10	12%	2	3%	169	10%

Source: Causes and Consequences of Health Care Intensity Patient Survey, national random sample of elderly Medicare beneficiaries, 2005.

Table 2. Logistic Regression of Preference to Seek Doctor Visit for Cough ($N = 2138$).

	Model 1		Model 2		Model 3		Model 4	
	B	*(SE)*	*B*	*(SE)*	*B*	*(SE)*	*B*	*(SE)*
Race and Ethnicity								
Black	0.86***	(0.13)	0.85***	(0.13)	0.74***	(0.13)	0.70***	(0.14)
Latino	1.15***	(0.23)	1.14***	(0.23)	0.97***	(0.23)	0.88***	(0.24)
Native American	0.56*	(0.27)	0.55*	(0.27)	0.48	(0.28)	0.50	(0.28)
white (ref)								
Demographic Characteristics								
Male	0.26**	(0.10)	0.27**	(0.10)	0.29**	(0.10)	0.32**	(0.11)
Age 75+ years	0.40***	(0.10)	0.39***	(0.10)	0.34***	(0.10)	0.32**	(0.10)
Health Need Characteristics								
Good SRH			0.09	(0.12)	0.12	(0.13)	0.14	(0.13)
Good SRMH			−0.25	(0.15)	−0.19	(0.16)	−0.24	(0.16)
Has medical condition			0.06	(0.10)	0.05	(0.10)	0.03	(0.11)
Predisposing Characteristics								
Finances important					0.12	(0.12)	0.15	(0.12)
Education 0–11 years					0.21	(0.14)	0.23	(0.14)
Education 12 years (ref)								
Education 13–15 years					0.09	(0.13)	0.07	(0.13)
Education 16 years					−0.24	(0.15)	−0.26	(0.15)
Social Factors								
Lives alone					0.06	(0.11)	0.05	(0.11)
Daily family or friend contact					−0.04	(0.11)	−0.02	(0.11)
At least weekly church or social activities					0.01	(0.11)	0.01	(0.11)

Table 2. *(Continued)*

	Model 1		Model 2		Model 3		Model 4	
	B	*(SE)*	*B*	*(SE)*	*B*	*(SE)*	*B*	*(SE)*
Health Beliefs and Attitudes								
Worries about health					0.38**	(0.15)	0.31*	(0.15)
Avoids the doctor					−0.51***	(0.11)	−0.48***	(0.11)
Enabling Characteristics								
Micro-Level Patient-Provider Relationship								
Has a usual source of care							0.49	(0.27)
High quality of care							0.19	(0.14)
Unmet desire for care							0.35*	(0.17)
Macro-Structural Healthcare Context								
Metropolitan area (ref)								
Micropolitan area							−0.45**	(0.17)
Small town							−0.33	(0.18)
Isolated rural							−0.20	(0.14)
PCP density ≤ 10th percentile							0.25	(0.20)
PCP density > 10th and < 50th percentile							−0.20	(0.18)
PCP density > 50th and < 90th percentile							0.02	(0.17)
PCP density > 90th percentile (ref)								
Intercept	−1.28***	(0.11)	−1.16***	(0.19)	−1.20***	(0.24)	−1.71***	(0.39)

Source: Causes and Consequences of Health Care Intensity Patient Survey, national random sample of elderly Medicare beneficiaries, 2005.
Note: Survey mode controlled in analyses, but not shown in table.
$^{*}p < 0.05$, $^{**}p < 0.01$, $^{***}p < 0.001$.

Table 3. Logistic Regression of Preference to Seek Specialist Referral for Cough ($N = 2138$).

	Model 1		Model 2		Model 3		Model 4	
	B	*(SE)*	*B*	*(SE)*	*B*	*(SE)*	*B*	*(SE)*
Race and Ethnicity								
Black	0.73***	(0.12)	0.70***	(0.13)	0.58***	(0.13)	0.53***	(0.13)
Latino	0.99***	(0.23)	0.97***	(0.23)	0.78***	(0.23)	0.67***	(0.24)
Native American	0.75**	(0.26)	0.73**	(0.26)	0.65*	(0.26)	0.66*	(0.27)
white (ref)								
Demographic Characteristics								
Male	0.31**	(0.09)	0.30**	(0.09)	0.33***	(0.10)	0.36***	(0.10)
Age 75 + years	−0.01	(0.09)	−0.03	(0.09)	−0.09***	(0.10)	−0.11	(0.10)
Health Need Characteristics								
Good SRH			−0.03	(0.12)	0.02	(0.12)	0.02	(0.12)
Good SRMH			−0.24	(0.15)	−0.14	(0.15)	−0.16	(0.15)
Has medical condition			−0.06	(0.10)	−0.08	(0.10)	−0.08	(0.10)
Predisposing Characteristics								
Finances important					0.13	(0.11)	0.15	(0.11)
Education 0–11 years					0.23	(0.13)	0.24	(0.13)
Education 12 years (ref)								
Education 13–15 years					−0.06	(0.12)	−0.09	(0.13)
Education 16 years					−0.10	(0.14)	−0.13	(0.14)
Social Factors								
Lives alone					0.14	(0.11)	0.13	(0.11)
Daily family or friend contact					−0.15	(0.10)	−0.13	(0.10)
At least weekly church or social activities					0.08	(0.10)	0.09	(0.11)

Table 3. *(Continued)*

	Model 1		Model 2		Model 3		Model 4	
	B	*(SE)*	*B*	*(SE)*	*B*	*(SE)*	*B*	*(SE)*
Health Beliefs and Attitudes								
Worries about health					0.57***	(0.14)	0.53***	(0.14)
Avoids the doctor					−0.17	(0.10)	−0.14	(0.10)
Enabling Characteristics								
Micro-Level Patient-Provider Relationship								
Has a usual source of care							0.25	(0.24)
High quality of care							0.15	(0.13)
Unmet desire for care							0.21	(0.16)
Macro-Structural Healthcare Context								
Metropolitan area (ref)								
Micropolitan area							−0.74***	(0.17)
Small town							−0.21	(0.16)
Isolated rural							−0.21	(0.13)
PCP density ≤ 10th percentile							0.28	(0.19)
PCP density > 10th and < 50th percentile							−0.05	(0.17)
PCP density > 50th and < 90th percentile							0.08	(0.17)
PCP density > 90th percentile (ref)								
Intercept	−0.78***	(0.10)	−0.51**	(0.18)	−0.71**	(0.23)	−1.03**	(0.37)

Source: Causes and Consequences of Health Care Intensity Patient Survey, national random sample of elderly Medicare beneficiaries, 2005.
Note: Survey mode controlled in analyses, but not shown in table.
$^{*}p < 0.05$, $^{**}p < 0.01$, $^{***}p < 0.001$.

care-seeking preferences for visiting a doctor and seeing a specialist. Our multivariate analysis consists of a series of nested multivariate logistic regression models that follow the sequencing of the behavioral model (Aday & Andersen, 1974; Andersen, 1995) plus social factors. This model suggests an assessment of the effects of race and ethnicity on care-seeking preferences, net of health need, predisposing characteristics and social factors, and enabling characteristics. Thus, Model 1 tests the effects racial/ethnic and demographic characteristics on care-seeking preferences, Model 2 adds health need characteristics, Model 3 adds predisposing characteristics and social factors, and Model 4 adds enabling characteristics. All models control for survey mode. We report unstandardized maximum likelihood coefficients, standard errors, and significance levels in our analytic models.

RESULTS

Sample Description

Table 1 indicates that white older adults exhibit lower preferences to seek doctor and specialist visits compared to all other racial and ethnic groups. In terms of health need, Black older adults have more reason to visit the doctor compared to all other groups; lower percentages of Black respondents reported good self-rated health and mental health, and a higher percentage reported having a medical condition that causes pain. If objective health need is related to care-seeking, then we would expect African Americans to exhibit greater desire to see doctors than other groups.

Finances are important for decisions to seek medical treatment for a majority of individuals in all groups (75%), but among racial and ethnic minorities financial strain plays a larger role in care-seeking decisions. Social relationships and engagement are high in the total sample and are fairly evenly distributed across groups; however, Native Americans have an exceptionally high percentage that report at least daily family or friend contact (74%) compared to the entire sample (64%), and Blacks are more likely to attend church or social activities weekly (75%) compared to the entire sample (68%). Respondents from all racial and ethnic minority groups are more likely to report worrying about their health compared to whites. The tendency to avoid going to the doctor is similar across groups (37%), with the exception of Native Americans, among whom almost half of the respondents avoid the doctor (48%). Nearly all of the respondents (96%) report having a usual source of care and all groups report similarly high quality of care (81%). Only 10% have unmet desire for care, and this is similar across groups. A majority of all respondents live in a metropolitan area (60%). Blacks are the least likely of all the groups to live in an area with low representation of primary care providers (15%).

Multivariate Analyses

Table 2 reports the results of multivariate logistic regression on our comprehensive set of factors related to health need, predisposing characteristics, social factors and enabling characteristics on care-seeking related to a lingering cough. In Model 1, we see Black, Latino, and Native Americans are all significantly more likely to say they would seek a doctor visit for a lingering cough compared to whites. In addition, men and the older elderly are more likely to prefer a doctor visit than waiting compared to women and the younger elderly. In Model 2, we see that none of the objective indicators of health need are related to preference for a doctor visit, and the racial and ethnic differences in care-seeking preference do not change. This indicates that the differences in care-seeking preferences we saw in the descriptive statistics are not explained by differences in objective health status.

Model 3 adds predisposing characteristics and social factors to the analyses. None of the socioeconomic or social relationship variables are significant, but health-related worry is significantly associated with greater preference for a doctor visit, while skepticism is significantly associated with lower desire for visiting a doctor. Notably, the addition of these factors slightly reduces, but does not eliminate, the significant positive associations of Black and Latino with greater desire to seek a doctor visit, but the positive association of Native American with care-seeking becomes nonsignificant. Model 4 additionally considers micro- and macro-level enabling characteristics. Having an unmet desire for care is positively related to preferences for a doctor visit, while living in a Micropolitan Area (a core urban area with 10,000–49,999 residents) compared to a Metropolitan Area (a core urban area of at least 50,000 residents) is related to lower desire for wanting a doctor visit. While all previous associations from Model 3 remain significant, we can see that the greater preferences among Latinos in particular are reduced in magnitude, indicating that unmet desire for care and living in smaller cities is responsible for some of their greater desire for visiting a doctor. In sum, the comprehensive factors related to health need, predisposing characteristics, social factors, and enabling characteristics account for some, but not all, of the positive association of Black and Latino with greater preferences for seeking a doctor visit for a lingering cough.

In Table 3, which shows the results from analyses of seeking a specialist referral, the overall patterns of results are similar to those regarding seeking a doctor visit. We therefore describe the results more broadly for this second outcome variable, discussing major patterns and points of departure. Again Black and Latino older adults demonstrate a greater preference for seeking care from a specialist compared to white older adults throughout the modeling sequence. In addition, Native American older adults also exhibit significantly greater preferences to seek care from a specialist. Unlike for preferences for a doctor visit, having a desire to avoid the doctor in general is not related to seeking specialist care. On the other hand, worrying about one's health is positively related to greater desire to see a specialist for a lingering cough. Overall, the story remains consistent across the two measurements of care-seeking preferences: Black, Latino, and Native Americans are more likely than whites to exhibit desire to seek healthcare, even after accounting for a comprehensive set of individual and social factors that generally account for racial differences in utilization.

DISCUSSION

Given the widespread and persistent disparities in use of healthcare in the United States, some scholars speculate that these differences may be due in part to racial and ethnic minorities' lower levels of care-seeking. Like others, we argue that care-seeking is not inherent to individuals, but is embedded in social contexts and stems from a lifetime of social experiences. We used the Behavioral Model of healthcare (Aday & Andersen, 1974; Andersen, 1995), as well as alternative measures of social relationships, health beliefs, healthcare, and system-level characteristics (Andersen, 1995), to investigate whether racial and ethnic differences in preferences for care-seeking among older adults remained after comprehensively accounting for these factors. Contrary to some previous research that suggests that racial and ethnic minorities have *lower* desire to seek care, in the current study we find that racial and ethnic minorities are *more* likely than white older adults to say they would seek doctor visits and specialist referrals. Further, we find that taking into account the comprehensive health need, predisposing characteristics, social factors or enabling healthcare system characteristics related to *using* healthcare does little to diminish differences in preferences for *seeking* care.

Our finding that Native American, Latino, and Black older adults are more likely to say they would seek doctor and specialist visits than their white counterparts represents a significant step forward in our understanding of the role of care-seeking in racial and ethnic disparities in healthcare. The comprehensiveness of our model resolves some of the inconsistencies found across investigations directly measuring racial and ethnic care-seeking preferences, which demonstrated that African Americans preferred both less (Ayanian et al., 1999; Martins et al., 2015) and more (Barnato et al., 2009; Diala et al., 2001; Schnittker et al., 2005) health and mental healthcare compared to whites. Inclusion of a broad set of variables helps to adjudicate whether racial and ethnic differences in preferences for care-seeking are real or artifact. We find that racial and ethnic differences in desire to seek care are persistent, and that all nonwhite groups exhibit *greater* intentions to seek care than whites. This finding underscores the notion that patient preferences are fundamental to both care-seeking and utilization, as shared decision-making and cultural competency guidelines suggest, but therefore we argue that these guidelines should be more attentive to the ways that individual decision-making about care may align with racial and ethnic identity.

We also find that health attitudes and the macro-structural context of healthcare are related to care seeking; particularly worrying about one's health, having skepticism toward doctors in general, and living in a small city rather than a large metropolitan area, explain some of the racial and ethnic variation in stated desire to seek care. Our finding that health-related worry is related to racial and ethnic differences in care-seeking, combined with the notion that it motivates preventive health behavior (Wolinsky & Johnson, 1991), suggests that this attitudinal factor may be a good place for further exploration in clinical decision-making guidelines. We also find that having skepticism toward doctors in general is related to racial and ethnic variation in seeking care. This finding is in line with other studies showing greater skepticism toward healthcare among racial and ethnic minorities (Born et al., 2004; Schnittker, 2004) and distrust in the system as a whole related to institutional racism and a historical legacy of mistreatment in medical research (Boulware, Cooper, Ratner, LaVeist, & Powe, 2003; Gamble, 1997). Finally, we find that compared to living in a large city, those living in a small city have lower preferences for care-seeking, and this accounts for a small part of the racial and ethnic difference among Black and Latino Americans. We speculate that this preference difference may relate to race discordance in patient-provider interactions (LaVeist et al., 2003) in small cities, as Black and Latino providers are more likely to be concentrated in large cities.

If a comprehensive accounting of the individual and social factors that explain healthcare utilization cannot account for racial and ethnic differences in preferences for care-seeking, then where do these differences come from? Today, research about care-seeking, preferences for care, and utilization disparities focuses on notions of improving cultural competence in the healthcare system (Anderson, Scrimshaw, Fullilove, Fielding, & Normand, 2003) and advocating for shared decision-making within the context of the clinical encounter (Kaplan, 1999; O'Connor, Llewellyn-Thomas, & Flood, 2004). Our findings, that despite persistent disparities in access to, use, and quality of healthcare, racial and ethnic minority older adults exhibit greater desire for seeking healthcare than whites, even after accounting for individual, social and structural factors, point to the need to more-carefully examine the broader social context of experiences related to race and seeking care outside of the clinical encounter. Below, we discuss three additional types of social determinants of care-seeking preferences that may align with racial and ethnic distinctions: unmeasured structural variables such as wealth, cultural models that people draw on in their interactions with healthcare institutions, and the ways that meanings individuals attach to situations may affect their assessments of illness-severity.

An emerging line of research finds that wealth exerts a unique effect on racial and ethnic health and healthcare disparities above and beyond other measures of SES (Alegría et al., 2002; Ostrove, Feldman, & Adler, 1999). Further, Braveman et al. (2005) suggest a reassessment of studies that fail to include measures of wealth, arguing that individuals who are evaluated on education and income alone are not socioeconomically comparable. One of the ways wealth influences healthcare decisions is its ability to buffer the effects of lost or temporarily low income, suggesting that wealth may be particularly important to the receipt of healthcare among groups clustered at the lower end of the SES spectrum (Robert & House, 1996). In fact, among those in the lowest income strata, wealth is the most important factor in explaining differences in health between whites and nonwhites (Wenzlow, Mullahy, Robert, & Wolfe, 2004). Wealth has not been widely used in health studies because of the difficulty in measuring it well (Juster, Smith, & Stafford, 1999); however, broad differences in wealth among racial and ethnic groups and its apparent importance in healthcare decision-making among low-income groups imply that it might explain some of the variation in care-seeking preferences, as well as the mismatch between desire to seek care and actual utilization.

We suggest that future research should also focus on specification of the cultural factors that may relate to racial and ethnic differences in care-seeking (Small, Harding, & Lamont, 2010). We argue that racial and ethnic minorities may be drawing upon similar cultural narratives in their interactions with the institutional context of the healthcare system (Shim, 2010). The fact that skepticism about doctors explained some of the racial and ethnic variation in desire to seek care in our models suggests that a history of disparate treatment from providers or distrust of the healthcare system in general may underlie desire or intentions to seek care (Musa, Schulz, Harris, Silverman, & Thomas, 2009; Sorkin et al., 2010; Van Houtven et al., 2005). We suggest that discriminatory experiences among racial and ethnic minorities may create a cultural narrative of inequity that frames interaction with the healthcare system. It may be that past and present injustice contributes to desire for more care to "compensate" for the rational expectation that they will receive inferior or discriminatory care. Future research should better conceptualize and measure the experiences contributing to this cultural narrative and the subsequent impact on preferences for, and actual seeking of care.

The meaning of illness may also vary according to individual circumstances surrounding the healthcare interaction, which have the potential to shape care-seeking differently for racial and ethnic minorities. Research on the mental health impacts of stressful events demonstrates that the circumstances surrounding interactions, particularly the amount of power and control people perceive themselves to have in situations, can make events appear more or less harmful (Simon, 1997). In healthcare, the patient-provider interaction is one site where "social power and inequality are made real" (Shim, 2010). In keeping with this assertion, racial and ethnic minorities report lower levels of trust and satisfaction in physicians (Boulware et al., 2003; LaVeist, Nickerson, & Bowie, 2000; Stepanikova, Mollborn, Cook, Thom, & Kramer, 2006), which is due, at least in part, to lack of racial concordance between patients and providers (LaVeist et al., 2003). In this way, we propose that feelings of powerlessness and lower trust in physicians among racial and ethnic minorities may affect assessments of illness-severity and also of desire to seek care. Indeed, LaVeist et al. (2003) demonstrate that race-concordant relationships with providers are associated with more utilization, as well as less delay in care-seeking and lower failure to use recommended services.

Though the findings we present address gaps in the literature on both care-seeking and racial disparities, they should be considered in light of two main limitations. First, our focus on a population of older adults allowed us to hone in more clearly on our variable of interest – preferences for seeking healthcare – without the potential confounding effects of insurance coverage. But, this limited focus on the elderly means that we cannot generalize these findings about care seeking to the young and middle aged adult population. Second, an important contribution of this study is that we conceptually separate intentions to *seek care* from measurement of actual *utilization of care*. Though sociologists have studied the social factors involved in care-seeking, many of the comprehensive studies of utilization that show racial disparities make assumptions about (less) care-seeking by racial and ethnic minorities. This study represents a first step in that we use a comprehensive model to empirically predict intentions for care seeking, which theoretically precede utilization; however, we do not measure utilization in this study, but rely on the theoretical relationship of intentions (to seek care) with (utilization) behavior.

Despite these limitations, this study represents a systematic analysis of the ways individual, social, and structural context may account for racial and ethnic differences in preferences for seeking medical care. Given the widespread racial and ethnic inequality in healthcare access and outcomes in the United States, some scholars speculate that utilization disparities may be due in part to a lower desire to seek healthcare among minorities. Contrary to these speculations, in the current study we find the opposite: racial and ethnic minorities are *more* likely to say they would seek healthcare than whites, suggesting that guidelines promoting the elicitation and understanding of patient preferences in the context of the clinical interaction is an important step toward reducing utilization disparities. These findings also underscore the notion that health policy should go further to address the broader social factors affecting preferences to seek care in the first place. Further, our existing theoretical models of factors affecting healthcare *utilization* do not account well for understanding healthcare *seeking* even when accounting for a wide array of social as well as individual factors. We call upon a rich sociological literature to complicate our understanding of the social determinants of care-seeking to include those that stem from unmeasured differences in wealth, cultural models based on experiences with the healthcare system, and individual meaning-making in the medical encounter.

REFERENCES

Aday, L. A., & Andersen, R. (1974). A framework for the study of access to medical care. *Health Services Research*, *9*(3), 208–220.

Adler, N. E., & Newman, K. (2002). Socioeconomic disparities in health: Pathways and policies. *Health Affairs*, *21*(2), 60–76.

Alegría, M., Canino, G., Ríos, R., Vera, M., Calderón, J., Rusch, D., & Ortega, A. N. (2002). Mental health care for Latinos: Inequalities in use of specialty mental health services among Latinos, African Americans, and non-Latino Whites. *Psychiatric Services*, *53*(12), 1547–1555.

Andersen, R. M. (1995). Revisiting the behavioral model and access to medical care: Does it matter? *Journal of Health and Social Behavior*, *36*(1), 1–10.

Anderson, L. M., Scrimshaw, S. C., Fullilove, M. T., Fielding, J. E., & Normand, J. (2003). Culturally competent healthcare systems: A systematic review. *American Journal of Preventive Medicine*, *24*(3), 68–79.

Anspach, R. R. (2010). Gender and health care. In C. E. Bird, P. Conrad, A. M. Fremont, & S. Timmermans (Eds.), *Handbook of medical sociology* (pp. 229–248). Nashville, TN: Vanderbilt University Press.

Archibald, M. E., & Rankin, C. P. (2013). A spatial analysis of community disadvantage and access to healthcare services in the U.S. *Social Science & Medicine*, *90*, 11–23.

Armstrong, K., Micco, E., Carney, A., Stopfer, J., & Putt, M. (2005). Racial differences in the use of BRCA1/2 testing among women with a family history of breast or ovarian cancer. *JAMA*, *293*(14), 1729–1736.

Asch, S. M., Sloss, E. M., Hogan, C., Brook, R. H., & Kravitz, R. (2000). Measuring underuse of necessary care among elderly medicare beneficiaries using inpatient and outpatient claims. *JAMA*, *284*(18), 2325–2333.

Ayanian, J. Z., Cleary, P. D., Weissman, J. S., & Epstein, A. M. (1999). The effect of patients' preferences on racial differences in access to renal transplantation. *The New England Journal of Medicine*, *341*(22), 1661–1669.

Baicker, K., Chandra, A., Skinner, J. S., & Wennberg, J. E. (2004). Who you are and where you live: How race and geography affect the treatment of medicare beneficiaries. *Health Affairs Web Exclusive*, doi:10.1377/hlthaff.var.33.

Barnato, A. E., Anthony, D. L., Skinner, J., Gallagher, P. M., & Fisher, E. S. (2009). Racial and ethnic differences in preferences for end-of-life treatment. *Journal of General Internal Medicine*, *24*(6), 695–701.

Bauer, H. M., Rodriguez, M. A., Quiroga, S. S., & Flores-Ortiz, Y. G. (2000). Barriers to health care for abused Latina and Asian immigrant women. *Journal of Health Care for the Poor and Underserved*, *11*(1), 33–44.

Bertakis, K. D., Azari, R., Helms, L. J., Callahan, E. J., & Robbins, J. A. (2000). Gender differences in the utilization of health care services. *Journal of Family Practice*, *49*(2), 147–152.

Bibbins-Domingo, K., Pletcher, M. J., Lin, F., Vittinghoff, E., Gardin, J. M., Arynchyn, A. ... Hulley, S. B. (2009). Racial differences in incident heart failure among young adults. *The New England Journal of Medicine*, *360*(12), 1179–1190.

Born, W., Greiner, A., Sylvia, E., Butler, J., & Ahluwalia, J. S. (2004). Knowledge, attitudes, and beliefs about end-of-life care among inner-city African Americans and Latinos. *Journal of Palliative Medicine*, *7*(2), 247–256.

Boulware, L. E., Cooper, L. A., Ratner, L. E., LaVeist, T. A., & Powe, N. R. (2003). Race and trust in the health care system. *Public Health Reports*, *118*(4), 358–365.

Boyer, C. A., & Lutfey, K. E. (2019). Examining critical health policy issues within and beyond the clinical encounter: Patient–provider relationships and help-seeking behaviors. *Journal of Health and Social Behavior*, *51*(1), S80–S93.

Braveman, P. A., Cubbin, C., Egerter, S., Chideya, S., Marchi, K. S., Metzler, M., & Posner, S. (2005). Socioeconomic status in health research: One size does not fit all. *JAMA*, *294*(22), 2879–2888.

Coulton, C., & Frost, A. K. (1982). Use of social and health services by the elderly. *Journal of Health and Social Behavior*, *23*(4), 330–339.

Cronin, K. A., Richardson, L. C., Jane Henley, S., Miller, J. W., Thomas, C. C., White, A., & Plescia, M. (2012). Vital signs: Racial disparities in breast cancer severity: United States, 2005–2009. In *Morbidity and mortality weekly report (MMWR)*. Washington, DC: Centers for Disease Control and Prevention.

de Boer, A. G., Wijker, W., & de Haes, H. C. (1997). Predictors of health care utilization in the chronically ill: A review of the literature. *Health Policy*, *42*(2), 101–115.

DeVoe, J. E., Fryer, G. E., Phillips, R., & Green, L. (2003). Receipt of preventive care among adults: Insurance status and usual source of care. *American Journal of Public Health*, *93*(5), 786–791.

Diala, C., Muntaner, C., Walrath, C., Nickerson, K. J., LaVeist, T. A., & Leaf, P. J. (2000). Racial differences in attitudes toward professional mental health care and in the use of services. *American Journal of Orthopsychiatry*, *70*(4), 455–464.

Diala, C., Muntaner, C., Walrath, C., Nickerson, K., LaVeist, T., & Leaf, P. (2001). Racial/ethnic differences in attitudes toward seeking professional mental health services. *American Journal of Public Health*, *91*(5), 805–807.

Diamant, A. L., Hays, R. D., Morales, L. S., Ford, W., Calmes, D., Asch, S., & Gelberg, L. (2004). Delays and unmet need for health care among adult primary care patients in a restructured urban public health system. *American Journal of Public Health*, *94*(5), 783–789.

DiMatteo, M. R. (2004). Social support and patient adherence to medical treatment: A meta-analysis. *Health Psychology*, *23*, 207–218.

DuBard, C. A., & Gizlice, Z. (2008). Language spoken and differences in health status, access to care, and receipt of preventive services among US Hispanics. *American Journal of Public Health*, *98*(11), 2021–2028.

Dunlop, D. D., Manheim, L. M., Song, J., & Chang, R. W. (2002). Gender and ethnic/racial disparities in health care utilization among older adults. *Journal of Gerontology: Social Sciences*, *47B*(3), S221–S233.

Ellison, C. G., & Levin, J. S. (1998). The religion-health connection: Evidence, theory, and future directions. *Health Education & Behavior*, *25*, 700–720.

Elwyn, G., Frosch, D., Thomson, R., Joseph-Williams, N., Lloyd, A., Kinnersley, P., & Barry, M. (2012). Shared decision making: A model for clinical practice. *Journal of General Internal Medicine*, *27*(10), 1361–1367.

Epstein, A. M., Weissman, J. S., Schneider, E. C., Gatsonis, C., Leape, L. L., & Piana, R. N. (2003). Race and gender disparities in rates of cardiac revascularization: Do they reflect appropriate use of procedures or problems in quality of care? *Medical Care*, *41*(11), 1240–1255.

Fiscella, K., Franks, P., & Clancy, C. M. (1998). Skepticism toward Medical care and health care utilization. *Medical Care*, *36*(2), 180–189.

Fiscella, K., Franks, P., Doescher, M. P., & Saver, B. G. (2002). Disparities in health care by race, ethnicity, and language among the insured: Findings from a national sample. *Medical Care*, *40*(1), 52–59.

Fiscella, K., Franks, P., Gold, M. R., & Clancy, C. M. (2000). Inequality in quality: Addressing socioeconomic, racial, and ethnic disparities in health care. *JAMA*, *283*(19), 2579–2584.

Freimuth, V. S., Crouse Quinn, S., Thomas, S. B., Cole, G., Zook, E., & Duncan, T. (2001). African Americans' views on research and the Tuskegee Syphilis Study. *Social Science & Medicine*, *52*, 797–808.

Gamble, V. N. (1997). Under the shadow of Tuskegee: African Americans and health care. *American Journal of Public Health*, *87*(11), 1773–1778.

Gaskin, D. J., Dinwiddie, G. Y., Chan, K. S., & McCleary, R. (2012). Residential segregation and disparities in health care services utilization. *Medical Care Research and Review*, *69*(2), 158–175.

Gee, G. C., & Ford, C. L. (2011). Structural racism and health inequities: Old issues, new directions. *DuBois Review*, *8*(1), 115–132.

Geronimus, A. T., Hicken, M., Keene, D., & Bound, J. (2006). Weathering' and age patterns of allostatic load scores among Blacks and Whites in the United States. *American Journal of Public Health*, *96*(5), 826–833.

Gone, J. P. (2007). 'We never was happy living like a whiteman': Mental health disparities and the postcolonial predicament in American Indian communities. *American Journal of Community Psychology*, *40*, 290–300.

Goodman, D. C., & Grumbach, K. (2008). Does having more physicians lead to better health system performance? *JAMA*, *299*(3), 335–337.

Gornick, M. E. (2003). A decade of research on disparities in medicare utilization: Lessons for the health and health care of vulnerable men. *American Journal of Public Health*, *93*(5), 753–759.

Griffith, D. M., Allen, J. O., & Gunter, K. (2011). Social and cultural factors influence African American men's medical help seeking. *Research on Social Work Practice*, *21*(3), 337–347.

Haggerty, J. L., Pineault, R., Beaulieu, M.-D., Brunelle, Y., Gauthier, J., Goulet, F., & Rodrigue, J. (2007). Room for improvement: Patients' experiences of primary care in quebec before major reforms. *Canadian Family Physician*, *53*(6), 1056–1057.

Hayward, M. D., Crimmins, E. M., Miles, T., & Yang, Y. (2000). The significance of socioeconomic status in explaining the racial gap in chronic health conditions. *American Sociological Review*, *65*, 910–930.

Hebert, P. L., Frick, K. D., Kane, L. R., & Marshall McBean, A. (2005). The causes of racial and ethnic differences in influenza vaccination rates among elderly medicare beneficiaries. *Health Services Research*, *40*(2), 517–537.

Hollinger, D. A. (2003). Amalgamation and hypodescent: The question of ethnoracial mixture in the history of the United States. *The American Historical Review*, *108*(5), 1363–1390.

Juster, F. T., Smith, J. P., & Stafford, F. (1999). The measurement and structure of household wealth. *Labour Economics*, *6*(2), 253–275.

Kaplan, R. M. (1999). Shared medical decision-making: A new paradigm for behavioral medicine—1997 presidential address. *Annals of Behavioral Medicine*, *21*(2), 3–11.

Katz, J. N. (2001). Patient preferences and health disparities. *JAMA*, *286*(12), 1506–1509.

Korenstein, D., Falk, R., Howell, E. A., Bishop, T., & Keyhani, S. (2012). Overuse of health care services in the United States: An understudied problem. *Archives of Internal Medicine*, *172*(2), 171–178.

LaVeist, T. A., Keith, V. M., & Gutierrez, M. L. (1995). Black/White differences in prenatal care utilization: An assessment of predisposing and enabling factors. *Health Services Research*, *30*(1), 43–58.

LaVeist, T. A., Nickerson, K. J., & Bowie, J. V. (2000). Attitudes about racism, medical mistrust, and satisfaction with care among African American and White cardiac patients. *Medical Care Research and Review*, *57*, 146–161.

LaVeist, T. A., Nuru-Jeter, A., & Jones, K. E. (2003). the association of doctor-patient race concordance with health services utilization. *Journal of Public Health Policy*, *24*(3/4), 312–323.

Levesque, J.-F., Pineault, R., Robert, L., Hamel, M., Roberge, D., Kapetanakis, C., Simard, B., & Laugraud, A. (2008). *Unmet health care needs: A reflection of the accessibility of primary care services?* Québec: Gouvernement du Québec.

Levine, R. S., Foster, J. E., Fullilove, R. E., Fullilove, M. T., Briggs, N. C., Hull, P. C., Husaini, B. A., & Hennekens, C. H. (2001). Black-White inequalities in mortality and life expectancy, 1933-1999: Implications for healthy people 2010. *Public Health Reports*, *116*(5), 474–483.

Lillie-Blanton, M., Martinez, R. M., & Salganicoff, A. (2001). Site of medical care: Do racial and ethnic differences persist? *Yale Journal of Health Policy, Law, and Ethics*, *1*(1), 15–32.

Long, S. K., King, J., & Coughlin, T. A. (2005). The implications of unmet need for future health care use: Findings for a sample of disabled medicaid beneficiaries in New York. *Inquiry*, *42*(4), 413–420.

Lum, Y.-S., & Chang, H.-J. (1998). The effect of medicaid coverage on use of health services by low-income elderly people. *Social Work Research*, *22*(1), 31–43.

Lynch, S. M. (2003). Cohort and life-course patterns in the relationship between education and health: A hierarchical approach. *Demography*, *40*(2), 309–331.

Mangione-Smith, R., Elliott, M. N., Stivers, T., McDonald, L., Heritage, J., & McGlynn, E. A. (2004). Racial/ethnic variation in parent expectations for antibiotics: Implications for public health campaigns. *Pediatrics*, *113*(5), e385–e394.

Martins, T., Ukoumunne, O. C., Banks, J., Raine, R., & Hamilton, W. (2015). Ethnic differences in patients' preferences for prostate cancer investigation: A vignette-based survey in primary care. *British Journal of General Practice*, *632*, e161–e170.

McCaul, K. D., Schroeder, D. M., & Reid, P. A. (1996). Breast cancer worry and screening: Some prospective data. *Health Psychology*, *15*(6), 430–433.

Mojtabai, R., Olfson, M., & Mechanic, D. (2002). Perceived need and help-seeking in adults with mood, anxiety, or substance use disorders. *Archives of General Psychiatry*, *59*(1), 77–84.

Musa, D., Schulz, R., Harris, R., Silverman, M., & Thomas, S. B. (2009). Trust in the health care system and the use of preventive health services by older Black and White adults. *American Journal of Public Health*, *99*(7), 1293–1299.

Mutchler, J. E., & Burr, J. A. (1991). Racial differences in health and health care service utilization in later life: The effect of socioeconomic status. *Journal of Health and Social Behavior*, *32*(4), 342–356.

Ngui, E. M., & Flores, G. (2007). Unmet needs for specialty, dental, mental, and allied health care among children with special health care needs: Are there racial/ethnic disparities? *Journal of Health Care for the Poor and Underserved*, *18*(4), 931–949.

Nyweide, D. J., Anthony, D. L., Chang, C.-H., & Goodman, D. (2011). Seniors' perceptions of health care not closely associated with physician supply. *Health Affairs*, *30*(2), 219–227.

O'Connor, A. M., Llewellyn-Thomas, H. A., & Flood, A. B. (2004). Modifying unwarranted variations in health care: Shared decision making using patient decision aids. *Health Affairs*, *23*, 63–72.

Ostrove, J. M., Feldman, P., & Adler, N. E. (1999). Relations among socioeconomic status indicators and health for African-Americans and Whites. *Journal of Health Psychology*, *4*(4), 451–463.

Pescosolido, B. (1992). Beyond rational choice: The social dynamics of how people seek help. *American Journal of Sociology*, *97*(4), 1096–1138.

Pescosolido, B. A., & Boyer, C. A. (1999). How do people come to use mental health services? Current knowledge and changing perspectives. In A. V. Horwitz & T. L. Scheid (Eds.), *A Handbook for the study of mental health: Social contexts, theories, and systems* (pp. 392–411). New York, NY: Cambridge University Press.

Pescosolido, B. A., & Kronenfeld, J. J. (1995). Health, illness, and healing in an uncertain era: Challenges from and for medical sociology. *Journal of Health and Social Behavior*, 5–33. (Extra).

Pescosolido, B. A., Tuch, S. A., & Martin, J. K. (2001). The profession of medicine and the public: Examining Americans' changing confidence in physician authority from the beginning of the 'health care crisis' to the era of health care reform. *Journal of Health and Social Behavior*, *42*(1), 1–16.

Pescosolido, B. A., Wright, E. R., Alegría, M., & Vera, M. (1998). Social networks and patterns of use among the poor with mental health problems in Puerto Rico. *Medical Care*, *36*(7), 1057–1072.

Phillips, K. A., Mayer, M. L., & Aday, L. A. (2000). Barriers to care among racial/ethnic groups under managed care. *Health Affairs*, *33*(11), 65–75.

Rumbaut, R. G. (2016). Pigments of our imagination: On the racialization and racial identities of "Hispanics" and "Latinos". In J. A. Cobas, J. Duany, & J. R. Feagin (Eds.), *How the United States racializes latinos: White hegemony and its consequences* (pp. 15–36). New York, NY: Routledge.

Ransford, H. E. (1986). Race, heart disease worry and health protective behavior. *Social Science & Medicine*, *22*(12), 1355–1362.

Robert, S. A. (1999). Socioeconomic position and health: The independent contribution of community socioeconomic context. *Annual Review of Sociology*, *25*, 489–516.

Robert, S., & House, J. S. (1996). SES differentials in health by age and alternative indicators of SES. *Journal of Aging and Health*, *8*(3), 359–388.

Schenck, A. P., Klabunde, C. N., & Davis, W. W. (2006). Racial differences in colorectal cancer test use by medicare consumers. *American Journal of Preventive Medicine*, *30*(4), 320–326.

Schnittker, J. (2003). Misgivings of medicine? African Americans' skepticism of psychiatric medication. *Journal of Health and Social Behaviors*, *44*(4), 506–524.

Schnittker, J. (2004). Social distance in the clinical encounter: Interactional and sociodemographic foundations for mistrust in physicians. *Social Psychology Quarterly*, *67*(3), 217–235.

Schnittker, J., Freese, J., & Powell, B. (2000). Nature, nurture, neither, nor: Black-White differences in beliefs about the causes and appropriate treatment of mental illness. *Social Forces*, *78*(3), 1101–1132.

Schnittker, J., Pescosolido, B. A., & Croghan, T. W. (2005). Are African Americans really less willing to use health care? *Social Problems*, *52*(2), 255–271.

Sedlis, S. P., Fisher, V. J., Tice, D., Esposito, R., Madmon, L., & Steinberg, E. H. (1997). Racial differences in performance of invasive cardiac procedures in a department of veterans affairs medical center. *Journal of Clinical Epidemiology*, *50*(8), 899–901.

Seeman, T. (1996). Social ties and health: The benefits of social integration. *Annals of Epidemiology*, *6*(5), 442–451.

Shim, J. K. (2010). Cultural health capital: A theoretical approach to understanding health care interactions and the dynamics of unequal treatment. *Journal of Health and Social Behavior*, *51*(1), 1–15.

Shuey, K. M., & Willson, A. E. (2008). Cumulative disadvantage and black-white disparities in life-course health trajectories. *Research on Aging*, *30*(2), 200–225.

Simon, R. W. (1997). The meanings individuals attach to role identities and their implications for mental health. *Journal of Health and Social Behavior*, *38*, 256–274.

Skinner, J., Weinstein, J. N., Sporer, S. M., & Wennberg, J. E. (2003). Racial, ethnic, and geographic disparities in rates of knee arthroplasty among medicare patients. *The New England Journal of Medicine*, *349*(14), 1350–1359.

Small, M. L., Harding, D. J., & Lamont, M. (2010). Reconsidering culture and poverty. *The Annals of the American Academy of Political and Social Science*, *629*(1), 6–27.

Smedley, B. D., Stith, A. Y., & Nelson, A. R. (2003). *Unequal treatment: Confronting racial and ethnic disparities in health care*. Washington, DC: Institute of Medicine.

Sorkin, D. H., Ngo-Metzger, Q., & Alba, I. D. (2010). Racial/ethnic discrimination in health care: Impact on perceived quality of care. *Journal of General Internal Medicine*, *25*(5), 390–396.

Stepanikova, I., Mollborn, S., Cook, K. S., Thom, D. H., & Kramer, R. M. (2006). Patients' race, ethnicity, language, and trust in a physician. *Journal of Health and Social Behavior*, *47*(4), 390–405.

Sternthal, M. J., Slopen, N., & Williams, D. R. (2011). Racial disparities in health: How much does stress really matter? *DuBois Review*, *8*(1), 95–113.

Suchman, E. A. (1965). Social patterns of illness and medical care. *Journal of Health and Social Behavior*, *6*(1), 2–16.

Umberson, D., Crosnoe, R., & Reczek, C. (2010). social relationships and health behaviors across the life course. *Annual Review of Sociology*, *36*, 139–157.

United States Census Bureau. (2013). Detailed years of school completed by people 25 years and over by sex, age groups, race and Hispanic origin: 2013. Retrieved from https://www.census.gov/hhes/socdemo/education/data/cps/2013/tables.html

Van Houtven, C. H., Voils, C. I., Oddone, E. Z., Weinfurt, K. P., Friedman, J. Y., Schulman, K. A., & Bosworth, H. B. (2005). Perceived discrimination and reported delay of pharmacy prescriptions and medical tests. *Journal of General Internal Medicine*, *20*(7), 578–583.

Ware, J. E., Keller, S. D., & Kosinski, M. (1998). *Sf-12: How to score the sf-12 physical and mental health summary scales*. Lincoln, RI: QualityMetric Incorporated.

Wenzlow, A. T., Mullahy, J., Robert, S. A., & Wolfe, B. L. (2004). *An empirical investigation of the relationship between wealth and health using the survey of consumer finances*. Institute for Research on Poverty: University of Wisconsin-Madison.

Williams, D. R. (2012). Miles to go before we sleep: Racial inequities in health. *Journal of Health and Social Behavior*, *53*(3), 279–295.

Williams, D. R., & Collins, C. (2001). Racial residential segregation: A fundamental cause of racial disparities in health. *Public Health Reports*, *116*(5), 404–416.

Williams, D. R., & Mohammed, S. A. (2009). Discrimination and racial disparities in health: Evidence and needed research. *Journal of Behavioral Medicine*, *32*, 20–47.

Wolinsky, F. D., & Johnson, R. J. (1991). The use of health services by older adults. *Journal of Gerontology: Social Sciences*, *45*(6), S345–S357.

Zola, I. K. (1973 [1967]). Pathways to the doctor: From person to patient. *Social Science & Medicine*, *7*(9), 677–689.

CHANGING PATTERNS OF FEMALE SMOKING: A COMPARISON OF WORKERS AND FULL-TIME HOMEMAKERS BY CLASS, RACE, AND COMMUNITY TYPE

William C. Cockerham, Bryant W. Hamby,
Shawn Bauldry and Patricia Drentea

ABSTRACT

This chapter compares smoking among American women employed outside the home with those of full-time homemakers at two points in time: 1979 and 2014.

Data are from the 1979 National Household Survey on Drug Abuse (NHSDA) and from the 2014 National Survey on Drug Use and Health (NSDUH). The NHSDA is the precursor to the present-day NSDUH and part of the same continuum of nationwide surveys on drug use. The analysis uses logistic regression models and the survey suite of commands in Stata 13 to include 1979/2014 sample weights and adjustments for the complex sample design.

Results show that smoking is most prevalent among homemakers in small communities. This outcome supports earlier studies citing smoking as a major causal factor for the decline in female life expectancy among

Health and Health Care Concerns among Women and Racial and Ethnic Minorities
Research in the Sociology of Health Care, Volume 35, 279–297

ISSN: 0275-4959/doi:10.1108/S0275-495920170000035014

less-educated white women in certain low-income and rural counties in the United States. The premise that female smoking is strongly associated with the workplace appears to be no longer true.

These data provide only a limited test of health lifestyle theory because many of the model's structural variables are not included. Otherwise the findings support the model.

This study finds that smoking is greatest among women who are full-time homemakers in medium and especially small towns. This is a new development and suggests the locus of smoking among women has moved away from its association with the job in cities to the home in less populated areas.

Keywords: Female smoking; workers; homemakers; class; race; and community

The purpose of this chapter is to compare smoking among American women employed outside the home with those of full-time homemakers at two points in time: 1979 and 2014. In 1979, some 30.1% of all women were estimated to smoke compared to 14.8% in 2014 (CDC, 2015). While the percentage of women smokers declined by half over this 35-year period, it is not clear within which social context – the workplace or the home – that female smoking remains most prevalent. Research on this topic helps us to clarify the social determinants of female cigarette use by identifying characteristics of women most likely to smoke. This is an important subject because smoking is associated with more diseases than any other health-related lifestyle practice and is the leading preventable cause of mortality in the United States.

Mortality rates among current smokers, for instance, are two to three times higher than among those who have never smoked (Carter, Abnet, Feskanich, & Freedman, 2015). Since 1950, deaths from lung cancer for women increased fivefold compared to men and for chronic obstructive pulmonary disease (COPD) nearly twofold (National Center for Health Statistics, 2014). The principal cause appears to be smoking cigarettes by women, given the well-established relationship between smoking and these diseases. These changes reflect the penalty large numbers of women have paid for smoking over time and is a clear sign of an adverse health legacy from the past. This development represents a "lag effect" in which heavy cigarette use led to death by a chronic disease several years after initiation (Annandale, 2016).

American women did not begin smoking in large numbers until World War II, when they entered civilian workplaces as replacements for men in the military (Hughes, 2003; Walsh, Sorensen, & Chapman, 1995). While never surpassing levels of male smoking, female smoking nevertheless increased dramatically in concert with the greater gender equality that came with paid employment outside the home. By 1965, about one-third of adult women were smokers. Thus, the initiation of widespread smoking among women was originally linked with the workplace. The various factors that went into promoting smoking among women workers, however, may no longer be operable today and a comparison of workers with full-time homemakers seems warranted.

FEMALE SMOKING: THE WORKPLACE VERSUS THE HOME

Prior to the 1940s, norms regarding gender and tobacco use in American society were clear: it was socially acceptable for men, but not women to smoke. Gentlemen were not supposed to smoke in the company of ladies, nor well-mannered women allow smoking in their presence, much less smoke themselves. As Walsh, Sorensen, and Leonard (1995, p. 151) put it: "gender was the decisive axis dividing smokers and nonsmokers." Public sentiment favored women staying home, having children, and taking care of the household. The norms governing gender relations reached back to Victorian times, which locked women into the private sphere of domestication and men into the public sphere of work (Collins, 2009).

World War II, as noted, began the long-term, massive migration of women into the labor force and their participation never returned to pre-war rates. The percentage of women working outside the home increased steadily from 33.9% in 1950 to 51.5% in 1979 and 57.7% in 2012 (U.S. Bureau of Labor Statistics, 2014). The movement of women into the marketplace was greatest during the 1970s and 1980s, and has since stabilized. Nevertheless, the majority of women now have the expectation of paid employment in adulthood (England, 2010).

Women have also expanded their work roles into occupations that were once largely male and act consistent with the norms of these occupations in order to be successful at what they do (England, 2010; Pinker, 2009). That is, the social roles of men and women used to be more rigid and predictable in that men typically behaved in certain distinct ways and women in others, but this is not necessarily the case when professional and occupational norms and tasks supersede traditional gender roles. With the women's movement and the shift of most adult women into the workplace, women's roles and behaviors have become more flexible than was formerly the case (England, 2010).

Consequently, women in the workforce who smoke may exhibit patterns of smoking similar to their male smoking counterparts as they adopt the same behaviors and share the stresses, strains, career and time pressures, and workloads of males in the same jobs. For some employed women, especially non-Hispanic whites, negative health practices are mimicking those of men (King, Marinous, Carnemolla, & Everett, 2009). There is a greater likelihood, for example, of female drinking in gender-balanced occupations than gender-typed jobs typical of women (Cho, 2004). That is, women who work around men drink more alcohol than women who work with other women and this may be the case for smoking as well.

Smoking was also considered by some women in the past as glamorous, as female Hollywood and television stars smoked on stage and screen, and served as role models in cigarette advertisements (Brandt, 2007). Smoking was likewise associated with the women's movement, as seen in the popularity of the Virginia Slims ads ("You've come a long way, baby!") showing successful modern women smoking (Brandt, 2007; Hughes, 2003; Walsh et al., 1995). These women smokers were depicted as thin, attractive, independent, fashionable, smart, and powerful. In this milieu, smoking a certain type of cigarette emerged as a form of cultural capital for young women (Haines, Poland, & Johnson, 2009). However, regardless of whether the increase in female smoking was due to greater gender equality, a general liberalization of norms concerning women's behavior, or a long history of smoking in the United States in which the use of cigarettes by men and women eventually became somewhat more similar, gender standards for smoking definitely changed (Pampel, 2001).

While women were finding meaningful work and entering more jobs and occupations, many had a "second shift," working for pay during the day and working for the family each evening (Hochschild, 1989). As Percheski (2008) and others (Maume, 2016) point out, the gendered nature of family life and childrearing has remained essentially intact even when women are employed outside the home. While we refer to family and household labor as the "second shift" for employed women, family demands aren't always confined to the evening hours, and nor is outside work confined to "first shift" hours.

Additionally, work-family/family-work conflict occurs either when family demands interfere with work obligations or when work demands interfere with family obligations. The experience and reaction to such conflict is gendered, with women having significantly greater responsibility for the home and children regardless of whether or not they hold a job (Mattingly & Sayer, 2006; Maume, 2016; Nomaguchi, Milkie, & Bianchi, 2005). While women have greater labor force participation and access to various types of jobs, they have disproportionately more work-family/family-work conflict and many are additionally subject to jobs of low quality, autonomy, and pay despite improvements in equality. There is research showing that the conflict resulting from work and family situations is associated not only with smoking, but also alcohol abuse, poor diet, lack of exercise, stress, hypertension, and depression (Allen & Armstrong, 2006; Nelson, Li, Sorenson, & Berkman, 2012).

There has also been a dramatic rise over time in divorce, childbearing outside of marriage, and single-parent families, most of which are female-headed households. Being a full-time parent with no spousal support is stressful for many women in these circumstances, who almost always must hold jobs to provide for themselves and their children. Single parents are also more likely to be smokers, even when accounting for gender differences. For example, among single parents, 29% were current smokers in 2013 compared to 15% of parents living in two-parent households, with single mothers more than twice as likely as mothers in two-parent households to be current smokers (Child Trends, 2014).

Many have also ended up in lower paying gender-segregated jobs, bumped up against glass ceilings when they entered male-dominated occupations, and found jobs they feminized losing prestige (Miller, 2009). They still coped with the "second shift" in which they continued to perform additional tasks outside of their place of employment as family and home caretakers (Nomaguchi et al., 2005). Some lost support from a male breadwinner through divorce or death and experienced the financial hardship of single parenthood. Thus women entering the work world in large numbers had stresses associated with many jobs that previously centered mostly on men and intensified problems associated with "second shift" responsibilities. At the same time, many women took up smoking which appears to explain much for those who have a poor health profile.

With the mounting scientific evidence that smoking is harmful to health and longevity, the proportion of men and women smokers declined. Although male smoking started falling in the 1970s, the percentage of female smokers did not seriously decrease until the 1980s and the rate of decline has been much slower than that of males. The reduction in smoking among women is somewhat offset by younger women talking up cigarettes as older women quit or die. Young female smokers are the segment of the population most resistant to stopping cigarette use (Hughes, 2003). For example, among young smokers between the ages of 12 and 17, the percentage of regular cigarette users in 2012 is about the same for females (6.3%) as males (6.8%) (National Center for Health Statistics, 2014). Among all smokers, the gap between men and women smokers has grown smaller with 18.8% of men smoking in 2014 compared to 14.8% of women (CDC, 2015).

Smoking also remains exceedingly more characteristic of people at the bottom of the social scale than at the top (Cockerham, 2013a; Pampel, 2001, 2002, 2005, 2009). This is seen in a growing number of studies originating at the county level in the United States where a decline in life expectancy among certain women has emerged in which smoking is identified as a prominent risk factor (Cockerham, 2014; Ezzati, Friedman, Kulkarni, & Murray, 2008; Montez & Zajacova, 2013; Wang, Schumacher, Levitz, Mokdad, & Murray, 2013). The women at greatest risk of early mortality are non-Hispanic whites with low levels of education and income living in less populated areas. Ezzati et al. (2008) found, for example, that decreasing female life expectancy was most prevalent for women in small towns in counties in the Deep South, Texas, Appalachia, and the lower Midwest. Cigarette smoking is important in these outcomes in that significantly more of it occurs among the less educated than the well-educated and among whites than blacks (Montez & Zajacova, 2013; Pampel, 2009; Syamial, Mazurek, & Dube, 2014).

There are not, however, many current studies examining the relationship between work and smoking. An exception is the Syamial et al. (2014) study that not only finds the physical and emotional health of women workers who smoke worse than that of male workers who use cigarettes, but that also that women in service occupations (e.g., police, food preparation, waitresses, and building maintenance) have the highest odds of being a current smoker, followed by female construction workers. Elementary and secondary school teachers were the least likely to smoke.

What this suggests is that employed women are generally more likely to smoke than full-time homemakers. However, jobs dominated by men, such as in manufacturing, are disappearing, with traditionally female occupations, like those of nursing, expanding which may lessen overall smoking associated with the workplace (Searcey, Porter, & Gebeloff, 2015). Additionally, many employers currently maintain smoke-free work environments, nonsmoking policies, and wellness programs that actively discourage employees from smoking. They may hire only nonsmokers. State and municipal laws also prohibit smoking in public places, thus adding to the stigmatization of the practice.

Women who stay home and take care of their residence and families, however, do not have to "fit in" to a male-dominated work world, be required to multitask between work and family, and are more likely to be in female-centered and more traditionally feminine roles of caring for others. As caretakers for their families, female homemakers, especially those who have children around them, may be less likely to smoke than those on the job in order to maintain their own health so they can perform caretaking duties (Pavalko, Gong, & Long, 2007). Smoking, being drunk, eating or serving unhealthy foods, abusing drugs, and similar negative practices jeopardize the health and well-being of their children, others dependent upon them, and themselves, and therefore should be less common behaviors for mothers and female caregivers –although there is research showing this is not necessarily the case among low-income families (Robinson & Kirkcaldy, 2007).

Despite caretaking roles, it may be that smoking is nevertheless concentrated more among homemakers than employed women in today's public anti-smoking environment. Past research shows that the homemaker role is relatively unstructured and invisible, has limited involvement with people outside the home, and carries with it a low sense of control because of economic dependency, the routine nature of the work, the strain of keeping house and taking care of others, and limited opportunities (Ross & Mirowsky, 2013). In such circumstances, women may be more prone to smoke in the privacy of their home than confront public censure in the workplace. In their study of non-Hispanic white women and early mortality, Montez and Zajacova (2013) found employment to have an "intriguing" role as women who worked had a greater life expectancy than those who were under-employed and unemployed. Smoking was depicted as a major contributor to premature female deaths.

Consequently, as previously noted, it is not clear whether female smoking is currently more prevalent in work environments on the job or at home and it is the objective of this study to help clarify this situation. Determining which social environment is more conducive to smoking helps us to better understand the dynamics of female smoking.

DATA AND METHODS

Our goal is to determine whether or not the association of the workplace with women's smoking has changed over time. Since we are dealing with two different cohorts of women at two differing points in time with respect to smoking, our strategy to determine social change in the aggregate is to analyze cross-section data from repeated surveys. According to Firebaugh (2008), two measurement points are required to estimate a changing-effects model in order to ascertain whether an association has changed from time 1 to time 2. In our study, data come from the 1979 National Household Survey on Drug Abuse (NHSDA) for time 1 and from the 2014 National Survey on Drug Use and Health (NSDUH) for time 2 (Center for Behavioral Health Statistics and Quality 2015; U.S. Department of Health & Human Services, 2015). The NHSDA is the precursor to the present-day NSDUH and is part of the same continuum of repeated nationwide surveys on drug use.

The 1979 NHSDA, collected by the Response Analysis Corporation, surveyed 7,224 respondents (83% response rate) via a multistage area probability sample of the contiguous United States, and collected information through personal interviews and survey questionnaires. The 2014 NSDUH, collected by the Research Triangle Institute, identified 67,901 respondents (71.2% response rate) via a multistage probability sample that included all 50 states and the District of Columbia, and collected data using computer-assisted self- and personal interviews.

For the 1979 baseline sample, men (N = 3,357) are excluded, along with people under the age of 18 (N = 1,037), races other than non-Hispanic whites and blacks (N = 208), students, the disabled, and women unable to work, unemployed, or retired (N = 419), and a small number of respondents missing data for income (N = 112) and smoking (N=4). Hispanics were excluded because of their relatively low number in the 1979 survey. These exclusions result in a sample of 2,087 female respondents in 1979. For the 2014 sample, those excluded were men (N = 26,322), people under the age of 18 (N = 6,690), races other than non-Hispanic whites and blacks (N = 5,686), women who reported that they did not have a job for any reason nor keep house full-time

($N = 4{,}221$), and did not report smoking status ($N = 7$). These exclusions result in a sample of 12,345 respondents in 2014.

Variables

The dependent variable is smoking status (smoker versus nonsmoker) as determined by the average number of cigarettes smoked daily. Respondents were categorized as smokers if they smoked an average of at least one cigarette a day. The primary independent variable of interest is whether respondents worked (full- or part-time) or kept house full-time. For the 1979 data we relied on one question determining work status at the present time and then, conditional on not working, another question asking the respondent which category of nonworker best describes the individual, including considering themselves to be a full-time housewife. For the 2014 data we relied on one question determining work status in the past week which included full-time work, part time work, those who held jobs but did not work in the past week, and reasons for not being part of the labor force, including keeping house full-time. Full-time workers, part time workers, and those who held a job but did not work in the past week were coded as workers, and those who indicated they were keeping house full-time were coded as homemakers.

The independent variables of secondary interest include race (non-Hispanic whites compared to non-Hispanic blacks), community type, and educational attainment. Community type is divided into three categories: (1) large urban areas, (2) small urban areas, and (3) nonurban areas. In the 1979 data these categories are determined by residence in a standard metropolitan statistical area (SMSA) consisting of one primary sampling unit (i.e., typically a large city), an SMSA consisting of more than one primary sampling unit (i.e., typically a smaller city or cities), and residence in a non-SMSA. In the 2014 data these categories are based on residence in a core-based statistical area (CBSA) with at least one million people, in a CBSA with less than one million people, and residence in a non-CBSA. Educational attainment is based on highest grade completed: (1) less than high school, (2) high school, (3) some college, and (4) 4-year college degree or higher.

In addition, we adjust for age, household income, and marital status in all of our models. The 2014 survey collected age as a categorical measure with 11 categories. We recoded the categories to midpoint ages and also included a square term due to a potential nonlinear association between age and smoking. The 1979 data had a continuous measure of age and a square term was also included similar to the 2014 data for ease of comparison. Household income takes four values that differ for 1979 and 2014. In the 1979 data the categories are: low (< \$7,000), below average (\$7,000–\$14,999), above average (\$15,000–\$24,999), and high (\$25,000+). In the 2014 data the categories are: low (< \$20,000), below average ($20,000–$49,999), above average ($50,000–$74,999), and high ($75,000 +). Marital status has four categories: (1) married, (2) widowed, (3) divorced or separated, and (4) never married. We explored the effects of number of children on smoking in the 2014 survey, but the results were not significant so we dropped number of children from the analysis.

Table 1 presents weighted descriptive statistics for all study variables for the 1979 and 2014 samples. In 1979, 36.5% of women respondents reported having smoked at least one cigarette a day. However, the percentage of women smoking fell to 22% in the 2014 sample. Similarly, the percentage who were full-time housekeepers dropped from 37.1% in the 1979 sample to 9.8% in 2014. The expansion of higher education during this time period is apparent – the percentage of women with a college degree climbed from 16% in 1979 to 37.9% in 2014, while the percentage of women in the two samples with a less than high school education fell from 20.6 to 4.9. Among the 1979 respondents, roughly equal percentages of respondents lived in the three different community types; however, in 2014 the majority lived in medium or large communities. This reflects a shift in the population away from small communities and into larger communities over this time period.

The percentage of white women in the sample was 89.2 in 1979 and 84.2 in 2014 as compared to percentages of 10.8 and 15.8, respectively, for black women. The income categories for women in the low and below average income groups were similar in the 1979 and 2014 samples, but those respondents in the above average income category declined during the two periods (from 31.5% to 18.6%, respectively). The high income group increased from 28.1 to 39.8 during the same period. The mean age in 1979 (40.1 years) was slightly greater in 2014 (42.8 years). Finally, while the majority of the sample was married, the percentage of those married decreased from 67.8% from 1979 to 53.1% in 2014, while those never married increased from 15.6% in 1979 to 26.8 in 2014.

Statistical Models

The analysis proceeds in three steps. First, we examine the bivariate associations between women's work status and smoking in 1979 and 2014. Second, we examine the associations between women's work status and smoking in 1979 and 2014 adjusting for the other covariates. Third, as we are interested specifically in the changing roles of women's social standing and surroundings, we examine whether there are any interactions between community type, education, and women's work status in predicting smoking in 1979 and 2014.

The analyses use logistic regression models and the survey suite of commands in Stata 13 to include the 1979/2014 sample weights and adjust for the complex sample design (StataCorp, 2013). Stata's margin command is used to

Table 1. Weighted Percentages and Means for Study Variables from the 1979 NSDAH and 2014 NSDUH.

	1979	2014
Cigarette Use		
Nonsmoker	63.6	78.0
Smoker	36.5	22.0
Work Status		
Works outside house	62.9	90.2
Homemaker	37.1	9.8
Education		
Less than high school	20.6	4.9
High school	40.9	26.3
Some college	22.6	30.9
College	16.0	37.9
Community type[a]		
Large	34.1	51.9
Medium	34.6	42.6
Small	31.3	5.5
Race		
White	89.2	84.2
Black	10.8	15.8
Income[b]		
Low	13.3	12.3
Below average	27.1	29.3
Above average	31.5	18.6
High	28.1	39.8
Age	40.1 (18–87)	42.8 (18–65)
Marital status		
Married	67.8	53.7
Widowed	7.1	3.5
Divorced or separated	9.3	16.0
Never married	15.6	26.8
N	2,085	12,345

[a]1979 Large: Self-representing SMSA, Medium: Non-self-representing SMSA, and Small: Not in a SMSA; 2014 Large: CBSA w/ 1 million+, Medium: CBSA w/ <1 million, and Small: Not in a CBSA.

[b]1979 Low: <\$7,000, Below average: \$7,000–\$14,999, Above average: \$15,000–\$24,999, and High \$25,000+; 2014 Low: <\$20,000, Below average: \$20,000–\$49,999, Above average: \$50,000–\$74,000, and High: \$75,000+.

construct predicted probabilities to facilitate the interpretation of interaction effects and variation in the strength of associations across the two surveys. A direct comparison of coefficients across models is not appropriate with logistic regression models (Long, 1997).

RESULTS

Bivariate associations for work status and smoking broken down by community type and educational attainment reveal some interesting differences between the two periods of our study In 1979, those who lived in the two larger community types were more likely to smoke than those in the smallest (37.0% and 41.0%, respectively, compared to 30.7%). However, by 2014, those living in the smallest community type showed no decrease in percentage of smoking (31.2%) compared to the 1979 time period, while there were significant declines in the rates of smoking of those within the two larger community types (the largest was down to 20.1% and medium to 23.2%). This suggests it may be that in less populated places, such as small towns and rural areas, female smoking has not declined appreciably over the course of 35 years. Furthermore, these associations are consistent with the county-level studies showing rising female mortality rates related to smoking in more sparsely populated places.

In both 1979 and 2014, women with less than a high school education were not only more likely to smoke than women with higher levels of education, but they were also smoking at the same level in both periods (39.2% in 1979 and 39.5% in 2014). Conversely, those in the other education categories had substantial decreases, with college-educated women reporting the greatest decrease (30.9% in 1979 compared to 10.9% in 2014).

Table 2 presents parameter estimates (odds ratios) from the logistic regressions of cigarette smoking. Models 1 and 5 include only work status for the 1979 and 2014 samples respectively. Keeping house is not a significant predictor of smoking in the 1979 sample, but is a significant predictor in the 2014 sample in which homemakers have 27% greater odds of smoking than workers. Models 2 and 6 introduce the remaining covariates. People living in large and medium sized communities are more likely to smoke in the 1979 sample; however, consistent with the bivariate results, this pattern no longer holds true by 2014. We observe the well-known education gradient in smoking in both 1979 and 2014. It is notable and consistent with the bivariate results that the estimated odds ratio of smoking among the least educated as compared with the most educated increases from twice as likely in 1979 to over four times as likely in 2014. In 1979 black women had 67% higher odds of smoking, but by 2014 they had 49% lower odds of smoking showing a significant racial reversal in cigarette use. This is a striking change and suggests black women have been

Table 2. Logistic Regression for Past Month Cigarette Use in the United States Using the 1979 NHSDA and 2014 NSDUH, Odd Ratios.

	1979				2014			
	Model 1	Model 2	Model 3	Model 4	Model 5	Model 6	Model 7	Model 8
Work Status (Works Outside House)								
Homemaker	0.82	0.93	0.85	1.03	1.27**	1.07	2.35**	0.42*
X Community Size								
Large			1.07				0.35**	
Medium			1.22				0.49*	
(Small)								
X Education								
Less than high school				0.97				5.85***
High school				0.87				2.55*
Some college				0.86				2.67*
(College)								
Community Size[a]								
Large		1.33 **	1.30	1.33$$		0.89	1.05	0.91
Medium		1.56**	1.46**	1.56**		0.88	1.01	0.89
(Small)								
Education								
Less than high school		1.99**	1.99**	1.94*		4.64***	4.59***	3.66***
High school		1.71*	1.71*	1.77*		3.62***	3.64***	3.47***
Some college		1.20	1.20	1.24		2.60***	2.61***	2.48***
Race								
(White)								
Black		1.67*	1.68*	1.67*		0.51***	0.51***	0.51***
Age		1.12***	1.12**	1.12**		1.16***	1.16***	1.16***
Age squared		1.00***	1.00***	1.00***		0.99***	0.99***	0.99***
income[b]								
(Low)								
Below average		0.86	0.85	0.86		0.84*	0.84*	0.85**
Above average		0.92	0.91	0.92		0.74**	0.74**	0.76*
High		0.97	0.97	0.96		0.61***	0.61***	0.62***
Marital status								
(Married)								
Widowed		1.31	1.31	1.31		2.47***	2.47***	2.45
Divorced or separated		1.65*	1.65*	1.64*		2.30***	2.29***	2.28***
Never married		0.93	0.92	0.93		1.92***	1.93***	1.90***
1979 $N = 2{,}087$								
2014 $N = 12{,}345$								

†$p < 0.10$, *$p < 0.05$, **$p < 0.01$. ***$p < 0.001$.

[a]1979 Large: Self-representing SMSA, Medium: Non-self-representing SMSA, and Small: Not in a SMSA; 2014 Large: CBSA w/ 1 million+, Medium: CBSA w/ <1 million, and Small: Not in a CBSA.

[b]1979 Low: <$7,000, Below average: $7,000$14,999, Above average: $15,000$24,999, and High $25,000+; 2014 Low: < $20,000, Below average: $20,000$49,999, Above average: $50,000 $74,000, and High: $75,000+.

more receptive than white women to smoking avoidance and cessation over time.

Among the remaining covariates, we observe a nonlinear association between age and smoking, in both 1979 and 2014, with middle-age women having the highest rates of smoking. Income was not a significant predictor of smoking in 1979, but in 2014, women in higher income categories had lower odds of smoking compared to those in the lowest income category. Finally, women who were divorced or separated were 66% and 130% more likely to smoke than married women in 1979 and 2014, respectively. Those who were never married did not differ from those who were married in 1979, but by 2014 they had about twice the odds of smoking as those who were married. Widows and married women show no significant differences in smoking in 1979, yet had 147% higher odds of smoking in 2014.

Models 3 and 7 of Table 2 introduce the interaction term of work status by community type, and models 4 and 8 introduce the interaction term of work status by education. As can be seen in Models 3 and 4, none of the interaction terms were significant in 1979; however, by 2014 models 7 and 8 show that both interactions were significant. To interpret the interactions we rely on graphs of predicted probabilities. Fig. 1 presents estimated predicted probabilities of cigarette smoking using the margins command in Stata. As a baseline, we illustrate the predicted probabilities for women who work outside of the home and homemakers from Model 6 (Fig. 1, Panel A) that shows little difference in smoking between homemakers and women who work outside the home.

Panel B of Fig. 1 illustrates the interaction of work status by community type (Model 7). This graph shows that women who are full-time homemakers and live in small communities have the highest probability of smoking of any female group. Consequently, higher rates of smoking in smaller communities and rural areas are driven by women in the home, and, as also shown in Panel B, to a lesser extent in medium-size communities. In large urban areas where female smoking has notably declined, the homemaker-worker distinction is more balanced.

Panel C illustrates the interaction of work status by education (Model 8). Women with a college education regardless of work status have the lowest predicted probabilities of all women to smoke ($p < 0.05$). However, among college-educated women only, those who do work outside the home have a higher predicted probability of smoking than those who keep house (even though they are less likely than women in all other categories of education to smoke). In other words, among college-educated women, those who have jobs are more likely to smoke than homemakers lending some support to the claim that women in higher level jobs may mirror similar males who smoke – despite the fact that college-educated women overall are less likely to smoke than women with lower levels of education. Conversely, women who keep house full-time with less than a high school education are significantly more likely to smoke than women in all other levels of education ($p < 0.05$). Women who

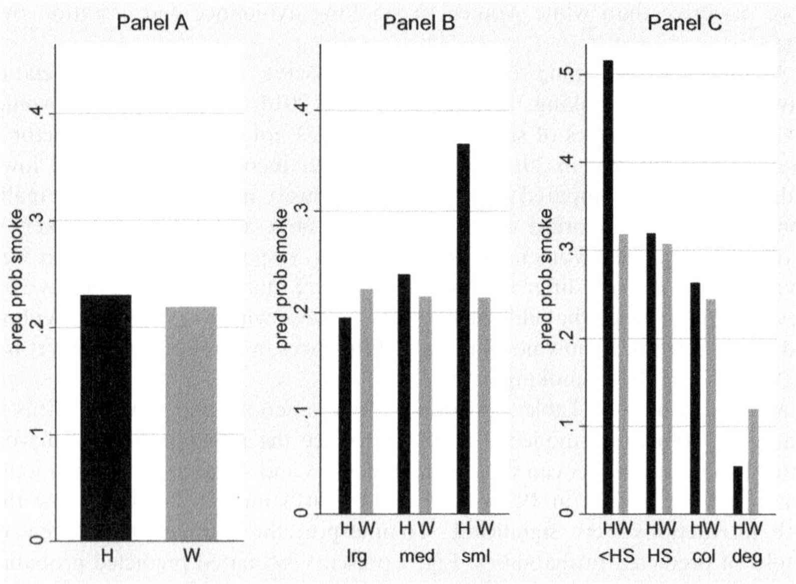

Fig. 1. Predicted Probabilities of Cigarette Use by Work Status, NSDUH 2014. *Note*: H = Homemaker, W = Worker.

work outside the high without a high school education do not differ significantly from those who have a high school diploma.

Overall, our results show that smoking is most prevalent among homemakers in small communities. This outcome clearly supports earlier studies citing smoking as a major causal factor for the decline in female life expectancy among less-educated white women in certain low-income and rural counties in the United States (Cockerham, 2014; Ezzati et al., 2008; Montez & Zajacova, 2013; Wang et al., 2013). The notion that female smoking is strongly associated with the workplace appears to be no longer true, with the exception of a subpopulation of college-educated women.

DISCUSSION

As of yet, there is no theoretical explanation in sociology that fully accounts for the change in female cohort smoking patterns found in this study. There is some support for diffusion theory that maintains widespread smoking generally begins in the upper class as a fashionable activity and overtime shifts downward throughout the class structure becoming concentrated at the bottom while it recedes in the higher echelons of society largely because of health concerns

(Pampel, 2002, 2005). Our literature review does not begin until the 1940s when female smoking spread into the working class (the middle stage of the theory) and our initial data point is not until 1979 when such smoking was slightly less than it was in the 1960s – the high watermark of women's cigarette use. So our findings are not a true test of diffusion theory although the pattern at the point we analyze data is consistent with the direction of the theory.

In his study of the experience of smoking, Hughes (2003) uses the term "habitus," that he, following Elias's perspective in *The Civilizing Process* ([1939] 1994), defines as an individual's "second nature" (specifically, learned standards of behavior), to describe how social considerations (tastes, tolerance thresholds, etc.) are imprinted on biological responses to tobacco. That is, social norms govern styles of tobacco use via the habitus. Hughes also observes that when a person becomes habituated to tobacco, he or she is addicted to it. Consequently, smoking cigarettes is not just a habitual activity consistent with a person's worldview, but a practice driven and reinforced by a physiological craving. This gives smoking a biological imperative that has to be satisfied through routine use in concert with prevailing social norms and the notion of the habitus helps explain this.

Whereas the concept of habitus may not in itself explain smoking changes in large female cohorts, it nevertheless has explanatory power as the centerpiece of health lifestyle theory that includes smoking as a class-based phenomenon (Cockerham, 2005, 2013a, 2013b). The best known use of habitus in sociology generally is found in the work of Pierre Bourdieu, 1977, 1984, 1990) to describe the cognitive map or mind-set of perceptions about the world that people use to routinely guide and evaluate their choices and behavioral options. A person's habitus originates through socialization and experience. The influence of social structures and conditions external to the individual are incorporated into the habitus, as well as the person's own inclinations, preferences, and interpretations. The dispositions that result typically reflect normative patterns of social behavior, but also encompass action that is habitual and even intuitive. The habitus is one of the reasons why social life is usually regular and predictable (Bourdieu & Wacquant, 1992).

The habitus is an important feature of health lifestyles that are defined as collective patterns of health-related behavior based on choices from options available to people according to their life chances (Cockerham, 2005, 2013a, 2013b). Health lifestyle theory holds that four categories of structural variables, namely: (1) class circumstances; (2) age, gender, and race/ethnicity; (3) collectivities (social networks of kinship, religion, politics, the workplace, etc.); and (4) living conditions (quality of housing, access to basic utilities, neighborhood facilities, public safety, etc.) provide the social context for socialization and experience that influence life choices and collectively constitute life chances in the model. The term "life choices" comes from Weber ([1922] 1978) and is a proxy for agency, while "life chances" refers to structures beyond the individual that influence the choices made and their probabilities for realization. While people have choices, those choices are constrained or enabled by their life chances – especially the resources or lack thereof that causes dispositions (a habitus) to act in certain ways as opposed to others that might be chosen. Health lifestyle theory recognizes that people have the capability of choosing their lifestyle, but their choices are limited by what is possible and strongly influenced by the style common to one's class position, gender, age, and the like via their habitus. It is based on the premise that health lifestyles are not the uncoordinated behaviors of socially disconnected individuals, but rather are personal routines that merge into a collective form characteristic of specific groups (e.g., a gender) and classes.

Health lifestyle theory is intended to provide a general model that explains the health-related practices of different social classes, races, genders, and so on. However, its use in this chapter is limited because many of the structural variables are missing. A measure of collectivities, for example, is only present in the form of the workplace (whether job holder or homemaker) and community type based on size by itself is an insufficient indicator of the effects of living conditions on health. Consequently, the range of variables in the NHSDA and NSDUH are not broad enough to test the theory.

Nevertheless, what this study contributes to the literature is the empirical finding that smoking is greatest among women who are full-time homemakers in medium and especially small towns. This is a new development and suggests that employee workplace wellness programs, anti-smoking policies in offices, stores, and public places, and the public stigma associated with smoking have been influential in reducing workplace smoking, particularly in cities. Full-time homemakers, in contrast to employed workers, are not subject to public scrutiny about what they do in their homes and the locus of smoking among women therefore seems to have moved away from its association with the job to the home in less populated areas. Full-time homemakers lack workplace constraints on smoking and their social context and class position may allow them to smoke with little or no stigma. We also found that female smokers tend to be non-Hispanic whites when compared to blacks, have the lowest levels of education and income, are middle-aged, and married.

The perspective on women's health advocating a "women's emancipation or equality thesis" which holds that an important aspect of the changing roles of women and the liberalization of gender-based norms has influenced them to mimic men's unhealthy behaviors in the workplace is not strongly supported by these data. The exception is college-educated women with jobs. Even though college-educated women as a whole smoke less than any other group of females in this study when controlling for education, among those who graduated from college – smokers are more likely to be found on the job and not at home.

Moreover, given the well-publicized dangers of second-hand smoking, it would logically be expected that having children in the home would offset the prevalence of smoking among homemakers, but this was clearly not the case with our data showing children made no difference whatsoever in smoking.

Research on a group of low-income mothers who smoke in the UK had the same outcome, with the mothers resistant to smoking cessation (Robinson & Kirkcaldy, 2007).

Thus, female smoking remains a major health problem in American society, although it is less common than in the past. This is seen in the increased mortality for women from lung cancer and COPD that is not matched or exceeded by men and whose origin lies in collective lifestyle changes in favor of smoking. Such a result attests to the power of gender as a structural variable influencing smoking. This study provides recent data on the smoking patterns of women and can serve as basis for future research, as more studies are needed to fully ascertain the contemporary gender dynamics of smoking.

ACKNOWLEDGMENTS

This study was supported by a grant from the National Institute of Minority Health and Health Disparities (U54MD008176).

REFERENCES

Allen, T. D., & Armstrong, J. (2006). Further examination of the link between work-family conflict and physical health: The role of health-related behaviors. *The American Behavioral Scientist*, *49*(9), 1204–1221.

Annandale, E. (2016). Health status and gender. In W. Cockerham (Ed.), *The New Blackwell companion to medical sociology* (pp. 97–110). Oxford, UK: Wiley-Blackwell.

Bourdieu, P. (1977). *Outline of a theory of practice*. Cambridge, UK: Cambridge University Press.

Bourdieu, P. (1984). *Distinction*. Cambridge, MA: Harvard University Press.

Bourdieu, P. (1990). *The logic of practice*. Stanford, CA: Stanford University Press.

Bourdieu, P., & Wacquant, L. J. D. (1992). *An invitation to reflexive sociology*. Chicago: University of Chicago Press.

Brandt, A. M. (2007). *The cigarette century: The rise, fall, and deadly persistence of the product that defined America*. New York, NY: Basic Books.

Carter, B. D., Abnet, C. C., Feskanich, D., Freedman, N. D., et al. (2015). Smoking and mortality – Beyond established causes. *New England Journal of Medicine*, *372*(7), 631–640.

Centers for Disease Control and Prevention. (2015). Current cigarette smoking among adults – United States, 2005–2014. *Morbidity and Mortality Weekly Report*, *64*(44), 1233–1240.

Child Trends Databank. (2014). *Parental smoking*. Retrieved from http://www.childtrends.org, Accessed February 20, 2016.

Cho, Y. (2004). Gender composition of occupation and industry and working women's alcohol consumption. *Journal of Studies of Alcohol*, *65*(3), 345–352.

Cockerham, W. C. (2013a). *The social causes of health and disease* (2nd ed.), Cambridge: Polity.

Cockerham, W. C. (2013b). Bourdieu and an update of health lifestyle theory. In W. Cockerham (Ed.), *Medical sociology on the move: New directions in theory* (pp. 127–154). Dordrecht: Springer.

Cockerham, W. C. (2014). The emerging crisis in American female longevity. *Social Currents*, *1*(3), 220–227.

Collins, G. (2009). *When everything changed: The amazing journey of American women from 1960 to the present*. New York, NY: Little, Brown.

Elias, N. ([1939] 1994). *The civilizing process*. Oxford: Blackwell.

England, P. (2010). The gender revolution: Uneven and stalled. *Gender & Society*, *24*(2), 149–166.

Ezzati, M., Friedman, A. B., Kulkarni, S. C., & Murray, C. J. L. (2008). The reversal of fortunes: Trends in county mortality and cross-county mortality disparities in the United States. *PLoS Medicine*, *5*, e66/001–e66/0011.

Firebaugh, G. (2008). *Seven rules for social research*. Princeton, NJ: Princeton University Press.

Haines, R. J., Poland, B. D., & Johnson, J. L. (2009). Becoming a 'real' smoker: Cultural capital in young women's accounts of smoking and other substance use. *Sociology of Health & Illness*, *31*(1), 66–80.

Hochschild, A. (1989). *The second shift: Working parents and the revolution at home*. New York: Viking.

Hughes, J. (2003). *Learning to smoke*. Chicago, IL: University of Chicago Press.

King, D. E., Marinous, A. G., Carnemolla, M., & Everett, C. J. (2009). Adherence to healthy life-style habits in US adults, 1988-2006. *American Journal of Medicine*, *122*(6), 528–534.

Long, J. S. (1997). *Regression models for categorical and limited dependent variables*. Thousand Oaks, CA: Sage.

Mattingly, M. J., & Sayer, L. C. (2006). Under pressure: Gender differences in the relationship between free time and feeling rushed. *Journal of Marriage and Family*, *68*(1), 205–221.

Maume, D. J. (2016). Can men make time for family? paid work, care work, work-family reconciliation policies, and gender equality. *Social Currents*, *3*(1), 43–63.

Miller, P. W. (2009). The gender pay gap in the U.S.: Does sector make a difference? *Journal of Labor Research*, *30*(1), 52–74.

Montez, J. K., & Zajacova, A. (2013). Explaining the widening education gap in mortality among U.S. white women. *Journal of Health and Social Behavior*, *54*(2), 166–183.

National Center for Health Statistics. (2014). *Health United States, 2013*. Washington, DC: U.S. Government Printing Office.

Nelson, C. C., Li, Y., Sorenson, G., & Berkman, L. F. (2012). Assessing the crelationship between work-family conflict and smoking. *American Journal of Public Health*, *102*(9), 1767–1772.

Nomaguchi, K. M., Milkie, M. A., & Bianchi, S. M. (2005). Time strains and psychological well-being: Do dual-earner mothers and fathers differ? *Journal of Family Issues*, *26*(6), 756–792.

Pampel, F. C. (2001). Cigarette diffusion and sex differences in smoking. *Journal of Health and Social Behavior*, *42*(4), 388–404.

Pampel, F. C. (2002). Inequality, diffusion, and the status gradient in smoking. *Social Problems*, *49*(1), 35–57.

Pampel, F. C. (2005). Diffusion, cohort change, and social patterns of smoking. *Social Science Research*, *34*(1), 117–139.

Pampel, F. C. (2009). The Persistence of educational differences in smoking. *Social Problems*, *56*(3), 526–542.

Pavalko, E. K., Gong, F., & Scott Long, J. (2007). Women's work, cohort change, and health. *Journal of Health and Social Behavior*, *48*(4), 352–368.

Percheski, C. (2008). Opting out? Cohort differences in professional women's employment rates from 1900 to 2005. *American Sociological Review*, *73*(3), 497–517.

Pinker, S. (2009). *The sexual paradox*. New York, NY: Scribner.

Robinson, J., & Kirkcaldy, A. J. (2007). 'You think that i'm smoking and they're not': Why mothers still smoke in the home. *Social Science & Medicine*, *65*, 641–652.

Ross, C. E., & Mirowsky, J. (2013). The sense of personal control: Social structural causes and emotional consequences. In C. Aneshensel, J. Phelan, & A. Bierman (Eds.), *Handbook of the sociology of mental health* (pp. 379–402). Dordrecht: Springer.

Searcey, D., Porter, E., & Gebeloff, R. (2015). As market evolves, health care opens paths, often for women. *New York Times* (February 23):A1, A12-13.

StataCorp (2013). *Stata statistical software: Release 13*. College Station, TX: StataCorp LP.

Syamial, G., Mazurek, J. M., & Dube, S. R. (2014). Gender differences in smoking among U.S. working adults. *American Journal of Preventive Medicine*, *47*(4), 467–475.

U.S. Bureau of Labor Statistics. (2014). *Current population survey*. Washington, DC: Department of Labor.

U.S. Department of Health and Human Services, National Institutes of Health and National Institute on Drug Abuse. (2015). National Household Survey on Drug Abuse, 1979: Inter-University Consortium for Political and Social Research (ICPSR) [distributor]. Retrieved from http://doi.org/10.3886/ICPSR06843.v4. Accessed onFebruary 13, 2015.

Walsh, D. C., Sorensen, G., & Leonard, L. (1995). Gender, health, and cigarette smoking. In B. Amick, A. Tarlov, S. Levine, & D. Walsh (Eds.), *Society and health* (pp. 131–171). New York, NY: Oxford University Press.

Wang, H., Schumacher, A. E., Levitz, C. E., Mokdad, A. H., & Murray, C. J. L. (2013). Left behind: Widening disparities for males and females in U.S. county life expectancy, 1985-2010. *Population Health Metrics*, *11*, 8. doi:10.1186/1478-7954-11-8

Weber, M. ([1922] 1978). *Economy and society* (Vol. 1). Berkeley, CA: University of California Press.

ABOUT THE EDITOR

Jennie Jacobs Kronenfeld is Professor Emerita in the Sociology Program, Sanford School of Social and Family Dynamics, Arizona State University. Her research areas are medical sociology and aging and the life course with special focus on health policy, health care utilization, and health behavior. She serves as editor of the research annual, Research in the Sociology of Health Care published each year by Emerald Press. She is coeditor of Health and Associate Editor In Chief, American Journal of Health Promotion. She has served in many roles with the American Sociological Association (ASA) including as Chair of the Medical Sociology Section and other positions in this group. She is currently serving as a council member with the Retired Sociologist Interest Group of the ASA. She has served as secretary-treasurer of the Medical Care section of the American Public Health Association. She is a past president of Sociologists for Women in Society.

INDEX

Printed and bound by CPI Group (UK) Ltd, Croydon, CR0 4YY

13/09/2026

14961058-0005